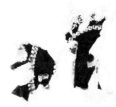

DIET, DEMOGRAPHY, AND DISEASE

Changing Perspectives on Anemia

FOUNDATIONS OF HUMAN BEHAVIOR

An Aldine de Gruyter Series of Texts and Monographs

SERIES EDITOR

Sarah Blaffer Hrdy

University of California, Davis

DIET, DEMOGRAPHY, AND DISEASE

Changing Perspectives on Anemia

Patricia Stuart-Macadam and Susan Kent

EDITORS

ALDINE DE GRUYTER

New York

About the Editors

Patricia Stuart-Macadam is Associate Professor of Anthropology at the University of Toronto.
Susan Kent is Associate Professor of Anthropology at Old Dominion University.

Copyright ©1992 Walter de Gruyter, Inc., New York

ALDINE DE GRUYTER
A division of Walter de Gruyter, Inc.
200 Saw Mill River Road
Hawthorne, New York 10532

The paper used in this publication meets the minimum requirements of American National Standard for Information Sciences—Permanence of Paper Printed Library Materials, ANSI Z39.48-1984.

Library of Congress Cataloging-in-Publication Data

Diet, demography, and disease : changing perspectives on anemia /
    Patricia Stuart-Macadam and Susan Kent, editors.
        p.   cm. — (Foundations of human behavior)
    Includes bibliographical references and index.
    ISBN 0-202-01189-5 (alk. paper)
    1. Iron deficiency anemia.   2. Paleopathology.   3. Physical
anthropology.   I. Stuart-Macadam, Patricia, 1951-   .   II. Kent, Susan,
1952-   .   III. Series.
    [DNLM: 1. Anemia—diet therapy.   2. Anemia—history.
3. Demography.   WH   155   D565]
RA645.I75D54   1992
616.1'52—dc20
DNLM/DLC   92-11086
for Library of Congress   CIP

Manufactured in the United States of America

10 9 8 7 6 5 4 3 2 1

To

JAMES MURRAY MACADAM

*You have more than fulfilled the vow you made to me on
September 20, 1975.*

P.L. S-M.

and

*to all those with anemia: may new views help
us understand old problems.*

S.K.

Contents

Part III. Commentary

Acknowledgments

There are a number of individuals we would like to sincerely thank for their assistance and encouragement during the preparation and production of this volume. First and foremost we thank the authors of the chapters, without whose hard work, patience, and general good cheer we could not have organized the book. We would particularly like to acknowledge the inspiration for the ideas presented in this volume provided by the innovative work of Dr. Gene Weinberg and Dr. George Wadsworth. We would also like to thank Dr. Roy Stuart who spent many hours editing the manuscripts and Dr. Steven Kent, a physician, who provided medical information and advice from the volume's prospectus to its final draft. The latter involved many a long discussion with the junior editor that went far beyond the duties of a younger brother. The senior editor would particularly like to thank James Macadam for his unfailing emotional and logistical support throughout the duration of the project. We also appreciate the valuable suggestions made by the extremely conscientious anonymous reviewer. Finally, we are most grateful to Richard Koffler, executive editor at Aldine de Gruyter, for his help and enthusiasm during every stage of the project. It was truly a pleasure to be able to work with him.

Patricia Stuart-Macadam
Susan Kent

Chapter 1

Anemia through the Ages: Changing Perspectives and Their Implications

Susan Kent

Anemia is a condition that has intrigued scientists and the public for over 3000 years. As early as 1500 B.C., an Egyptian manual of therapeutics, the *Papyrus Ebers*, described a disease characterized by pallor, dyspnea, and edema that may have been an anemia of some type (Stuart-Macadam 1989). By A.D. 1640, Lazarus Riberus recommended the use of iron as a remedy for what probably was anemia (Stuart-Macadam 1989). Until the nineteenth century, chronic anemia was known as chlorosis, or "green sickness," in reference to the pallor that characterized severe cases. Today, anemia continues to intrigue scientists from a variety of disciplines. It is currently considered to be one of the most common maladies afflicting humankind (Arthur and Isbister 1987). Anemia appears to have been equally prevalent in many prehistoric populations, as evidenced by pathologic bone changes called porotic hyperostosis (see Stuart-Macadam, this volume, Chapter 5). The frequency of porotic hyperostosis seems to have increased in skeletal populations from a few cases identified in the Paleolithic and Mesolithic to many cases in the Neolithic and post-Neolithic to the twentieth century.

Diet, Demography, and Disease: Changing Perspectives of Anemia examines both past and modern occurrences of anemia in view of recent studies from a variety of disciplines. By combining information from medicine, microbiology, physical anthropology, archaeology, and nutrition, it is possible to understand the causes and consequences of low iron levels, as well as their distribution and frequency in past and present populations.

Prior to the nineteenth century, chronic anemia, "chlorosis, or green sickness, was attributed to unrequited passion. Medieval Dutch painters portrayed the pale olive complexion of chlorosis in portraits of young women. Young Shakespearean heroines and heros, disappointed by love, were smitten with the green sickness" (Farley and Foland 1990:89). Rather than attribute anemia to unrequited love, modern medicine generally attributes it to poor diets that fail to replenish iron loss due to injury, destruction of red blood cells, physiological factors, or dietary iron inhibitors (Kent 1992).[1] One of today's solutions to reduce the frequency of "green sickness," or, more properly, acquired anemia, is to increase the dietary intake of iron. This is accomplished by iron fortification of many cereal and grain products in a number of Western countries, as well as the use of prescription and nonprescription iron supplements worldwide. The volume uses an interdisciplinary approach to explore the relationship between anemia and diet and disease by questioning whether the frequency of noninherited anemia is primarily caused by a diet deficient in iron. The implications of the conclusions from the chapters in this book go far beyond understanding modern distributions of low iron levels to include interpreting and explaining past, as well as predicting future, distributions.

Dietary Iron-Deficiency Anemia or Anemia of Chronic Disease?

Technically, anemia is defined as a subnormal number of red blood cells per cubic millimeter (mm^3), subnormal amount of hemoglobin in 100 ml of blood, or subnormal volume of packed red blood cells per 100 ml of blood. There are a number of hematological tests of varying sensitivity and specificity that can be used to identify anemia in modern populations (Kent and Stuart-Macadam 1992). Although many kinds of anemia exist, only two of the most common acquired types, iron deficiency and anemia of chronic disease, are the subject of this volume.

It has been estimated that approximately 30% of the world's population of nearly 4.5 billion are anemic; at least half of these (500–600 million people) are thought to have iron-deficiency anemia (Cook and Lynch 1986). In developing nations, 40 to 100% of specific subpopulations are anemic (DeMaeyer and Adiels-Tegman 1985). Even in affluent Western nations, 20% of menstruating females are thought to be iron deficient (Arthur and Isbister 1987:172; although recent surveys indicate that these figures may be too high for the United States, Dallman 1987; Dallman et al. 1984; Centers for Disease Control 1986).

The fact that iron-deficiency anemia will probably ensue if a diet is severely deficient in iron over a long period of time has led to the common practice of attributing most occurrences of low iron levels to dietary causes. However, a number of scientists studying the precise amount of iron loss through sweat, urine, stools, and other secretions conclude that it "is unusual for iron deficiency to occur from dietary deficiency alone" (Daly 1989:131; also see Aruthur and Isbister 1987; Wadsworth 1975 and this volume). In the absence of blood loss or parasites, even the most frugal diets rarely result in iron-deficiency anemia because most water and natural foods contain small amounts of iron (Wadsworth, this volume, Chapter 3). According to Arthur and Isbister (1987:173), a review of previous studies of anemia indicates "iron deficiency is almost never due to dietary deficiency in an adult in our community [i.e., Western society]." This is because the average person requires very little iron intake to replace that lost through sweat, menstruation, and urine because as much as 90% of the iron needed for the formation of new blood cells is derived from recycling senescent red blood cells (Hoffbrand 1981).[2] In addition, individuals suffering from iron deficiency absorb significantly more iron from the same diet and excrete significantly less iron than nondeficient individuals. That is, "the intestine can adjust its avidity to match the body's requirement" of iron (O'Neil-Cutting and Crosby 1987: 491; see note 1). The presence of porotic hyperostosis (skeletal evidence of anemia—see Stuart-Macadam, this volume, Chapter 5) in nonhuman primates, such as chimpanzees, gorillas, orangutans, and various species of Old World monkeys, including baboons (Hengen 1971), reinforces the unlikelihood that an impoverished diet is the irreducible cause since it is improbable that such diverse species of primates would all suffer from impoverished diets. A more probable etiology of porotic hyperostosis in these primates is the anemia of chronic disease/inflammation since such diverse species all can potentially suffer from a range of diseases known to produce low iron levels. This alternative model of the etiology of anemia is explored in detail in the following chapters.

Because of similarities in the hematological presentation of iron-deficiency anemia and the anemia of chronic disease, they can be difficult to differentiate. Studies indicate that misdiagnosis has occurred wherein dietary iron-deficiency anemia was identified when, in fact, the anemia was the result of chronic diseases or inflammation. The difficulty of interpretation lies in the fact that both types of anemia are characterized by subnormal hemoglobin levels, although levels are often lower in iron-deficiency anemia. Moreover, both types of anemia are associated with subnormal serum iron and transferrin saturation levels (Table 1). However, in contrast to dietary iron deficiency anemia, anemia of chronic dis-

Table 1. Comparison of Anemia of Dietary Iron Deficiency and Anemia
of Chronic Disease Laboratory Values

Anemia	Hemoglobin	Serum Iron	% Saturation	Serum Ferritin
Iron deficiency	Decreased	Decreased	Decreased	Decreased
Chronic disease	Decreased	Decreased	Decreased	Normal–raised

ease can be, but is not always, hypochromic (pale red blood cells with
reduced hemoglobin content) or microcytic (small red blood cells;
Reizenstein 1983:43). Serum ferritin levels are one of the most reliable
criteria with which to distinguish iron-deficiency anemia from the
anemia of chronic disease because storage iron is held within the ferritin
molecule (Table 1).[3] Serum ferritin is subnormal in individuals with
dietary iron-deficiency anemia and is normal to elevated in individuals
with anemia of chronic disease (Bothwell et al. 1979; Cook 1980:83–85;
Henry 1984; Noyes 1985).

The reliability of serum ferritin surpasses that of free erythrocyte
protoporphyrin and other tests sometimes thought to be diagnostic in
discriminating the etiology of anemia (Zanella et al. 1989). Serum ferritin
is a particularly reliable measurement because it reflects changes in iron
stores before they are completely exhausted or, in the case of overload,
increased (e.g., Cook and Skikne 1989; Finch and Huebers 1982). There
are now numerous studies of various protocols that show that serum ferritin is an accurate measure of iron stores, second only to actual bone
marrow aspirations (e.g., Burns et al. 1990; Guyatt et al. 1990; Thompson
1988). In fact, it was noted that previous "studies in younger subjects
have consistently shown the usefulness of serum ferritin in the diagnosis
of iron-deficiency anemia, and suggested that serum ferritin is more
powerful than other blood tests. . . . Our results are consistent with these
findings: in elderly patients with anemia, serum ferritin determination is
by far the best test for diagnosis of iron deficiency" (Guyatt et al.
1990:208; also see Cook and Skikne 1982). The reason is that serum ferritin "closely reflects total body iron stores. This assay is a very sensitive
indicator of iron deficiency, even before anemia or changes in erythrocyte
indices are manifest. For this purpose it is much preferable to SI, TIBC,
and T-Sat [i.e., serum iron, total iron binding capacity, and transferrin
saturation]. . . . patients with malignancy or inflammatory disorders . . .
[that is chronic diseases] the serum ferritin concentration is increased"
(Stein 1990:1076). Moreover, research is beginning to show that "Traditional tests of serum iron and TIBC may be useful but currently are not

recommended for indirect measurement of iron stores [i.e., measurement in the absence of a bone marrow biopsy]" (Beissner and Trowbridge 1986:88–90). More recently, it has been noted that "a wide range of values for transferrin saturation and total iron-binding capacity is consistent with either iron deficiency anemia or anemia of chronic disease. . . . The two disorders can be distinguished by the serum ferritin level, iron stain of a bone marrow specimen for hemosiderin, or both" (Farley and Foland 1990:92).[4]

In spite of these findings, serum ferritin is not always monitored in studies of anemia (although it is becoming more common). Because it is not possible to conclusively distinguish dietary iron-deficiency anemia from the anemia of chronic disease without serum ferritin and/or bone marrow aspirations, diet has been assumed to be the cause of low iron levels when chronic diseases/infections are in fact responsible. For example, "Out of 29 patients 'diagnosed' as having iron deficiency anaemia, only 11 patients in fact had true iron deficiency when reviewed by the authors. Most patients had the anaemia of chronic disease that was misdiagnosed as iron deficiency. There is a strong clinical impression amongst hematologists that this problem of misdiagnosis is not unique to hospital based specialists but also applies more widely" (Arthur and Isbister 1987:172; also see Cook et al. 1971:601). Another example is a study that found that almost 50% of infants classified as dietary iron deficient were instead found to have occult gastrointestinal blood loss, without anatomic lesions, which was the source of their anemia (Fairbanks and Beutler 1988:208).

Hypoferremia as a Defense against Disease

One of the most intriguing facets of iron metabolism is the association between hypoferremia, or a decrease in circulating iron, and the body's defense against pathogens (see Weinberg, this volume, Chapter 4). A number of studies demonstrate the role of hypoferremia as a defense against pathogens that require iron for proliferation, but cannot store it in a nontoxic form. They, therefore, are required to extract iron from their host. In response, the body lowers the availability of iron by reducing serum iron levels. It does so by shifting circulating iron to storage, which is visible hematologically by a drop in hemoglobin, serum iron, and transferrin saturation levels and a rise in serum ferritin levels. Minor infectious diseases are associated with this drop in circulating iron levels and concomitant increase in storage iron. Moreover, inflammation is reduced in anemic individuals. "Mild nutritional iron deficiency significantly reduced the severity of adjuvant induced joint inflammation assessed by histology, microfocal radiography, and subjective scoring" (Andrews et al. 1987:859). A number of studies have shown that iron may be a limiting nutrient to the growth and replication of cancer cells as well (Stevens 1990:177). Therefore, the body's ability to lower iron levels is an important deterrent to the development and proliferation of cancer cells.[5]

Perhaps one of the most convincing and well-controlled examples of hypoferremia as a body's defense in action against pathogens was observed over a period of 30 days. Researchers analyzed the blood of healthy, well-nourished, and nonanemic infants both before and after they were immunized with live measles virus (Olivares et al. 1989). After immunization, hemoglobin, serum iron, and transferrin saturation levels fell significantly, whereas serum ferritin levels rose significantly as the body shifted circulating iron to storage. These levels persisted for 14 to 30 days, while the body produced hypoferremia, or low levels of circulating iron, in an attempt to make iron less available. Even "in those infants with prior evidence of normal iron status, the viral process induced changes indistinguishable from iron deficiency" (Olivares et al. 1989:855). The authors noted that changes in the white blood cells mimicked a bacterial infection as did changes in iron levels—that is, in both cases rapid proliferation of the virus mimicked the rapid proliferation of bacteria (Olivares et al. 1989). The body was unable to differentiate between the proliferation of bacteria and the proliferation of the virus and responded in a similar manner by producing hypoferremia.

Other research supports the association between mild infectious diseases and anemia. One example, is a study of 1347 outpatient children in whom there was a strong association among fever, elevated erythrocyte sedimentation rate (ESR, which is indicative of disease), and anemia as measured by hemoglobin levels (Jansson et al. 1986). These authors concluded that "The results show that anemia was commonly associated with the usually mild infections that are typically seen in a pediatric primary care setting. The anemia could be inferred to be . . . unrelated to iron deficiency in most cases" (Jansson et al. 1986:424).

A number of studies also indicate a protective role in the shifting of circulating iron to storage. For example, in contrast to nonanemic Turkana from Kenya, mildly anemic Turkana who consume little meat, poultry, or other heme iron have a lower incidence of infectious diseases such as various parasitic infections and malaria, brucellosis, and diarrhea—particularly amebiasis (Murray et al. 1980a). Among the Maasai of Kenya, anemic individuals have significantly lower incidence of amoebic dysentery. Examination of cow's milk drunk by Maasai "showed that it not only had a concentration of iron below the minimum necessary for the growth of *E histolytica* [an amoebia] but also contained partly saturated lactoferrin and transferrin, which may actively compete with the parasite in the colon for ambient iron" (Murray et al. 1980b:1351; also see Murray and Murray 1977 and Murray et al. 1976). When associated with malaria and other infections, serum ferritin levels are generally increased in anemic children (Adelekan and Thurnham 1990). This indicates that iron stores are present, despite the lowered serum iron, transferrin saturation, and hemoglobin levels. Thus, the anemia is definitely not the result of dietary inadequacies.

Inflammation causes a proliferation of various types of white blood cells, including neutrophils. The neutrophils produce the iron-binding lactoferrin protein during inflammatory conditions, which can significantly enhance the capacities of macrophages and monocytes to destroy specific invaders as part of the host's defense system (Lima and Kierszenbaum 1987). The result is the binding of available iron to deprive microorganisms of this essential nutrient, i.e., the anemia of chronic disease (also see Cole et al. 1976). In one sense, this response may be seen as a case of mistaken identity wherein the body does not discriminate between microorganism proliferation and inflammatory or chronic diseases such as rheumatoid arthritis or cancer cell proliferation. However, the response is appropriate since rapidly reproducing tumors and other neoplastic cells also have high iron requirements. While it is recognized that reduced iron availability will not necessarily completely suppress microorganism invasion, nor is it necessarily the only defense the body has to fight pathogens, hypoferremia as a normal nonspecific immunologic defense against microorganism invasion is overlooked more often than are other defenses the body activates to fight invaders.[6]

In the anemia of chronic disease, the body removes circulating iron to storage in an attempt to reduce its availability to the bacteria, parasites, or neoplasia (cancer) infecting the body. Weinberg details the mechanisms involved in Chapter 4 of this volume. The anemia of chronic disease/inflammation, then, can be seen as a nonspecific defense the body employs against invading pathogens, neoplasia, and inflammation (see Chapter 4, but also see notes 5–7).[7]

How can we account for a similar response of body defenses to such dissimilar processes as infection, neoplasia, and chronic inflammatory diseases? It is suggested that the rapid proliferation of cells may cause the body to respond with hypoferremia. In other words, the processes that inhibit iron availability in response to an invading pathogen might be stimulated by the rapid proliferation that is characteristic of these pathogens. However, rapid proliferation of cells also occurs as the result of conditions unrelated to microorganisms, such as neoplastic disease, viral infections, and inflammation. The rapid proliferation of neoplastic cells creates a need for iron. The body fights back with a number of mechanisms designed to divert circulating iron to storage and by surrounding tumor cells with macrophages that can ingest lactoferrin-bound iron; however, these are often not effective against the iron-accumulating mechanisms of the tumor (Weinberg 1983:230). It is suggested that the body does not discriminate on the basis of the cause of the proliferation, i.e., bacterial, viral, parasitism, or neoplasia proliferation, but responds in a similar manner—by reducing the available iron. Hypoferremia in the form of the anemia of chronic disease results.

This does not deny the fact that severely anemic individuals with hemoglobin levels below 4–5 g/100 ml are at great risk and need iron supplementation. Instead, it indicates that mild anemia (hemoglobin levels above 7 g/100 ml) may not be the cause of the high mortality rates or morbidity found in many developing nations but may instead result from the body's attempt to protect itself (see Wadsworth, this volume, Chapter 3). In fact, a comprehensive review of *in vitro* and *in vivo* research in humans and animals led Farthing (1989:50) to conclude the following:

> Certainly there is no evidence to suggest that patients with iron deficiency suffer the devastating infective complications of the well-defined immunodeficiency syndromes either congenital or acquired. This would appear to be true even in patients with severe iron deficiency and profound anaemia (haemoglobin <5 g/dl).
>
> These clinical observations, however, detract in no way from the fundamental importance of iron in maintaining the integrity of immune function, and its wider involvement in many basic cellular processes in all body tissues. However, like many other macro- and micronutrients that have global and multiple functions in cell metabolism extremes of deficiency can often be tolerated with relative ease. Thus perhaps one should conclude that despite the essential nature of iron in many processes including those performed by the immune system, survival in a surprisingly healthy state is possible even in the extremes of deficiency and excess.

Iron Overload

To gain a different perspective of the relationship between iron and disease, we can examine the effects of hyperferremia, or too much iron (detailed in Kent et al. 1990, n.d.). If the anemia of chronic disease is a nonspecific defense against infection and inflammation, then the opposite, or too much iron, should result in an increase of infection and inflammation. Numerous studies show that this is precisely what occurs—hyperferremia stimulates pathogen growth.

For example, the incidence of serious bacterial infections increases significantly when normal infants are given intramuscular iron-dextran. In one study, "When the iron administration was stopped the incidence of disease in Polynesians decreased from 17 per 1,000 to 2.7 per 1,000 total births" (Barry and Reeve 1973:376; also see Barry and Reeve 1977). Other research substantiates the association between an increased incidence of bacteria, such as *Escherichia coli* sepsis and others, and the administration of intramuscular iron-dextran in neonates (Becroft et al. 1977; Masawe et al. 1974; Oppenheimer et al. 1986b). Malarial infection greatly increased in infants with higher transferrin saturation levels, leading researchers to conclude that hypoferremia provides a protective role against malaria (Oppenheimer et al. 1986a). Infants receiving high-iron infant formula had a significantly higher risk of contracting salmonellosis than breast-fed infants because "it may be that maintaining a relatively low concentration of iron in the neonatal gastrointestinal tract is one of nature's strategies for protecting infants from bacterial infections during the critical first few months of life. Commercial iron-supplemented infant formula, on the other hand, contains from 12 to 19 mg of iron per liter and would provide the intestinal flora of infants fed these products with from 8 to 12 times more iron than is available to breast-fed infants" (Haddock et al. 1991:1000).

Some diseases result in highly elevated transferrin saturation levels, which make iron much more accessible to pathogens. In diseases such as leukemia, patients have been observed with sera that was 96–100% saturated (normal is 16–50%). As a consequence, leukemia patients are unusually susceptible to infection. In one study, 78% of 161 leukemia patients who died did so as a result of infection and *not* as a result of the leukemia directly (Kluger and Bullen 1987:258).

Anemia and Performance

Iron is required to catalyze various aspects of the humoral and cell-mediated immune systems, DNA synthesis, electron transport, redox reactions, brain neurotransmission, and for tissue oxygen delivery (Neilands 1981; Weinberg 1984; Gidding and Stockman 1988; Youdim et al. 1989; Yehuda and Youdim 1989). In addition, iron is necessary for normal growth and physical and cognitive performance (Dallman 1989). These facts may have influenced some people to conclude that normal iron levels are essential for normal performance. Whereas individuals with extremely low iron levels obviously cannot perform at an optimal level, how do more moderate cases of mild anemia affect individuals' mental and physical capabilities? Although iron-deficient individuals have a lower maximum work capability and endurance (Lozoff and Brittenham 1987; Gardner et al. 1977; Scrimshaw 1990, 1991), we can question how much of that poor performance is related to dietary iron deficiency and how much is related to poor calorie, vitamin, and protein intake and/or parasitic or other disease.

As detailed in Kent (1992), there has been much research concerning anemia and performance. However, the anemia is not always specified and the underlying disease(s), particularly parasites, are often cured as part of the study. Intake of calories, protein, and vitamins are also improved in some of the studies designed to investigate performance and anemia. Performance results of anemic persons with parasitism and other diseases are not directly comparable to results of the later nonanemic, nondiseased individuals who were given an antihelminthic drug (e.g., Pollitt et al. 1989). Ingestion of oral iron can stimulate the appetite and there is often a weight gain associated with higher hemoglobin levels (Kent et al. 1990). This overall improvement in nutrition has been suggested as the cause of the improved mental facilities (Wadsworth, this volume, Chapter 3). Furthermore, a number of studies that indicate improved performance after administration of iron have been reanalyzed. These reanalyses show that changes noted were sometimes not statistically significant, did not always include a control group, or were ambiguous in what prompted the improvements noted (see Lozoff and Brittenham 1987; Johnson and McGowan 1983). For example, based on four studies Seshadri and Gopaldas (1989) claim that iron deficiency negatively impacts cognitive functions in preschool and school age children. However, commentators on the article raise serious problems with each of the studies, ranging from the identification of anemic versus nonanemic children (based only on hemoglobin levels with a cutoff value of 110 g/liter) to uncontrolled confounding variables such as the presence of parasites and potential bleeding, the addition of folate acid to the diet, and general "flaws in internal validity and construct validity" of the research (Walter 1989; Heywood 1989).

The problem here, as noted throughout this volume, is the separation of cause and consequence; anemia as a physiological problem or as a defense.[8] No one denies that someone severely deficient from blood loss will perform poorly compared to a healthy person. However, such severly deficient individuals are not usually part of the performance test groups reported in the literature. More mild anemia may be significantly but spuriously associated with poor mental and physical performance, the causal association being between disease and poor achievement or between insufficient calories and achievement. That is, is it the increase in iron per se that is causing the improvement in skills or is it the improvement in overall health and nutrition, particularly the elimination of disease or the addition of needed calories and protein? Some nutritionists are suggesting that the association between iron and performance may be noncausal and the result of other factors not monitored in most research designed to study this. For example, according to Lozoff et al. (1991:692):

> *None of the studies available to date prove that iron deficiency caused the children's lower test scores in infancy and at five years of age.* Establishing a cause-and-effect relation between two factors on the basis of correlational data depends on documenting a reliable association between them, confirming that the . . . relation is neither spurious nor fortuitous—that is, that the association cannot be explained by some other factor or by chance alone. Recent research on the relation between iron-deficiency anemia in infancy and children's behavior meets the first criterion of reliable association, but not the others. A prospective study would be needed to demonstrate that the behavior of infants with iron deficiency was not different from that of nondeficient infants before the onset of the deficiency. Even if pre-existing behavioral differences were absent, other conditions closely associated with iron deficiency could account for the observed alterations in behavior. A deficiency of one nutrient suggests that the intake of calories or other nutrients might also be inadequate. . . . It is also difficult to be sure that the children never had a recurrence of iron deficiency after the initial study. . . .
>
> In contrast, differences in the home environment are likely. . . . [The] available measures of the home environment are too crude to dismiss the possibility that differences among families accounted for the difference in scores. In fact, it seems probable that there were other important differences in the degree of stimulation and type of care the children received. *Thus, as with several other risk factors, such as low birth weight, elevated blood lead levels, and generalized undernutrition, a worse developmental outcome in infants with iron deficiency may be inextricably linked to perinatal and environmental factors* (emphasis added).

Elsewhere, after a thorough review of the literature, Lozoff (1990:122) wrote "In any case, poorer developmental outcome in iron deficiency [in infants] may be inextricably linked to environmental disadvantage." The persistence of the dietary model for anemia and its impact on performance results from the general popularity of the dietary model among both scientists and the public and from a lack of alternative hypotheses (i.e., such as the one proposed here: that anemia results from chronic disease that affects performance) Therefore, in spite of the previous statements, Lozoff et al. (1991) revert back to the traditional conclusion that diets need to be altered to rectify performance levels in disadvantaged children. They state: "Despite such unresolved issues [as those quoted above], the results of this study indicate that relatively severe and chronic iron deficiency in infancy may serve as a convenient marker for any associated factors that contribute to poor developmental outcome but are harder to identify during routine pediatric care. . . . The possibility that earlier detection of iron deficiency or longer treatment [with iron supplements] might be effective in preventing developmental disadvantage needs to be assessed. . . . However, given the findings to date that lower test scores persist, a vigorous effort to prevent iron deficiency is the safest approach" (Lozoff et al. 1991:692–693; also see Lozoff 1989).

Although most of the following authors would certainly agree that prevention of anemia is necessary, they would disagree on the method of prevention. Most of the chapters in this volume indicate that the anemia identified is from chronic disease in the cases they describe. Administrating iron supplements would not be prudent in these cases. Iron supplementation and fortification should occur only when it is firmly established that anemia is (1) actually severe, and (2) the direct result of blood loss, or, more rarely, of an exceedingly inadequate diet, although such diets would not be common except under extreme conditions of abject poverty and actual starvation, war, or similar situations that do unfortunately exist in some parts of the world today. Otherwise, prescribing iron may not achieve the desired results and may, in fact, produce higher rather than lower morbidity.

Obviously this is a controversial view, particularly for nutritionists and others trained to hold that dietary iron deficiency, rather than infections/ inflammations underlying the anemia of chronic disease, is a major cause of low performance and high morbidity in populations around the world. This book presents an alternative model with alternative prophylactic and curative methods suggested by that model. The point of disagreement is not in the underlying belief that anemia is an indication that something is wrong, be it poor diet or the presence of disease. Instead, the contention is in the cause, and therefore the cure, of the anemia. In the former dietary case, anemia is seen as a symptom of the problem that needs to be corrected and in the latter as a defense against the problem and, as a defense, one that should not be altered unless it turns into a life threatening situation, most common from blood loss accompanying many parasitic infections.

Recent Perspectives on Anemia and Diet, Demography, and Disease

The present volume challenges past explanations of anemia and its consequences by exploring the relationship between diet, demography, disease, and anemia. Authors see chronic diseases and inflammations as more often responsible for the frequency of low iron levels than diet. Demography, in particular sedentism and aggregation, is implicated as a major factor in producing increased bacterial and parasitic diseases leading to anemia. Although most of the authors in this book might agree with those readers who claim that anemia in developing countries is one of the most common conditions found, with far reaching consequences that make it a major public health concern, they may not agree on the nature and etiology of that anemia—that is, dietary-induced, disease-induced, or a combination of both. Determining the cause of anemia, i.e., whether it is a disorder or a defense, is critical before establishing programs to eradicate it. In one case, diet needs to be modified, perhaps including iron supplementation and food fortification; and in the other case, the causes of high levels of infectious/inflammatory diseases, such as poor sanitation and overcrowding, need to be eliminated. Authors build on the foundations of previous anthropological, medical, and microbiological knowledge to explore the validity and implication of the anemia of chronic disease in a variety of past and present contexts. The chapters tend to be cross-cultural, cross-temporal, or both, providing a greater depth and breadth of information than most papers examining acquired anemia. Their use of interdisciplinary data results in a holistic view of anemia. The conclusions are essential to consider when modeling past morbidity and for endeavors to eradicate modern and future health problems.

The chapters can be grouped into three categories—theoretical/topical issues, case studies, and commentary. Garn in Chapter 2 presents the traditional views of inherited and acquired anemias and provides a backdrop for the following chapters, which offer alternative views based on recent research. For example, Wadsworth (Chapter 3) examines the iron content of food and the body's need for and use of iron. He concludes that an association between the nature of diet and the etiology of anemia has not yet been proven and, therefore, diet cannot usually be implicated as a cause of acquired anemia. Weinberg (Chapter 4) demonstrates the link between low iron levels and the body's defense against disease, a response that is unrelated to diet. Several chapters provide a detailed history and review of traditional perspectives of anemia (e.g., see Chapters 2–5), so one is not presented in this chapter. Instead, a brief overview of each chapter is followed by a discussion from the perspective of the anemia of chronic disease/inflammation and its implications.

Theoretical and Topical Explorations

Garn provides an excellent baseline discussion for the book in Chapter 2 by outlining traditional views of past incidences of anemia (i.e., porotic hyperostosis) and modern incidences of both acquired and inherited anemias. The difficulties in using hemoglobin/hematocrit values in determining health or disease is reviewed in this chapter and the factors influencing these values are detailed, including smoking, obesity, and altitude. Garn furthermore reviews criticisms of the association between porotic hyperostosis and acquired anemia. He also examines the theory of genetic hemoglobin differences between racial groups. Finally, he discusses the role of diet as a factor responsible for the relatively high frequency of anemia found worldwide. Each of the following chapters in this section addresses one of the issues introduced by Garn (Wadsworth looks at diet and anemia; Weinberg discusses hypoferremia as a defense against disease; and Stuart-Macadam examines porotic hyperostosis and acquired anemia).

Garn points out that low hemoglobin levels have been attributed to genetic differences between different populations or races. However, a problem with the view of racially determined genetic differences, in which Blacks have lower hemoglobin values as a norm than Whites, is the difficulty in identifying absolute racial categories. This is especially true in the case of Black and White Americans because of the considerable gene flow that has occurred between the two groups (i.e., people are often categorized as Black even if the majority of their ancestors were White). In fact, more sophisticated studies, which include serum ferritin in the parameters monitored, are beginning to show that hemoglobin differences between Blacks and Whites (and American Indians) are much smaller than previously thought. Even more importantly, most surveys used to support claims of racial differences in hemoglobin levels were never intended to answer that question and therefore were not designed to address it. In addition, some differences that occur may be attributed to mild cases of thalassemia, which is associated with different sub-populations not necessarily restricted to Black populations (Yip et al. 1984; Expert Scientific Working Group 1985).

The cause of lower values among Blacks than Whites, even when factoring out differences in income, might result from a number of sociological reasons that exist for one subgroup (or race) to be subjected to poorer living conditions and more bodily insults than another, particularly in a society where racism is unfortunately all too common. There is some hematological evidence for this contention—later studies that included serum ferritin measurements show that whereas Blacks have lower hemoglobin levels, they concomitantly have higher serum ferritin levels, indicative of infectious diseases (Blumenfeld et al. 1988; Haddy et al. 1986:1084). This is noted by Garn (Chapter 2) who states that while Blacks have, on an average, lower hemoglobin levels, they also have, on an average, higher serum ferritin levels. Low hemoglobin and high serum ferritin levels are the diagnostic criteria for the anemia of chronic disease, an acquired and not genetic condition. More Blacks may suffer from infectious diseases and the associated anemia of chronic disease because of poverty, overcrowding, inadequate shelter, poor medical care, stress from being in a minority position, etc. This conclusion is supported by the fact that other impoverished and/or discriminated minorities in North America also tend to have lower hemoglobin values. For example, the prevalence of anemia among Chinese-Canadians was similar to Black Americans and dissimilar to White Americans (Chan-Yip and Gray-Donald 1987). Female Spanish-speaking Americans (Hispanics or Mexican-Americans) between the ages of 20 and 44 had a statistically higher frequency of anemia than Whites or Blacks, although the etiology of the anemia was not determined (Looker et al. 1989). Thus, lower hemoglobin levels appear not to be a Black-associated trait, but a minority- and poverty-associated trait.

Wadsworth discusses the worldwide distribution of low hemoglobin levels in Chapter 3, noting that most occurrences are not severe (i.e., values are above 7.0 g/100 ml). He outlines three basic properties of human physiology: (1) the body tends to conserve iron, (2) the amount of iron absorbed increases in anemic individuals and decreases in normal individuals, and (3) the higher the rate at which red blood cells are produced, the greater the amount of iron that enters the body. Thus, women who lose iron through menstruation will absorb twice as much iron as men. These properties combine so that the body's daily requirement for iron is met almost entirely by internal sources, regardless of diet. Moreover, Wadsworth points out that many, if not most, natural foods contain some iron and that many are further fortified with iron in most Western countries. Considering this, and the fact that a small amount of iron is available in most drinking water, Wadsworth concludes that diet has been given too much importance as a cause of anemia.

If diet and genetics do not account for the high incidence of anemia found worldwide, then what does? Weinberg, in Chapter 4, presents microbiological and medical data that show that hypoferremia, or low circulating iron levels, is a natural, nonspecific defense the body employs against disease. He demonstrates the link between hypoferremia and infectious disease—specifically, microorganisms require iron to proliferate but have no mechanism to store it. Microorganisms, therefore, must acquire iron from the host. Through a number of mechanisms including fever, lactoferrin, macrophages, suppression of intestinal absorption, etc., the body reduces the availability of iron in an attempt to combat microbial and neoplastic invasion. Weinberg reviews numerous studies that consistently show that iron overload promotes infectious disease and neoplasia, and that hypoferremia prevents them. He details the specific mechanisms involved in the iron withholding defense against disease and the cultural practices inhibiting that defense. The succeeding chapters directly or indirectly use the concepts presented in Weinberg's chapter to evaluate traditional views of anemia and to present new interpretations.

The role of anemia in past populations is investigated by Stuart-Macadam in Chapter 5. She convincingly establishes the association between acquired anemia and porotic hyperostosis. Stuart-Macadam further demonstrates that although inherited anemias can create porotic hyperostosis, this does not, pro forma, mean that acquired anemias cannot. Radiographs of crania exhibiting porotic hyperostosis show a number of similarities to radiographs of crania of living individuals with acquired anemia. Stuart-Macadam identifies three types of factors that influence the distribution of porotic hyperostosis: (1) temporal, (2) geographic, and (3) ecological variables. Temporally, the incidence of porotic hyperostosis increases from the Upper Paleolithic to the Neolithic. Geographically, porotic hyperostosis increases in frequency in areas closer to the equator. Ecologically, the incidence of porotic hyperostosis varies depending on the setting. In other words, porotic hypereostosis is more common in some sites than others that are located in different ecological settings but are occupied by the same people during the same time period. In each case, the role of anemia of chronic disease as a defense against disease is shown to be a major factor causing porotic hyperostosis. This is particularly true in areas where high pathogen loads occur, such as sedentary aggregated villages. In fact, for most situations where there is a high occurrence of porotic hyperostosis, the frequency of anemia can be better explained by a heavy pathogen load than by an inadequate diet.

Case Studies

This section examines in-depth the incidence of anemia in specific past and present societies. Authors evaluate and support many of the conclusions of the chapters in the theoretical and topical section. The chapters illustrate methods to distinguish between iron-deficiency anemia and the anemia of chronic disease in modern and prehistoric populations.

In Chapter 6, Kent and Lee discuss the hematology of !Kung hunter–gatherers of the Kalahari Desert at a time (1969) when the population maintained a nomadic to seminomadic, dispersed life-style and then again in 1987 when they lived in sedentary communities. The longitudinal data on the !Kung provide an opportunity to test the validity of the hypothesis that hypoferremia, rather than invariably being symptomatic of inadequate diets, can instead be a defense against disease in sedentary situations with high pathogen loads. The !Kung have undergone a number of transformations since 1969, particularly sedentism. The major dietary changes in 18 years are the heavy consumption of mealie meal (maize) flour and a concomitant substantial reduction in the amount of wild plants consumed. Despite these changes, meat still forms part of their diet in a roughly equivalent amount to that consumed before, although more meat is from domestic animals than before. A hematological follow-up study was conducted in 1987 in the same area and, in some cases, with the same individuals as the 1969 study. Lee noted that morbidity appeared to be higher in the 1987 population.

In spite of a similar meat intake, serum iron and transferrin saturation levels were lower in 1987. These levels were more similar to those found at Chum!kwe (a sedentary !Kung settlement in Namibia where health is known to be very poor) than to the levels observed when the group was living a more nomadic and dispersed life-style 18 years earlier. In fact, Kent and Lee point out that the 1987 Dobe population with a roughly adequate iron intake had a higher percentage of adults with subnormal serum iron and transferrin saturation values than did Chum!kwe adults with an acknowledged deficient diet. Concomitantly, a number of Dobe individuals had high normal to elevated serum ferritin levels in 1987, which is an indirect measure of hypoferremia in action. Since dietary intake of iron has not changed to the point of being nonnutritious in the intervening 18 years, whereas the health status has changed appreciably, the difference in hematologic values over the 18 years is probably due to a hypoferremic response to chronic, infectious diseases as a consequence of the newly sedentary life-style of the !Kung, rather than the result of changes in diet per se.

Ubelaker investigates the occurrence of porotic hyperostosis in Ecuador through time in Chapter 7. His data span 7000 years, during which time people shifted from a dispersed nomadic hunting–gathering way of life to an aggregated sedentary farming life-style. The data show that increased porotic hyperostosis coincides with decreased life expectancy and increased dental hypoplasia and periosteal new bone formation, but *not* with dietary changes (including an increased reliance on maize). In fact, skeletal remains exhibit evidence of porotic hyperostosis at some late sites containing numerous terrestrial faunal remains and maritime shell and fish resources in addition to cultigens. Conversely, skeletal remains at other sites where maize was a larger component of the diet have less porotic hyperostosis. A number of indirect measures of the frequency of infectious diseases provide evidence that porotic hyperostosis is found in sedentary aggregated communities with high pathogen loads, irrespective of diet. Parasitic infestations, particularly hookworm, probably also contribute to the frequency and distribution of porotic hyperostosis through time in Ecuador.

The relationship between porotic hyperostosis and parasites is further explored by Reinhard in Chapter 8. He presents a detailed analysis of prehistoric cases of anemia, diet, and disease using coprolite data collected from the southwestern region of the United States. Obvious dietary differences between Archaic hunter–gatherers and later Anasazi farmers have been invoked to explain an observed increase in porotic hyperostosis through time. However, demographic changes also occurred between the two periods—later people became much more sedentary and aggregated. As discussed in the other chapters in this section, sedentism and aggregation promote infectious diseases and this is seen in Reinhard's coprolite data. The frequency of parasites in coprolites increases from Archaic peoples to the Anasazi. There is a greater species richness (but not diversity) and a greater prevalence of parasites in the horticulturalists' than in the hunter–gatherers' coprolites. Importantly, Reinhard demonstrates that the incidence of porotic hyperostosis in skeletal populations and the incidence of maize consumption (as inferred from coprolite data) vary independently. The amount of bone in coprolites, from which the consumption of meat is inferred, also varies independently of the frequency of porotic hyperostosis. However, heavy infestation of parasites seems to covary with high percentages of porotic hyperostosis in skeletal populations. This shows that diet is not an influential factor in the distribution of porotic hyperostosis in prehistoric skeletal remains from the Southwest, but that the frequency instead results from sedentism and aggregation, and the poor sanitation and high morbidity that accompany the heavy pathogen loads characteristic of such a life-style.

Changing Perspectives and Their Implications

Together, the following chapters imply one inescapable conclusion—that we may in some cases have confused anemia resulting from dietary deficiencies with anemia resulting from chronic diseases/infections. This confusion has complicated our attempts to understand past and present causes of anemia and to alleviate present high levels of morbidity as defined by the frequency of anemia. One unifying theme of the previous chapters is that acquired low iron levels are not necessarily the result of inadequate diets. As a consequence, there exists a need to reexamine the commonly held belief of the public and some scientists that dietary iron supplements are necessary, even in the absence of complaints or symptoms (e.g., Parks, et al. 1989; Palti et al. 1987; and others). Such beliefs have resulted in government subsidy programs such as the Women, Infants, and Children (WIC) program for mothers and children at risk that allows mothers to purchase only iron-fortified infant formula as part of their policy. Also as a result of this belief, vitamins containing large doses of iron are popular among different groups (e.g., vitamins for pregnant women, older people, athletes, and/or individuals under stress). A number of products, flour, for example, are routinely enriched with iron. The conclusion one reaches after reading the following chapters is that it is necessary to question this common practice of massive, indiscriminate iron fortification and supplementation. However, to alter the mindset of the public will not be easy, even if it means the possibility of reducing morbidity. Policies formulated on the belief that most anemia results from dietary-induced iron deficiency may actually be perpetuating morbidity levels rather than eliminating them.

Although not all the following authors embrace the view that disease may be more important than diet in promoting anemia, they all recognize the need to include disease as a possible factor when interpreting their data on anemia. A holistic, interdisciplinary approach to past and present causes and distributions of anemia provides new avenues of inquiry into diet, demography, and disease, thereby increasing the possibility of reducing morbidity worldwide.

Often it seems reasonable to attribute the most obvious point about a phenomenon to its cause. The most obvious point about iron levels is that an extremely deprived diet can ultimately lead to acquired anemia. It is debatable whether such diets actually exist now or in the past except where people are literally starving to death under conditions of war, severe drought, or modern cash crop policies, which sacrifice subsistence farming (as is found in parts of Central and South America, Africa, and Asia). It is important to note that this volume deals with the amount of iron ingested and not with vitamins, protein, carbohydrates, fats, and other necessary components of a healthy diet.[9] We are not referring to populations that are starving to death, but to the other populations in which anemia is also prevalent. In fact, none of the authors in this book would state that diet is never a factor in causing acquired anemia. Instead, their work shows that the cause of anemia—whether diet or disease—must be demonstrated rather than simply assumed. Such a demonstration would require evidence that the anemia does not result from other actors now known to lower iron levels, such as hypoferremia as a body's defense against disease. As part of that evidence, hematological studies need to include analyses of several measures, particularly serum ferritin. Hemoglobin levels do not appear to be the most reliable indicators of health because they can be influenced by a number of cultural practices, such as smoking (Chapters 2, 4, and 6).

Kent and Lee (this volume) demonstrate how iron-deficiency anemia can be distinguished from anemia of chronic disease in modern populations. Relying on any single hematological index, such as hemoglobin values, out of the context or to the exclusion of the others can be misleading. Ubelaker and Reinhard both demonstrate how iron-deficiency anemia can be distinguished from the anemia of chronic disease in past populations also through the use of different lines of evidence, such as settlement patterns, skeletal pathologies indicative of infection, and coprolites, in addition to the presence of porotic hyperostosis. To accomplish this, diets need to be carefully reconstructed using faunal and botanical remains. Moreover, settlement patterns need to be determined using regional site size and distribution information. This is not an impossible goal and has, in fact, been done in the Southwest on the basis of coprolite data (Reinhard, this volume) and on the basis of various kinds of archaeological data, including faunal, botanical, and demographic (Kent 1986). Ubelaker (this volume) also illustrates how the etiology of porotic hyperostosis in skeletal populations can be determined using data from Ecuador.

A number of important implications can be drawn from the following chapters. First and foremost is the importance of constantly reevaluating theories as more data become available. Fever was once thought to be a problem associated with illness that needed to be eradicated. It is now known that fever aids in the defense of the body against infections (Jampel et al., 1983; Kluger and Rothenburg 1979). We propose that like fever, slightly to moderately low iron levels not associated with dietary insufficiency are also not a cause of disease but a defense against disease.

Second, it is imperative to be aware of our assumptions. Western society sometimes assumes that "you cannot have too much of a good thing," i.e., that iron additives improve health whether or not an individual actually physiologically needs them. In contrast, numerous studies indicate that more iron can be detrimental to health.

Third, it is necessary to test all interpretations against competing hypotheses. If diet alone is considered to be the probable cause of, for example, porotic hyperostosis, then the inevitable conclusion is that diet was at least partially responsible for the porotic hyperostosis. When multiple hypotheses are considered, the data, in many cases, fit the model of low hemoglobin levels associated with the anemia of chronic disease because of its role in warding off infections rather than the model of dietary iron-deficiency anemia. This is particularly true, for example, in areas where porotic hyperostosis exists in the skeletal population even though studies show that the intake of dietary iron was at least minimally acceptable (e.g., prehistoric Southwest, eastern United States, Alaskan Inuit or Eskimos, coastal California and elsewhere; Kent 1986, 1992; Nathan 1966; Powell 1988:48–58; Walker 1986).

Fourth, we need to reexamine the widespread policy of iron fortification of food from the perspective of acquired anemia presented here (see also Kent et al. 1990). If low iron levels are a function of the body's nonspecific immune system and that system is thwarted by the ingestion of large amounts of iron through fortified food and iron supplements, morbidity may actually increase rather than decrease. In other words, are we helping the microorganisms and hurting ourselves?

The chapters that follow do not necessarily agree in all details, but they do agree with the overall view that traditional concepts of acquired anemia need to be reexamined in the light of new data and changing ideas. The reader will find the following contributions provocative and

stimulating in their demand for a reassessment of the causes and consequences of acquired anemia in the past, the present, and the future.

Acknowledgments

I am most grateful for the excellent advice I received concerning this
chapter and would like to sincerely thank Drs. Patty Stuart-Macadam,
Gene Weinberg, George Wadsworth, Sara Quandt, R. Stuart, and an
anonymous reviewer for Aldine Press for their valuable comments and
suggestions. In addition, I am grateful to my brother, Dr. Steve Kent, a
physician, for his medical advice. I am, however, solely responsible for
any inadequacies of this chapter.

Notes

1. The consumption of large amounts of certain items inhibits the absorption
of dietary iron, causing individuals who are otherwise consuming more than adequate amounts of iron to be deficient (e.g., see Bindra and Gibson 1986). Iron
inhibitors include tannin (i.e., in tea), dietary fiber, coffee, calcium phosphate, soy
protein, phytates found in bran, and nuts, such as walnuts, almonds, peanuts,
hazelnuts, and Brazil nuts (Macfarlane et al. 1988; Monsen 1988; Munoz et al.
1988) The larger the amount of phytate consumed, the less iron is absorbed
(Hallberg et al. 1989). A diet may contain sufficient iron for the replacement of
normal physiological losses, but inhibitory factors can limit the absorption of that
iron. In these cases, people need to eat fewer food items that inhibit iron absorption rather than eat more iron-rich food.

In addition, moderate to heavy consumption of fish has been associated with a
significantly increased laboratory bleeding time among both males and females,
presumably resulting in significantly more blood loss and lower iron stores
(Herold and Kinsella 1986; Houwelingen et al. 1987; Sullivan 1989). This probably
explains why young women who habitually ate fish as their major source of protein had levels of serum ferritin and anemia similar to those of strict vegetarians
consuming iron-inhibitory substances (Worthington-Roberts et al. 1988).

There also are dietary iron enhancers that increase normal iron absorption. Absorption increases as a result of consumption of heme and nonheme iron together
in the same meal or as a result of the ingestion of enhancers, such as ascorbic acid,
alcohol, and, in some circumstances, citrate (Hallberg et al. 1989; Rodriguez et al.
1986; Clydesdale 1983). Thus, we can see that the amount of iron ingested per se
is not directly related to levels of anemia. Occult blood loss and iron absorption
are as important in fostering iron-deficiency anemia as is the actual amount of
dietary iron ingested.

2. Healthy 70-kg adult males lose approximately 1 mg of iron daily through
excretion by the skin and the gastrointestinal and urinary tracts (Bothwell, et al.

1989). As a consequence, required replacements are only 1 mg daily. Children lose only about 0.5 mg daily but their required replacement is approximately 1 mg daily to compensate for the needs of rapid growth. A Swedish study showed that the average woman loses between 0.6 and 0.7 mg through menstruation; 95% of women lose an average of *less* than 1.4 mg per day (Fairbanks and Beutler 1988:205). Nutritionists are beginning to recommend that average menstruating women absorb only 1.4 mg iron daily to replace losses (Monsen 1988:786).

Absorption of dietary iron varies according to the iron source and the iron-status of an individual. Iron-deficient males absorb 20% more nonheme iron found in vegetables and 21% more heme iron found in red meat than iron-replete males; normal males absorb less (Cook 1990:304). The same adaptability applies to iron loss. Normal males lose about 0.9 mg of iron per day. In contrast, hypoferremic males lose only about 0.5 mg per day and hyperferremic males lose about 2.0 mg per day (Finch 1989).

3. Between 0.7 and 1.5 g of iron in the body is found in storage (Bezkorovainy 1989). Storage iron occurs in either a diffuse soluble form as ferritin, an intracellular protein, or as hemosiderin, an insoluble aggregate form of ferritin (Bezkorovainy 1989). Ferritin is formed when apoferritin (an iron-free protein) combines with freed iron from the breakdown of hemoglobin in senescent red blood cells (Simmons 1989:14). Hemosiderin represents the end point of the intracellular storage iron pathway. Hemosiderin granules are actually denatured, partly degraded, aggregated molecules of ferritin (Bezkorovainy 1989). A small amount of ferritin occurs in plasma, which then provides a useful measure of an individual's iron stores.

4. A study of 301 patients showed that "iron deficiency was correctly diagnosed by serum iron in 41%, TIBC in 84%, %Sat [transferrin saturation] in 50%, and ferritin in 90%" (Burns et al. 1990:240).

5. This can be seen in studies of specific types of cancer. For instance, the etiology of colon cancer has been linked to free radicals, which play an important role in carcinogenesis (Babbs 1990; also see Bacon and Britton, 1990, for a study of the role of free radicals in hepatic cancer as evidenced from experimental iron overload in nonhuman animals). This etiology explains why there is an increased incidence of colon cancer in people who ingest a high meat diet that provides more iron or who ingest a low fiber diet that allows for greater fecal concentration of iron. It also explains the incidence of colon cancer among suffers from chronic ulcerative colitis—the condition makes heme iron available from chronic bleeding and may result in prescribed iron supplementation of the diet to correct for chronic blood loss and consequent iron deficiency anemia (Babbs 1990:198). Other researchers have found significant correlations between parenteral supplementation of iron and the augmentation of tumor yield and oral iron and the augmentation of tumor incidence (Nelson et al. 1989). According to Babbs (1990:198) one of several important measures to reduce the risk of colon cancer is "recommending a lower iron diet and fewer iron supplements in adult men and postmenopausal women, who are at greater risk of developing colon cancer and do not have physiologic requirements for iron." This suggestion has been made for other types of cancer (see Weinberg, Chapter 4 for a discussion of cancer and iron).

6. Other reasons for the relationship between viral and secondary bacterial infections, for example, include (1) viral depression of normal neutrophil and macrophage activity, (2) viral impairment of chemotactic factors critical to host defense in early bacterial invasion, and (3) enhancement of colonization of both

gram-positive and gram-negative bacteria through the alteration of cell surface, thereby permitting bacteria to propagate within the intestine rather than being flushed harmlessly through the system (Kent 1986). Phagocytic cell dysfunction and virus-induced immunosuppression, particularly of the lymphocytes, also increase host susceptibility to secondary microbial invasion (Babiuk 1984).

7. There has been some contradictory reports of macrophage activation in anemic experimental subjects. Many studies indicate iron increases microbicidal action; however, there are some reports that suggest that iron actually inhibits such action, as pointed out by Scrimshaw (1991). Weinberg offers several explanations for the apparent contradiction. One "reason for such incongruity might relate to the specific intracellular location of the pathogen. Trypanasomes multiply in the cytoplasm of the macrophage whereas leishmania reside in phagolysosomes; and ... [other bacteria] live in phagosomes that do not fuse with lysosomes" (Weinberg 1992:41). He further suggests that another "possible reason for opposing effects of iron in various systems might be associated with the tissues in which the macrophage is localized" (Weinberg 1992:41). Nonetheless, his conclusion, as outlined in Chapter 4, is that low iron levels are a defense the body employs against disease.

8. A similar problem of distinguishing cause and effect can be seen in studies of the immunological system and anemia. Some investigators claim their studies illustrate that anemia causes an impairment in the immunological system that affects the body's ability to ward off disease (e.g., Vyas and Chandra 1984). Others claim their studies illustrate that anemia improves immunity from disease (Murray and Murray 1977). For instance, despite *in vitro* studies that show experimentally that there is a decrease in bactericidal capabilities in neutrophils, *in vivo* studies of human infections show "no noticeable increase ... in respiratory, gastrointestinal, or in [general] morbidity, either in the few days before the initiation of iron therapy, or in the subsequent 15 days of close clinical and laboratory follow-up, confirming previous observations that iron deficiency anemia, even when severe, does not appear to compromise immune mechanisms to the extent of allowing ominous clinical manifestations" (Walter et al. 1986). Of course, this observation does not necessarily apply to extremely severe cases where there is insufficient iron to perform basic metabolic functions. Such extremely severe anemia is often the consequence of parasitic infection and/or bleeding, rather than due to diet.

9. Studies do show that poor protein and energy intake will stunt children's growth and adversely affect mental development (Grantham-McGregor et al. 1991).

References

Adelekan, D., and David Thurnham. 1990. Plasma ferritin concentrations in anemic children: Relative importance of malaria, riboflavin deficiency, and other infections. *American Journal of Clinical Nutrition* 51:453–56.

Andrews, F.J., C.J. Morris, E.J. Lewis, and D.R. Blake. 1987. Effect of nutritional iron deficiency on acute and chronic inflammation. *Annals of the Rheumatic Diseases* 46:859–865.

Arthur, C.K., and J.P. Isbister. 1987. Iron deficiency: Misunderstood, misdiagnosed and mistreated. *Drugs* 33:171–182.

Babbs, C. 1990. Free radicals and the etiology of colon cancer. *Free Radical Biology and Medicine* 8:191–200.

Babiuk, L. 1984a. Viral-bacterial synergistic interactions in respiratory infections. In E. Kurstak (ed.), pp. 431–443. *Applied Virology*. New York: Academic Press.

Bacon, B., and R. Britton. 1990. The pathology of hepatic iron overload: A free radical-mediated process? *Hepatology* 11:127–137.

Barry, D.M., and A.W. Reeve. 1973. Iron injections and serious gram-negative infections in Polynesian newborns. *New Zealand Medical Journal* 78:376.

Barry, D.M., and A.W. Reeve. 1977. Increased incidence of gram-negative neonatal sepsis with intramuscular iron administration. *Pediatrics* 60:908–912.

Becroft, D.M., M.R. Dix, and K. Farmer. 1977. Intramuscular iron-dextran and susceptibility of neonates to bacterial infections. *Archives of Diseases of Childhood* 52:778–781.

Beissner, R., and A. Trowbridge. 1986. Clinical assessment of anemia. *Postgraduate Medicine* 80(6):83–95.

Bezkorovainy, A. 1980. *Biochemistry of Nonheme Iron*. New York: Plenum Press.

Bezkorovainy, A. 1989. Biochemistry of nonheme iron in man. *Clinical and Physiological Biochemistry* 7:1–17.

Bindra, G., and R. Gibson. 1986. Iron status of predominantly lacto-ovo vegetarian East Indian immigrants to Canada: A model approach. *American Journal of Clinical Nutrition* 44:643–652.

Blumenfeld, N., M. Fabry, B. Thysen, and R. Nagel. 1988. Red cell density is sex and race dependent in the adult. *Journal of Laboratory and Clinical Medicine* 112:333–338.

Bothwell, T., R. Charlton, J. Cook, and C. Finch. 1979. *Iron Metabolism in Man*. Oxford: Blackwell Scientific Publications.

Bothwell, T., R.D. Baynes, B.J. MacJarlane, and A.P. MacPhail. 1989. Nutritional iron requirements and food iron absorption. *Journal of Internal Medicine* 226:357–365.

Burns, E., S.N. Goldberg, C. Lawrence, and B. Weinz. 1990. Clinical utility of serum tests for iron deficiency in hospitalized patients. *American Journal of Clinical Pathology* 93:240–245.

Centers for Disease Control. 1986. Declining anemia prevalence among children enrolled in public nutrition and health programs: Selected states, 1975–1985. *Morbidity and Mortality Weekly Report* 35 (36):565–567.

Chan-Yip, A., and K. Gray-Donald. 1987. Prevalence of iron deficiency among Chinese children aged 6 to 36 months in Montreal. *Canadian Medical Association Journal* 136:373–378.

Cole, M., A.R. Mestecky, J. Prince, S. Kulhavy, A., and McGhee, J.R. 1976. Studies with human lactoferrin and *Streptococcus mutans*. In *Microbial Aspects of Dental Caries* Stiles HM, Loesche W and O'Brien T, eds. pp. 359–373. Washington, D.C.: Information Retrieval, Inc.

Cook, J. (ed.). 1980. *Iron*. New York: Churchill Livingston.

Cook, J. 1990. Adaptation in iron metabolism. *American Journal of Clinical Nutrition* 51:301–308.

Cook, J., and S. Lynch. 1986. The liabilities of iron deficiency. *Blood* 68:803–809.

Cook, J., and B. Skikne. 1989. Serum ferritin: A possible model for the assessment of nutrient stores. *American Journal of Clinical Nutrition* 35:1180–1185.

Cook, J., J. Alvarado, A. Gutnisky, M. Jamra, J. Labardini, M. Layrisse, J. Linares, A. Loria, V. Maspes, A. Restrepo, C. Reynafarje, L. Sanchez-Medal, H. Velez, and F. Viteri. 1971. Nutritional deficiency and anemia in Latin America: A collaborative study. *Blood* 38:591–603.

Clydesdale, F. 1983. Physicochemical determinants of iron bioavailability. *Food Technology* 37:133–144.

Dallman, P. 1987. Has routine screening of infants for anemia become obsolete in the United States? *Pediatrics* 80(3):439–441.

Dallman, P. 1989. Iron deficiency: Does it matter? *Journal of Internal Medicine* 226:367–372.

Dallman, P., R. Yip, and C. Johnson. 1984. Prevalence and causes of anemia in the United States, 1976 to 1980. *American Journal of Clinical Nutrition* 39:437–445.

Daly, M. 1989. Anemia in the elderly. *American Family Physician* 39(3):129–136.

DeMaeyer, E., and M. Adiels-Tegman. 1985. The prevalence of anaemia in the world. *World Health Statistics Quarterly* 38:302–316.

Expert Scientific Working Group. 1985. Summary of a report on assessment of the iron nutritional status of the United States population. *The American Journal of Clinical Nutrition* 42:1318–1330.

Fairbanks, V., and E. Beutler. 1989. Iron. In *Modern Nutrition in Health and Disease*. M. Shils and V. Young, eds., pp. 193–226. Philadelphia: Lea & Febiger.

Farley, P., and J. Foland. 1990. Iron deficiency anemia: How to diagnose and correct. *Postgraduate Medicine* 87(2):89–101.

Farthing, M.J. 1989. Iron and immunity. *Acta Paediatric Scandinavia Supplemental* 361:44–52.

Finch, C.A. 1989. Introduction: Knights of the oval table. *Journal of Internal Medicine* 226:345–348.

Finch, C.A. and H. Huebers. 1982. Perspectives in iron metabolism. *New England Journal of Medicine* 306(25):1520–1528.

Gardner, G., V.R. Edgerton, B. Senewiratne, et al. 1977. Physical work capacity and metabolic stress in subjects with iron deficiency anemia. *American Journal of Clinical Nutrition* 30:910–917.

Gidding, S., and J. Stockman. 1988. Effect of iron deficiency on tissue oxygen delivery in cyanotic congenital heart disease. *American Journal of Cardiology* 61:605–607.

Gould, S.J. 1977. *Ever Since Darwin: Reflections in Natural History*. New York: W.W. Norton.

Grantham-McGregor, S.M., C.A. Powell, S.P. Walker, and J.H. Himes. 1991. Nutritional supplementation, psychosocial stimulation, and mental development of stunted children: The Jamaican Study. *The Lancet* 338:1–5.

Guyatt, G., C. Patterson, M. Ali, J. Singer, M. Levine, I. Turpie, and R. Meyer. 1990. Diagnosis of iron-deficiency anemia in the elderly. *American Journal of Medicine* 88:205–209.

Haddy, T., O. Castro, S. Rana, and R. Scott. 1986. Iron status and liver function in healthy adults: A multiracial pilot study. *Southern Medical Journal* 79: 1082–1085.

Haddock, R., S. Cousens, and C. Guzman. 1991. Infant diet and salmonellosis. *American Journal of Public Health* 81:997–1000.

Hallberg, L., M. Brune, and L. Rossander. 1989. Iron absorption in man: Ascorbic acid and dose-dependent inhibition by phytate. *American Journal of Clinical Nutrition* 49:140–144.

Hengen, O.P. 1971. Cribra orbitalia: Pathogenesis and probable etiology. *Homo* 22:57–77.

Henry, J. 1984. *Clinical Diagnosis and Management by Laboratory Methods*, 17th ed. Philadelphia: W.B. Saunders.

Herold, P.M., and J.E. Kinsella. 1986. Fish oil consumption and decreased risk of cardiovascular disease. *American Journal of Clinical Nutrition* 43:566–598.

Heywood, A. 1989. Comment on Impact of iron supplementation on cognitive functions by Seshadri and Gopaldas. *American Journal of Clinical Nutrition* 50:685.

Hoffbrand, A.V. 1981. Iron. In *Postgraduate Hematology*. A.V. Hoffbrand and S.M. Lewis, eds., pp. 35–42. London: William Heinemann Medical Books.

Houwelingen, R.V., A. Nordoy, E. van der Beek, U. Houtsmuller, M. de Metz, and G. Hornstra. 1987. Effect of a moderate fish intake on blood pressure, bleeding time, hematology, and clinical chemistry in healthy males. *American Journal of Clinical Nutrition* 46:424–436.

Jampel, H., G. Duff, R. Gershon, E. Atkins, and S. Durum. 1984. Fever and immunoregulation. *Journal of Experimental Medicine* 157(4):1229–1238.

Jansson, L.T., S. Kling, and P.R. Dallman. 1986. Anemia in children with acute infections seen in a primary care pediatric outpatient clinic. *Pediatric Infectious Diseases* 5:424–427.

Johnson, D., and R. McGowan. 1983. Anemia and infant behavior. *Nutrition and Behavior* 1:185–192.

Kent, S. 1986. The influence of sedentism and aggregation on porotic hyperostosis and anemia: A case study. *Man* (N.S.) 21:605–636.

Kent, S. 1992. Iron deficiency and other acquired anemias. In *The Cambridge Historical, Geographical, and Cultural Encyclopedia of Human Nutrition*. K. Kipple, ed. Cambridge: Cambridge University Press.

Kent, S., and P. Stuart-Macadma. 1992. Iron. In *The Cambridge Historical, Geographical, and Cultural Encyclopedia of Human Nutrition*: edited by K. Kipple, ed. Cambridge: Cambridge University Press.

Kent, S., E. Weinberg, and P. Stuart-Macadam. 1990. Dietary and prophylactic iron supplements: Helpful or harmful? *Human Nature* 1(1):55–81.

Kent, S., E. Weinberg, and P. Stuart-Macadam, n.d. The etiology of the anemia of chronic disease. Submitted for publication.

Kluger, M.J., and J.J. Bullen. 1987. Clinical and physiological aspects. In *Iron and Infection*. J.J. Bullen and E. Griffiths, eds., pp. 243–282. London: John Wiley.

Kluger, M., and B. Rothenburg. 1979. Fever and reduced iron: Their interaction as host defense response to bacterial infection. *Science* 203:374–376.

Lima, M.F. and F. Kierszenbaum. 1987. Lactoferrin effects on phagocytic cell function. *Journal of Immunology* 139:1647–1651.

Looker, Anne, C. Johnson, M. McDowell, and E. Yetley. 1989. Iron status: Prevalence of impairment in three Hispanic groups in the United States. *American Journal of Clinical Nutrition* 49:553–558.

Lozoff, B. 1989. Methodologic issues in studying behavioral effects of infant iron-deficiency anemia. *Journal of Clinical Nutrition* 50:641–654.

Lozoff, B. 1990. Has iron deficiency been shown to cause altered behaviour in infants? In *Brain, Behaviour, and Iron in the Infant Diet*. J. Dobbing, ed., pp. 107–131. London: Springer-Verlag.

Lozoff, B., and G. Brittenham. 1987. Behavioral alterations in iron deficiency. *Hematology/Oncology Clinics of North America* 1(3):449–464.

Lozoff, B., E. Jimenez, and A. Wolf. 1991. Long-term developmental outcome of infants with iron deficiency. *New England Journal of Medicine* 325(10):687–694.

Macfarlane, B., W. Bezwoda, T. Bothwell, et al. 1988. Inhibitory effect of nuts on iron absorption. *American Journal of Clinical Nutrition* 47:270–274.

Masawe, A.E., J.M. Muindi, and G.B. Swai. 1974. Infections in iron deficiency and other types of anaemia in the topics. *Lancet* 2:314–317.

Monsen, E. 1988. Iron nutrition and absorption: Dietary factors which impact iron bioavailability. *Journal of the American Dietetic Association* 88:786–790.

Munoz, L, B. Lönnerdal, C. Keen, and K. Dewey. 1988. Coffee consumption as a factor in iron deficiency anemia among pregnant women and their infants in Costa Rica. *American Journal of Clinical Nutrition* 48:645–651.

Murray, M.J., and A. Murray. 1977. Starvation suppression and refeeding activation of infection: An ecological necessity? *Lancet* 1:123–125.

Murray, M.J., N. Murray, and M. Murray. 1976. Somali food shelters in the Ogaden famine and their impact on health. *Lancet* 1:1283–1285.

Murray, M.J., A. Murray, and C.J. Murray. 1980a. An ecological interdependence of diet and disease? *American Journal of Clinical Nutrition* 33:697–701.

Murray, M.J., A. Murray, and C.J. Murray. 1980b. The salutary effect of milk on amoebiasis and its reversal by iron. *British Medical Journal* 280:1351–1352.

Nathan, H. 1966. Cribra orbitalia: A bone condition of the orbit of unknown nature: Anatomical study with etiological considerations. *Israel Journal of Medical Science* 2:171–191.

Neilands, J.B. 1981. Iron absorption and transport in microorganisms. *Annual Review of Nutrition* 1:27–46.

Nelson, R.L., S.J. Yoo, J.C. Tanure, G. Andrianopoulos, and A. Misumi. 1989. The effect of iron on experimental colorectal carcinogenesis. *Anticancer Research* 9:1477–1482.

Noyes, W. 1985. Anemia as a result of insufficiency in the production of red cells.

In *Hematology and Oncology.* Marshall Lichtman, ed., pp. 23–28. New York: Grune & Stratton.

Olivares, M., T. Walter, M. Osorio, et al. 1989. Anemia of a mild viral infection: The measles vaccine as a model. *Pediatrics* 84(5):851–855.

O'Neill-Cutting, M., and W. Crosby. 1987. Blocking of iron absorption by a preliminary oral dose of iron. *Archives of Internal Medicine* 147:489–491.

Oppenheimer, S.J., S.B. MacFarlane, J.B. Moody, et al. 1986a. Effect of iron prophylaxis on morbidity due to infectious disease: Report on clinical studies in Papua New Guinea. *Transactions of the Royal Society of Tropical Medicine and Hygiene* 80:596–602.

Oppenheimer, S.J., F.D. Gibson, S.B. MacFarlane, et al. 1986b. Iron supplementation increases prevalence and effects of malaria: Report on clinical studies in Papua New Guinea. *Transactions of the Royal Society of Tropical Medicine and Hygiene* 80:603–612.

Palti, H., B. Adler, J. Hurvitz, D. Tamir, and S. Freier. 1987. Use of iron supplements in infancy: A field trial. *Bulletin of the World Health Organization* 65(1):87–94.

Parks, Y.A., M.A. Aukett, J.A. Murray, P.H. Scott, and B.A. Wharton. 1989. Mildly anaemic toddlers respond to iron. *Archives of Disease in Childhood* 64:400–401.

Pollitt, E., P. Hathirat, N. Kotchabhakdi, L. Missell, and A. Valyasevi. 1989. Iron deficiency and educational achievement in Thailand. *American Journal of Clinical Nutrition* 1989:687–697.

Powell, M. 1988. *Status and Health in Prehistory: A Case Study of the Moundville Chiefdom.* Washington, D.C.: Smithsonian Institution Press.

Reizenstein, P. 1983. *Hematologic Stress Syndrome: The Biological Response to Disease.* New York: Praeger Scientific.

Rodriguez, M.C., M.S. Henriquez, A.F. Turon, F.J. Novoa, J.G. Diax, and P.B. Leon. 1986. Trace elements in chronic alcoholism. *Trace Elements in Medicine* 3:164–167.

Scrimshaw, N. 1990. Functional significance of iron deficiency. In *Functional Significance of Iron Deficiency.* C. Enwonwu, ed., pp. 1–13, Nashville, TN: Meharry Medical College.

Scrimshaw, N. 1991. Iron deficiency. *Scientific American* 265:46–52.

Seshadri, S., and T. Gopaldas. 1989. Impact of iron supplementation on cognitive functions in preschool and school-aged children: The Indian experience. *Journal of Clinical Nutrition* 50:675–686.

Simmons, A. 1989. *Hematology: A Combined Theoretical and Technical Approach.* Philadelphia: W.B. Saunders.

Stein, J. 1990. *Internal Medicine.* Boston: Little, Brown.

Stevens, R. 1990. Iron and the risk of cancer. *Medical Oncology and Tumor Pharmacother* 7(2/3):177–181.

Stuart-Macadam, P. 1989. Nutritional deficiency diseases: A survey of scurvy, rickets, and iron-deficiency anemia. In *Reconstruction of Life from the Skeleton.* M. Iscan and K. Kennedy, eds., pp. 201–222. New York: Liss.

Sullivan, J. 1989. The iron paradigm of ischemic heart disease. *American Heart Journal* 117:1177–1188.

Thompson, Warren. 1988. Comparison of tests for diagnosis of iron depletion in pregnancy. *American Journal of Obsetetrics and Gynecology* 159:1132–1134.

Vyas, D., and R.K. Chandra. 1984. Functional implications of iron deficiency. In *Iron Nutrition in Infancy and Childhood*. A. Stekel, ed., pp. 45–59. New York: Raven Press.

Wadsworth, G. (1975). Nutritional factors in Anaemia. *World Review of Nutrition and Diet* 21:75–150.

Walker, P. 1986. Porotic hyperostosis in a marine-dependent California Indian population. *American Journal of Physical Anthropology* 69:345–354.

Walter, T. 1989. Comment on Impact of iron supplementation on cognitive functions by Seshadri and Gopaldas. *American Journal of Clinical Nutrition* 50:685.

Walter, T., S. Arredondo, M. Arevalo, and A. Stekel. 1986. Effect of iron therapy on phagocytosis and bactericidal activity in neutrophils of iron-deficient infants. *American Journal of Clinical Nutrition* 44:877–82.

Weinberg, E. 1983. Iron in neoplastic disease. *Nutrition and Cancer* 4:223–233.

———. 1984. Iron withholding: A defense against infection and neoplasia. *Physiological Reviews* 64:65–102.

Weinberg, E. 1992. Roles of iron in function of activated macrophages. *Journal of Nutritional Immunology* 1(1):41–63.

Worthington-Roberts, B., M. Breskin, and E. Monsen. 1988. Iron status of premenopausal women in a university community and its relationship to habitual dietary sources of protein. *American Journal of Clinical Nutrition* 47:275–279.

Yehuda, S. and M. Youdim. 1989. Brain iron: A lesson from animal models. *American Journal of Clinical Nutrition* 50:681–629.

Yip, R., S. Schwartz, and A. Deinard. 1984. Hematocrit values in White, Black, and American Indian children with comparable iron status. *American Journal of Diseases in Childhood* 138:824–827.

Youdim, M., D. Ben-Shachar, and S. Yehuda. 1989. Putative biological mechanisms of the effect of iron deficiency on brain biochemistry and behavior. *American Journal of Clinical Nutrition* 50:607–617.

Zanella, A., L. Gridelli, A. Berzuini, et al. 1989. Sensitivity and predictive value of serum ferritin and free erythrocyte protoporphyrin for iron deficiency. *Journal of Laboratory and Clinical Medicine* 113(1):73–78.

Part I

THEORETICAL EXPLORATIONS

Chapter 2

The Iron-Deficiency Anemias and Their Skeletal Manifestations

Stanley M. Garn

Anemia (literally "no blood") is a condition characterized by a decreased number of red blood cells, decreased hemoglobin concentrations, or both. Apart from disorders of the blood-forming system and exposure to certain toxins and renal disorders, anemia is commonly due to parasitization, caloric insufficiency, inadequate intakes of iron and zinc, and the presence of dietary factors that limit the availability of dietary iron and zinc. With anemia, defined in terms of decreased hemoglobin concentration (g/dl) and decreased red cell volume (9% vol), there is pallor, lassitude, and decreased learning ability at all ages and decreased growth and delayed sexual maturation. From existing population data, we would expect that past populations in areas of single-grain dependence or where wheat and other grain phytates were considerable would show evidence of anemia. However, the skeletal manifestations of anemia—including marrow cavity enlargement and decreased cortical mass—have not been well studied. Furthermore, it is difficult to relate the clinical condition of "anemia" to the skeletal manifestations (subperiosteal pits and lacunae), often but incorrectly termed "osteoporosis." If individual skeletal remains so characterized can be shown to have marrow cavity enlargement in the tubular bones and decreased bone mass relative to volume, the putative relationship could be confirmed. Moreover chronic renal disease, with anemia due to failure of erythropoiesis, could be a useful working model. Individuals with excessive iron intake and *hemosiderosis* provide an alternative (and opposite) model to test, as do populations ingesting animal blood and those consuming heart, liver, or kidneys on a daily basis.

Introduction

Hundreds of years ago the term *anemic* (i.e., without blood) was applied to individuals with pallor, lassitude, and shortened attention span.
Such individuals resembled, more or less, those who had lost blood in
battle, following accidents or after the crude surgery of the time. So the
word anemia came into the language, but only in the last century has it
been realized that anemia is a symptom and not a disease in itself.

Now we measure the percentage of red blood cells in the blood, as the
hematocrit (Hct). We also measure the concentration of the blood pigment
hemoglobin (Hgb). These two measurements, percent packed cell volume
and hemoglobin concentration expressed as grams per deciliter, provide
information on both excesses and deficiencies of the hematologic system,
including those of dietary and nutritional origin.

Our attention here is primarily devoted to deficiencies in red cell number and in hemoglobin content and the "anemias" of dietary, nutritional,
and parasitic origin. However, the excesses also merit notice, for high
altitude, exposure to atmospheric pollutants, excessive iron intake, and
even a high level of athletic performance all complicate the interpretation
of hematologic data.

Some Causes of "Anemia"

There are many reasons why Hgb and Hct may be low, beginning with
overt blood loss and covert blood loss from ulcers and neoplasms of the
gastrointestinal system. Menstrual blood loss can be a factor, and exposure to chemicals that cause hemolysis. "Anemias" may also stem
from deficiencies in the blood-forming tissue, from renal disease and
from the inability resorb and reuse iron. However, the anemias we are
concerned with here are primarily those attributable to insufficient
dietary iron and zinc, and to other dietary factors that may limit the
availability of Fe and Zn.

There is also folate-deficiency anemia (so-called pernicious anemia),
and certain other anemias of dietary origin. Most of the time, however,
low levels of hemoglobin or a low hematocrit can be traced to an insufficient iron intake or to dietary factors (like wheat phytate) or excessive
fiber that limit the amount of Fe or Zn that can be absorbed. These are of
particular interest to archaeologists concerned with the effects of agricul-

ture and the varied consequences of dependence on rice, corn, wheat, barley, and other grains.

"Who Is "Deficient," "Low," and "Normal" in Hgb and Hct?

Hemaglobin concentrations and percent packed-cell volumes have been used for many years, because they are so simple to determine. Prior to the advent of photoelectric colorimeters, hemoglobin concentration was read off visually against a printed color standard. A hand-operated two-tube centrifuge allowed blood samples to be "spun down" in capillary tubes and the hematocrit was then read across a percentage nomogram. Once, no physician's office was so poorly provided as to lack the basic equipment. Now the doctor sends the blood sample out to a clinical laboratory instead.

So hemoglobin and hematocrit "standards" came into early use, and such standards can be found in most medical textbooks (cf. Nelson et al. 1969) and in manuals for nutrition surveys (ICNND 1963). However, these traditional standards often leave much to be desired, simply because of their antiquity. For the most part they simply provide indications of the "normal range" for infants, adolescents, and adults, often grouping all above age 20 in the latter category. Some tables further list particular cut-off values designated as "low" and "deficient," respectively.

It is difficult to ascertain where the standard values originally came from (cf. Wintrobe 1974), since they have been handed down from hematology textbook to hematology textbook, in the process called cannibalization. Rarely have the terms "low" and "deficient" been accorded quantification, and in some published standards these terms are used interchangeably (see Figure 1). In apology it is stated that the published values are the result of long experience and that there is considerable normal variation.

Further complications occur at even moderate altitude (i.e., below 1 mile or 2 km). Since blood cell concentrations are higher where the air pressure is less, a correction constant is often added to the textbook standards for Hgb and Hct. Thus, the standards used for the nutritional evaluation of Navajos in Greasewood, NM are the standards of the ICNND Nutrition Survey Manual minus an altitude correction.

Since we now have hematologic data on tens of thousands of infants, children, and adults from the Ten-State Nutrition Survey (TSNS), the Pre-School Nutrition Survey, and from NHANES I and NHANES II, it is pos-

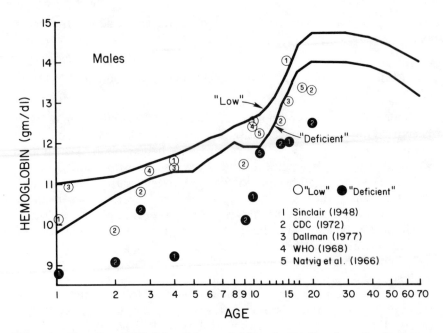

Figure 1. "Low" and "deficient" hemoglobin values taken from the literature
plotted against the 5th and 85th centiles calculated from NHANES I.
Particularly for infants and children, traditional textbook cutoff values may
be viewed as unrealistically low (cf. Garn et al. 1981c,d; Johnson et al. 1978).

sible to calculate percentiles from such massive data for use as standards.
Here the 15th percentile is a useful statistical definition of "low" and the
5th percentile constitutes a useful cut-off value for "deficient." These cor-
respond more or less to the −1 and −2 SD limits, since Hgb and Hct distributions are approximately Gaussian and without kurtosis except
during adolescence (when there is a mixture of early-maturing and late-
maturing individuals) (see Figure 2, and Garn et al. 1981).

From the Ten-State, Pre-School Nutrition Survey, and NHANES
hematologic data, it is clear that many of the traditional cut-off values for
"low" are remarkably low, compared with the median values in the
recent surveys. Fully 50% of the boys and girls and younger men and
women in these surveys may be designated as "low" in Hgb and Hct by
the commonly used textbook standards (and a still larger proportion of
older adults).

Now it can be argued that population data on Hgb and Hct constitute

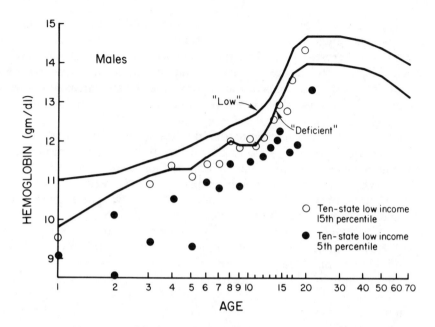

Figure 2. Fifth centile (black dots) and 15th centile values (open dots) for low-income children and adults in the Ten-State Nutrition Survey plotted against the 5th and 15th centiles for the NHANES I National Probability Sample. Hemoglobin values for the impoverished are systematically far below national expectancy (Garn et al. 1981c).

an inadequate basis for hematologic norms and standards, since some of the people in these surveys were indeed iron deficient and therefore "at risk." So it is customary to use additional data on serum transferrin levels, percent transferrin saturation, and serum iron to identify and eliminate those at-risk individuals from the survey data sets. One can then modify or adjust the population data, excluding those with low transferrins, etc. Various workers have therefore developed tables showing suggested values for "deficient" and "low" hemoglobins and hematocrits (cf. Garn et al. 1981a,b,c; cf. Lowe et al. 1975).

There are still complications and additions to note. Pregnant women should be listed by trimester of pregnancy, not lumped as a group. Older men and women (defining "older" as over 40 for men and over 50 for women) deserve separate attention, especially those in the eighth decade and above. For adolescents, maturational level is also critical. A 15-year-old boy who is developmentally mature should be 1 g/dl higher in Hgb than a still immature adolescent of exactly the same age.

For those who plan to employ hematologic data in a critical fashion, these newer "suggested" values of Hgb and Hct do merit attention, along with the further need to identify those with low and deficient transferrin levels. There is still the problem of altitude and altitude correction, for use in Colorado, New Mexico, and Arizona, the elevated areas of Central America, the Andes, the Himalayas, and Tibet. Then there are the hemoglobinopathics.

Moreover, there is also need to identify those whose hematologic levels are unacceptably *high*, excluding athletes and similarly trained individuals (whose elevated hematologic values result from their "fitness"). What is unacceptably high, as distinct from statistically high, is at present somewhat difficult to define, since obesity, emphysema, and chronic exposure to dust and lint also enter the picture. Smoking, that is cigarette smoking, at a one-pack level or above also pushes up Hgb and Hct levels (complicating interpretations at all levels). Probably, smokers have higher hematologic levels because part of their hemoglobin is carboxyhemoglobin, without ability to transfer oxygen to the tissues. In any event, smokers should be separated from nonsmokers in data analysis, even for subteens in many cultures (where smoking may begin at age 10 or even earlier).

So textbook norms for Hgb and Hct must be used with appropriate caution, especially the cut-off values for "low" and "deficient" hemoglobin concentrations and packed cell volumes. Though newer suggested cut-off values for "low" and "deficient" are more appropriate than the long-used standard values found in many hematology texts and most older pediatric textbooks, there is the further need in population surveys to give particular attention to serum transferrin, transferrin saturation, and iron saturation to know who is truly at risk for iron-deficiency anemia and who may be unacceptably high (cf. Perry et al. 1992).

Validating Hematologic Levels

From mass-survey nutritional data—TSNS, PNS, NHANES—it is abundantly clear that growing individuals with higher hematologic levels are at an advantage. Boys and girls who are taller and heavier for their age do have higher Hgb and Hct levels. Conversely, those with higher Hgb and Hct levels are also taller and heavier. Even within the accepted range of "normal" (or the 15th and 85th percentiles), higher hematologic levels do appear to be auxogenic. Conversely, lower levels

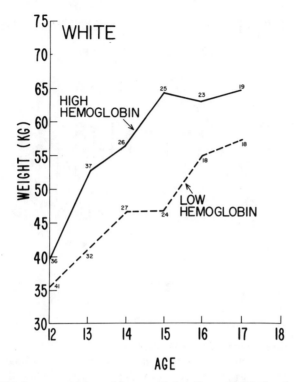

Figure 3. Weight comparisons of boys with low hemoglobin levels ($p \leq 15$) and high hemoglobin levels ($p \geq 85$). Boys with higher Hgb levels average 5 kg higher, in part because they are developmentally advanced (cf. Figure 4).

of Hgb and Hct (even within the range of "normal") appear to be growth depressing, though it is often difficult to separate cause from effect (see Figures 3 and 4).

Socioeconomic effects on Hgb and Hct

Hemoglobin and hematocrit levels, expressed as g/dl and percent cell volume, both increase with increasing socioeconomic status (SES) and with its components—income, education, and occupation. High SES infants, children, adolescents, and adults tend to have higher Hgb and Hct levels than do their low-SES age peers. The magnitude of the hematologic

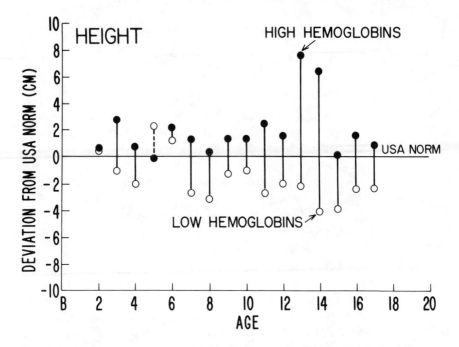

Figure 4. Stature comparisons of White boys with high Hgb levels (black dots) and low Hgb levels (open dots). High Hgb levels are associated with greater stature during growth, especially during the period when the mixture of early maturers and late maturers exaggerates the stature differences (cf. Figure 5).

differences is a function of sample size, and the contrasting SES cuts. Accordingly, the differences between the high-income and low-income segments of the Ten State Nutrition Survey partially sampled in Table 1 is only illustrative (and there are additional factors to consider).

Why the poor have lower Hgb and Hct levels than the affluent is not certain, though diet and living conditions and knowledge of nutrition all play a role. Parallel dietary data generally show lower iron intakes for the poor, and the poor are less likely to employ dietary supplements. The impoverished are more likely to be parasitized, and they have more recurrent infections as demonstrated by their globulin levels. However, education does have an independent bearing on hematologic levels, as shown in income matched samples. (Maternal knowledge of nutrition is

Table 1. Socioeconomic Effects on Hemoglobin
Levels (g/dl) in White Females[a]

Age	Low Income		High Income	
	N	Median	N	Median
2	29	11.5	18	11.8
4	47	12.2	17	12.2
6	64	12.2	15	12.5
8	60	12.6	19	12.6
10	85	12.8	22	13.1
12	63	12.8	27	13.5
14	45	13.1	22	13.5
16	49	13.4	26	13.6
20	128	13.4	193	13.5
30	189	13.3	255	13.3
40	187	13.6	197	13.5
50	132	13.3	346	13.6
60	122	13.5	286	13.8
70	124	13.7	155	13.7
80	46	13.1	52	13.5

[a] All data derived from the Ten State Nutrition Survey of 1968–1970. See also Owen et al. (1973) for the Pre-School Nutrition Survey.

more important than income when it comes to the hemoglobins and hematocrits of the children.)

The data of the Ten-State Nutrition Survey also reveal a geographical effect, independent of income and maternal education, described at length in the C.D.C. report (1972). Income by income, or education by education hemoglobins and hematocrits were higher in the northern states than in the southern states participating in that massive study.

SES effects on hematologic levels may be far larger in the third-world countries where the income and education range is greater than in the United States, and where iron-deficiency and folate-deficiency anemias are common, and where intestinal parasites plague most villagers and where water supplies are contaminated.

Fatness, Hgb, and Hct

At all ages, from infancy onward, fatter children, adolescents, and adults do have higher Hgb and Hct levels and vice versa. Comparing the lean and the obese, the differences in packed-cell volume and hemo-

globin concentration are considerable (see Figure 5 and Table 1). Why
fatter boys and girls and adolescents and fatter adults have higher Hgb
and Hct levels is not clear. The parsimonious explanation is that fatter
individuals probably eat a little more and so ingest more iron. Conversely, and by this line of reasoning, leaner, i.e., less fat—children and adults
may eat less and so ingest less iron. However, it is not certain that this
food-volume explanation is a sufficient answer.

Extremely fat, obese, and morbidly obese adolescents and adults may
have remarkably high Hgb and Hct levels, a function of their respiratory
problems and problems of oxygen transport, so it may be that the fatness–hematologic relationship has a further physiological basis. Conversely, the low Hgb and Hct values in the lean and undernourished may

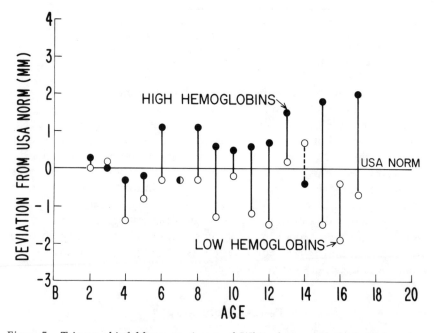

Figure 5. Triceps skinfold comparisons of White boys with high Hgb value
(solid dots) and low Hgb values (open dots). At all ages, and in both sexes
fatness increases with hemoglobin levels and the obese have higher Hgb and
Hct values than do the lean (Garn and Petzold 1982; Garn and Ryan 1982).

Table 2. Hemoglobin Differences between Obese and Lean Individuals in NHANES I

Age Group	Total N[a]	Males (g/dl)	Z	Females (g/dl)	Z
Infants (1–3)	396	0.30	0.33	0.12	0.10
Children (4–11)	808	0.22	0.26	0.20	0.20
Adolescents (12–17)	499	0.09	0.08	0.10	0.21
Adults (17–84)	4438	0.31	0.25	0.21	0.18
Total (1–84)	6091	0.28	0.23	0.19	0.17

[a] Total number of lean and obese individuals in that age category. All Z-scores are age and sex specific. For details see Garn and Clark (1975), Garn and Ryan (1982, 1983), and Lowe et al. (1975).

be purely dietary in nature, they may suggest actual problems in iron absorption, or they may also be partly physiological (see Figure 3 and Table 2).

The Question of Black–White Differences in Hgb and Hct Levels

While it has been long assumed that "normal" Hgb and Hct levels are the same for all populations, assuming adequate nutrition and iron nutrition in particular, a number of studies prior to 1950 did indicate lower hematologic levels in American Blacks (Milam et al. 1946; Eads et al. 1949). The parsimonious explanation was nutritional, since the Blacks were of lower SES and dietary records suggested poorer nutrition for them. (cf. Looker et al. 1990)

However, beginning in 1975, data from major surveys indicated that Blacks had lower Hgb and Hct levels (by nearly 1 g/dl or 3% in Hct) even after income-matching and adjustments for dietary differences (Garn et al. 1975, 1976a; Garn and Clark, 1976). Data from the Ten-State Nutrition Survey, the Pre-School Nutrition Survey, and NHANES I all agreed in this respect (see also Owen et al. 1973; Garn and Ryan 1983). Even iron-supplemented athletes reiterated the Black–White differences (see Garn et al. 1975, Figure 4). Equally obese Black and White women differed by nearly 1.0 g/dl in Hgb (Garn et al. 1982, 1983). Similar Black–White differences during pregnancy were revealed in the data from the National Collaborative Perenatal Study (NCPP). Tens of thousands age-matched, income-matched, and weight-matched pregnant Black women were lower in Hgb and Hct than their white peers (Garn et al. 1976b, 1987a,b, and Table 3). Similar differences were found in age-matched chronic renal disease, dialysis and transplant patients despite their generally low hematologic levels (Garn et al. 1976c and Figure 6).

Throughout, there have been repeated attempts to reexplain the Black–White Hgb difference as purely environmental and/or dietary. To this end, Jackson et al. (1991) argue that "common recent African origins for all modern humans, as suggested by the fossil and molecualar data, as well as our close biochemical affinities with chimpanzees and gorillas, suggest that biologically significant differences among populations of contemporary humans are unlikely."

Though the question has remained open, several recent studies have confirmed the Black–White differences in Hgb as very close to 0.7 g/dl (i.e., 0.7 SD units). The Touro Infirmary group showed such differences even after corrections for hemoglobinopathies and dietary differences (Bazzano 1986). This group therefore concludes that "even after the iron supplementation, the racial differences in hemoglobin and hematocrit

Table 3. Magnitude of Black–White Hemoglobin Difference after Matching for SES, Diet, Hemoglobinopathies, etc.

Author(s)	Sample	Description	Summary
Garn et al. (1975)	Ten State Nutrition Survey	27,144 subjects aged 1–80	Difference ≤ 0.9 g/dl with SES matching and iron supplementation
Garn et al. (1980)	NHANES I	2996–3778 pairs selected on a national probability basis	Income and education-adjusted difference at 0.7 g/dl
Garn et al. (1976b)	National Collaborative Perinatal Project	24,514 consecutive pregnant women	0.7 g/dl difference after age and SES matching
Bazzano (1986)	Hammond, La Study Sample	Up to 1001 Black and White children aged 5–9	0.7 g/dl difference after SES and diet matching, excluding abnormal hemoglobins
Perry et al. (1992)	NHANES II	N = 2982 subjects, aged 3–45 complete with ferritins	0.9 g/dl difference after SES and diet corrections

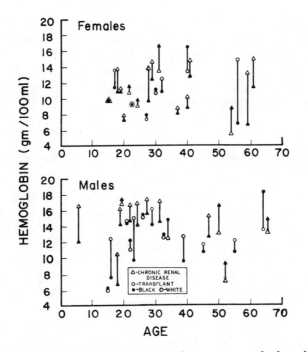

Figure 6. Comparison of hemoglobin levels in age-matched and condition-matched Black and White chronic renal disease and transplant patients. Despite all of the medical interventions and complications, 60% of these black patients exhibit lower Hgb values than their White peers. (cf. Mayor et al. 1976).

levels of the children with normal MCV (>75 fl) or normal MCH (>26.6 pg) still remained. This result strongly suggests that the racial difference cannot be attributed either to the nutritional iron status and/or high prevalence of single gene thalassemia abnormality in the black population" (Bazzano 1986:56).

A still more recent reanalysis of the NHANES II data also confirms a Black–White difference of the same order, after corrections or adjustments for SES, diet, and ferritin levels (Perry et al. 1992). They write as follows: "Despite their lower hemoglobin levels, blacks had higher serum ferritin levels than whites. These results suggest that the difference in hemoglobin levels between blacks and whites in the U.S. is the result of factors other than iron intake and iron status."

While the possibility will exists that some aspect of diets may still explain the hematologic differences (even in higher-income blacks), the original findings reported in the *Journal of the National Medical Association* in 1975 continue to hold. The question therefore arises as to whether differences in red cell enzymes may be involved in oxygen transport or whether 13.43 g/dl of hemoglobin in Blacks is as efficient in oxygen transport as 14.33 g/dl in Whites (here taking the NHANES data as reanalyzed by Perry et al. 1992) (see Table 3).

Anemia during Pregnancy and Its Effects on the Conceptus

Though lower hemoglobin and hematocrit levels are associated with diminished vitality at all ages, they have particular implications during pregnancy—to all fetal outcomes. With a low Hgb or a very low Hct, corrected for pregnancy level of course, gestation length tends to be restricted, fetal growth limited, prematurity more common, and neonatal death more frequent. Hematologic status during pregnancy is therefore especially important to the next generation and (as a risk factor) far more important to the conceptus than to the mother herself. These generalizations apply with equal force to White paras and Black paras, though the hematologic levels that are indicative of excessive risk are different.

Why low hemoglobin concentrations and low packed cell volumes during pregnancy are so critical to the fetus is not certain, but some working assumptions can be stated. First, and as we well know, the fetus is far more vulnerable to injury, a consequence of cellular differentiation and rapid cell proliferation. Second, a poor hematologic status in the mother does not stand alone as an isolated risk factor, but is commonly associated with generally poorer nutrition and lesser body fat reserves. It is tempting to suggest that diminished oxygen transport is involved, thinking of reduced reproductive capacity reported at high altitudes, but again this is not certain.

However, it is also important to note that the disadvantages of a low Hgb or a low Hct, with respect to pregnancy outcomes, are also repeated when Hgb and Hct are *high*. At high levels of hemoglobin concentration or when the percent packed cell volume is high, unfavorable pregnancy outcomes are similarly increased. Taking all unfavorable pregnancy outcomes into account, the relationship to hematologic status is curvilinear and U-shaped. It is bad for the baby if maternal Hgb and Hct are low and equally bad when they are high. At the middle of the range of hemoglobins or hematocrits the prevalence of unfavorable pregnancy outcomes is least. By analogy, and assuming that the fetus is the most sensitive reflection of hematologic status, the middle of the hematologic range may be

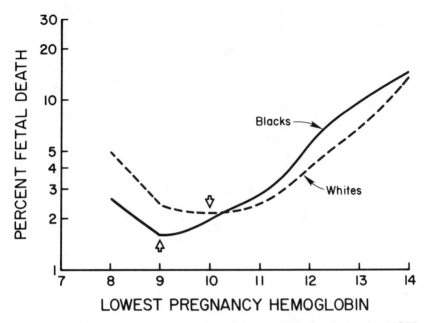

Figure 7. Fetal loss as related to maternal hemoglobin levels in the NCPP. Minimal fetal loss is associated with a Hgb of 9 g/dl in Black mothers and 10 g/dl in White mothers. Fetal mortality increases dramatically in those women who do not undergo hypervolemia during pregnancy (cf. Garn et al. 1981).

viewed as most salubrious, at all points in the life cycle. However, the poorer fetal outcomes associated with high Hgb and Hct levels may be a special case—reflecting failure of the normal blood volume expansion during pregnancy, i.e., hypervolemia (see Figures 7 and 8).

Cigarette Smoking and Hematologic Levels

Various nondietary factors affect hemoglobin and hematocrit levels by increasing oxygen requirements, interfering with oxygen transport, or both. So hematologic values become higher at high altitude, they are higher in trained athletes, they are higher in the morbidly obese and they are higher in individuals (and groups) exposed to atmospheric pollution of the particulate type. Hemoglobin and hematocrit levels are also higher in individuals exposed to carbon monoxide, including both traffic policemen and cigarette smokers, since some of the hemoglobin in their blood is carboxyhemoglobin.

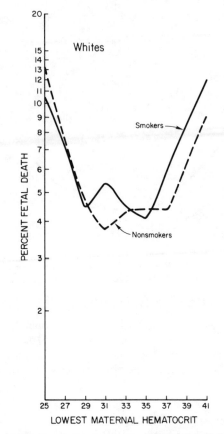

Figure 8. Fetal mortality in relation to maternal hematocrit. In both smokers and nonsmokers, fetal mortality is at its minimum in the maternal Hct range of 30–36% and increases dramatically at both lower and higher hematologic levels (cf. Garn et al. 1981).

The fact that smokers have higher hemoglobin levels is important, since the usual colorimetric measures do not distinguish between the two types of hemoglobin. In general, carboxyhemoglobin levels are proportional to cigarette usage and type of smoking, but in nonlinear fashion (see Garn 1978a). Moreover, there is a surprisingly direct dose–response relationship between maternal cigarette usage during pregnancy and the 4 hour hemoglobin and hematocrit levels of their neonates. The higher the levels of cigarette usage during pregnancy (expressed as cigarettes/day or half-packs/day), the higher the hematologic levels in their neonates (see Figure 9). This is equally true for term neonates and for preterm neonates, though the latter tend to lower Hgb and Hct values throughout.

In a way, this fetal response to maternal smoking resembles the fetal response to high altitude.

Sex and Age Differences in Hgb and Hct

During infancy and childhood, hematologic levels in boys and girls are much the same in all cultures. During early adolescence, however, hemoglobin levels begin to increase in boys, stabilizing (by the later teens) at a level about 1 g/dl higher than in girls. The adolescent increase in males is earlier in those who are early maturing and later in those who are late maturing. While it has been argued that the adolescent and adult sex difference in hematologic status is purely dietary (males eat more than females, even on a per kilogram basis), a specific effect of masculinizing hormones is far more tenable. Certainly, both Hgb and Hct decrease after castration. In any event, the pinker or ruddier coloration of males reflects their higher red blood counts and their greater surface vascularity, noted by the early Egyptians and depicted in tomb paintings.

Although men continue to have higher hemoglobin and hematocrit levels than do women, through most of the adult decades, the long-term trends for the two sexes are in opposite directions. Men tend to diminish in Hgb and Hct fairly early. In contrast, women tend to increase in Hgb and Hct for many years, until they, too, eventually begin to diminish.

One can only guess at the reasons why middle-aged men decrease in hematologic status while women continue to increase. The diminution in the male may reflect decreased testosterone secretion, decreased activity, or both. The continued increase in hemoglobin levels and percent packed cell volumes in women may be variously attributed to decreased menstrual blood loss, decreased blood volume, and a decrease in the water content of all tissues, literally a drying-out (see Figures 1 and 2 and Table 4).

Hematological Changes after the Seventh Decade

In both men and women, hemoglobin and hematocrit values eventually peak and then begin to decline. This peak and later decline are scarcely evident in those textbook hematologic norms where all adults are often

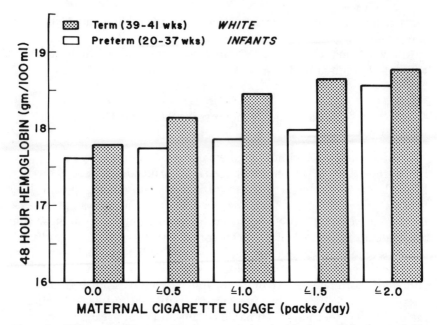

Figure 9. Effect of maternal cigarette usage (packs/day) on 48 hr hemoglobin levels in their progeny. Both in preterm neonates (white bars) and term neonates (shaded bars) the 48 hr Hgb increases in dose–response fashion in relation to maternal smoking level.

grouped together regardless of age. However, it is very evident in the mass-survey data from the Ten-State Nutrition Survey, NHANES, and in data from the Baltimore Aging Study, the Bogalusa Heart Survey, and the Tecumseh, Michigan Community Health Survey. It is also evident that men peak and begin to decline in Hgb and Hct at an earlier age than do women, a situation not unique to these red cell measures, but characteristic of serum cholesterol, serum triglycerides, etc.

   Why these hematologic measures reach a peak and then decline is not certain, but there are a variety of possible explanations. One explanation for the decline may rest in the decreased food intake of older people, with iron intake decreasing in proportion. A second but closely related explanation is that iron intake may decrease more than caloric intake, due to a lesser consumption of animal flesh and heart, liver, and kidney tissues by the elderly. Indeed, decreased iron intake due to dietary alterations is a logical explanation for the age-associated decline in Hgb and Hct but not for the timing.

Table 4. Life Cycle Changes in Hemoglobin Levels (g/dl)[a]

	Males		Females	
Age	N	Median	N	Median
1	64	11.1	64	11.7
2	81	12.0	96	11.9
3	130	12.0	96	11.9
4	142	12.2	142	12.3
5	190	12.5	161	12.4
6	217	12.5	205	12.4
7	272	12.6	231	12.7
8	272	12.8	229	12.8
9	263	12.8	250	12.9
10	286	13.0	253	12.8
11	272	13.1	250	13.0
12	270	13.3	238	13.0
13	251	13.4	212	13.3
14	198	13.9	175	13.3
15	172	14.2	174	13.3
16	164	14.6	163	13.4
17	137	14.9	138	13.5
20	518	15.3	779	13.4
30	665	15.2	125	13.4
40	605	15.1	899	13.5
50	610	15.2	900	13.5
60	575	14.9	757	13.8
70	502	14.8	694	13.8
80	240	14.4	306	13.3

[a] Data calculated for White participants in the Ten State Nutrition Survey of 1968–1970; compare with Johnson et al. (1978) for NHANES I and Johnson and Abraham (1979).

A decrease in activity level is another possible cause, activity (caloric expenditure) decreasing in both sexes over time. As we know, high levels of activity and athletic fitness are associated with higher hematologic levels. So a reduction in activity may underlie some of the age-associated decrease in Hgb and Hct. But why would reduced activity show up disproportionately later in women than men?

At some point in time, decreased hematopoietic activity must be involved, i.e., decreased activity of the blood-forming tissues. We know that red marrow is gradually replaced by yellow (fatty) marrow in the bones, but why does Hgb and Hct fall off so late? Is the blood of older individuals more and more a population of older corpuscles, less frequently replaced, and with oxygen-carrying power less than the RBC (red blood count) might suggest?

Finally, one may well ask whether the age-associated decrease in Hgb and Hct is a direct measure of "aging" or a predictor of demise. Do those who drop more in Hgb and Hct die earlier? Does a really low Hgb (say well under 10 g/dl or even less) predict the end of life? As a parallel question, will iron supplementation raise hematologic levels in the elderly and thus prove life sustaining? This is of interest to the gerontologic set ("Geritol" is advertised and sold as an iron supplement). Would prune juice (4 mg/serving) or clams (7.5 mg/serving) prove to be a life extender for the aged, or would such foods and over-the-counter supplements overly load the liver with iron and do more harm than good?

The question may be restated. Is the age-associated decrease in Hgb and Hct physiologic or symptomatic of iron deficiency? Would iron supplementation and intervention prove life-extending or possibly the reverse?

Iron Intake and Iron-Deficiency Anemia

Iron-deficiency anemia was the first of the anemias to be understood, and the first to respond to supplementation. So we are urged to include "iron-rich" foods in our diets, including liver, heart, and kidneys (cf. Appendix I). The targeted value is about 20 mg of iron per day, and if the diet is insufficient, then supplementation with iron salts must be considered.

There are a few metabolic conditions in which excessive iron stores accumulate, but these are rare. There are a few situations in which dietary iron may be excessive, the best known stemming from South African "bush" beer home-brewed in rusted petroleum tins. There are also dietary excesses leading to excessive iron storage in the liver, as in early alcoholism, but these are a separate consideration.

Cultural and technological factors can affect the iron as well as the zinc content of the diet. The iron in water supplies may be partly available, giving an advantage to rusty water and old iron pipes and plumbing. Iron leached from cooking vessels may be biologically available, and iron from spaghetti sauce long simmered in cast-iron pots may provide useful dietary iron. The Iron age and the advent of iron cookware may have improved iron nutrition as compared with earlier traditions of food preparation in stoneware and pottery.

Many of the world's peoples now, and earlier, cannot or could not achieve a daily intake of 20 mg of iron. Most grains are rather low in iron, especially corn, wheat, and rice (often below 2 mg per serving). One would expect that people who had excessive dependence on corn, wheat, or rice would show evidence of iron-deficiency anemia. Beans and other legumes are, in general, better sources of iron than most grains but it takes a lot of beans or chickpeas to provide 2 mg of iron a day. Spinach is a better source of iron than many of our leafy vegetables, but at 2 mg a serving it takes a lot of spinach to ingest 20 mg/day.

Probably, diggers and grubbers and seed eaters were better off iron-wise, though few seeds quite equal sunflower seeds in iron content (7 mg/serving) or even peanuts (3 mg/serving). The iron content of sunflower seeds becomes important when compared with the far lower iron content of maize, which largely replaced sunflower seeds in prehistoric Indian diets.

Dietary Factors That Interfere with Iron Absorption

Iron-deficiency anemia may occur, in the presence of adequate iron intakes, if other dietary components interfere with absorption. This can be demonstrated when dietary fiber is in excess, and it may also stem from the excessive use of alcoholic beverages. However, the type case occurs when wheat or other grain phytates are in excess, as in populations highly dependent on boiled wheat (in North Africa and the Middle East). In North Africa, Egypt, and in Iran (to cite three specific examples) growth failure, dwarfism, and markedly delayed sexual maturation are common. Iron and iron–zinc supplementation has reversed the growth retardations in therapeutic trials (cf. Ronaghy et al. 1969).

This discovery has major implications to past populations in North Africa and the Middle East, where wheat (typically boiled wheat) has long been the staple. It also applies in principle to other grain sources, including barely, and opens possibilities for study wherever wheat and barley agriculture provided a staple grain supply to replace the more varied diets during the Mesolithic.

Geophagia and Pica and Dietary Iron

Dietary iron may be restricted in its availability by particular foods or drinks or by nonnutritive additions to the diet or by the sheer volume of soluble and insoluble fibers. Excessive use of alcoholic beverages and excessive dietary fiber are two examples, and so is geophagia (literally "eating dirt").

Many people, even in the United States today, regularly consume clay. Some, currently resident in Michigan or Minnesota, send back home for the familiar Georgia clays of their childhood. Geophagia is widespread and we can only guess as to what proportion of people were clay eaters in earlier times.

Clay, especially the finer clays, bind iron so that it is unavailable. (Some other clays are actually sources of iron, not commonly counted in dietary assessments but contributory.) So we must consider geophagia in its various forms and starch-eating and flour-eating among the dietary practices that may lead to an insufficient iron intake and iron-deficiency anemia even when the iron content of the diet is seemingly adequate.

Parasites and Such

We Are Not Alone is the title of a once-popular novel by James Hilton. The same statement, "We are not alone," also describes the fact that most of the people, in most of the world, share their life and lot with parasites of various shapes and sizes. From highly macroscopic yard-long tapeworms to the pinworms our grandmothers worried about, to round worms and flat worms, people share their daily bread with parasites—unselfishly and without meanness of spirit, but at a loss of 1–4 mg/Fe per day (WHO Report 1975).

Some of these unbidden guests hop over or move over from kith and kin, significant others, and "loved ones." Some are the uninvited gifts of animals, domestic or wild, husbanded or hunted. Some come from animal flesh eaten in the raw or inadequately cooked state. Some are present in streams, lakes, and pools, or in the annual floodings. Some enter the food supply from the feces of others, as when "nightsoil" is used as fertilizer or simply by hand-to-mouth communication.

Among the widely distributed parasites are also the malarial parasites, of varied virulence, but they all serve to deplete iron stores to a greater or lesser degree. Fleas and ticks may have minimal effects, but the intestinal parasites far more. Where population densities are high, where the ground is warm, and where aquatic snails abound, parasitization is nearly inevitable. The Anasazi, we now know, were heavily parasitized, (and probably anemic).

Most of our ancestors were parasitized, often heavily, a problem that remained with us until fairly recently and still remains where people and animals comingle, and where the eggs or parasites easily enter into the food supply, or where animal and insect vectors abound. Probably all of the people in neolithic villages were generous hosts, and the advent of village life led to decreased iron stores and iron-deficiency anemia. Even hunters in cold climates were not exempt, getting their parasites from the hunted, and communicating parasites to each other in their crowded dwellings.

One should also make note of the many diarrheas, reducing dietary iron in proportion to their frequency, and the chronic (amoebic) diarrhea, that yield to intensive drug treatment now. They are part of our heritage, still common in tropical areas and a familiar risk for travelers from the north.

Assessing the Iron Nutrition of Past Populations

Assessing the nutritional status of past populations *ex cathedra* is not particularly difficult, if appropriate assumptions are made. If the imagined caloric intake is set high enough and if dietary diversity is also assumed, then the presumed diet would have met or exceeded United States, Canadian, and W.H.O. recommendations for energy intake and essential nutrients. With more imagination, substituting fish for fatty-animal flesh, and insisting on trimmed cuts of game animals, it can be made a low-cholesterol/low-fat "healthy" diet by the stroke of a pen. Yet many a past population must have existed on a lower than recommended caloric intake and a more restricted food range. Moreover, the small body size of most of the skeletons from past suggests a less-than-textbook caloric intake, a greater energy expenditure, or recurrent episodes of nutritional deficiency, or all three (cf. Garn and Leonard 1990).

With respect to iron nutrition in past populations, the working assumptions are critical. Given enough mammalian flesh and accepting heart, spleen, liver, and kidneys as regular food items, a daily intake of 18–20 mg of iron might also be assumed. However, when most of the calories come from grain or tubers, the recommended iron allowance is unlikely to be met, and far lower daily iron intakes must be hypothesized. Add the action of wheat and other phytates and the effects of high-fiber diets and parasitization, the *available* iron would then be scarcely adequate for health.

One might still accord hunting populations good marks for iron intake, and hunters and grubbers and diggers and gatherers a reasonable approximation to the RDAs. People who ate small animals and smaller squirmy things, organs and all (and chewing the bones for their marrow) were probably equally well provided with dietary iron. However, the advent of cultivated grains, and then excessive dependence on grains, would have changes the levels of iron intake to levels we would consider questionable for health. Besides these agriculturists would have remained together and defecated together and shared parasites together, adding greater iron losses to lesser iron intakes. Excessive maize dependence, excessive rice dependence, excessive wheat dependence, and excessive dependence on yams and mealies all would have made iron-deficiency anemias more common.

We have a special example when pasteurized cows' milk became available so cheaply that it become uneconomic to breast feed. The result was bigger babies, an advantage, and an increased incidence of iron-deficiency anemias in infancy, a disadvantage. To a lesser but not unimportant extent, the shift in this century from iron cookware and iron pipes has also decreased iron intakes somewhat. (Replacing galvanized iron milk cans and processing equipment with stainless steel has also decreased dietary zinc.)

One may therefore seek, in the skeletal remains, evidence of dietary change and iron nutrition in particular, while recognizing variables other than dietary iron. The shift from hunting and gathering to major dependence on grain in the Middle East, the Far East, Central America, and the Southwest is one dietary shift to explore. The shift from sunflower seeds (7 mg of iron per serving) to ground maize (0.2 mg per serving) in parts of North America commends itself for study.

However, it is often impossible to separate iron nutrition from protein nutrition in areas of single-grain dependence, where the grains were low in iron but with limiting amino acids and where caloric intakes were also low. So Central America, from Mexico southward, may not be definitive, even in archaeological time. New Guinea is an area of low iron intake (at least since the yam became a staple), but protein intakes are also low there, and fat intakes disproportionately low, and there is malaria. (cf. Tracer, 1991)

Of course, it is difficult to reconstruct past diets from archaeological evidence even where there are kitchen-middens and piles of bones. One can demonstrate the presence of fish or sea-going mammals, rodents, or ungulates but not the daily intake of fish or game. Still, a high dependence on animal flesh, hunted or domesticated, contrasts with a high dependence on grain and little else. Legumes bear watching (as noted in Appendix I on iron content of different foods) and especially when beans are cooked in iron pots.

Skeletal Manifestations of Anemia

Many anemias are reflected by changes in the skeletal mass, due to a widening of the marrow cavity (as seen in radiographs) and—in consequence—decreased bone mass relative to bone volume. This is evident in the leukemias, in individuals with sickle-cell disease, in Mediterranean anemia (due to hemoglobin ε), in pernicious (folate deficiency) anemia, and the like. However, the radiographic manifestations are not diagnostic, and may easily be confused with bone loss due to protein–calorie malnutrition (PCM) and bone loss due to malabsorption states and to osteogenesis imperfecta. Radiographs do reveal diminished cortical mass and mass/volume, but they do not identify the cause. (Garn, 1970)

Diminished bone mass relative to bone volume, diminished trabecular bone, and thinning and diminution of the plate-like structures are commonly referred to as *osteoporosis* (literally porous bone). Sometimes a further descriptive term is added, as in *involutional osteoporosis* (as found in older individuals). Again, osteoporosis is not easily distinguished from osteopoenia, meaning "deficient bone," but it is a commonly used and popular clinical term. (cf. Garn, 1970)

Some osteologists have also applied the term "osteoporosis" to the pits and lacunae seen in archaeological specimens, particularly on the frontal bone and around the orbits. Their osteological etymology cannot be criticized, for the pits and lacunae are indeed porosities or holes in the bones. However, there is no definitive evidence as yet that these cranial and calvarial manifestations are related to "osteoporosis" as radiologically defined, or to bone loss as seen in the tubular bones or the vertebrae, especially the lumbar vertebrae and the femur. Yet the possibility can easily be tested, using cadaver material or already skeletalized material from anatomical museums and archaeological sites.

Cadavers of older individuals and especially alcoholics are likely to evidence the radiological manifestations of osteoporosis. (Alcoholics show osteoporosis as a result of combined low protein and low calcium intakes.) Accordingly, one would look for pits and lacunae on the defleshed skulls of such individuals to test for a possible association.

If the pits and lacunae on the skull are indeed related to bone loss, one would expect that archaeological specimens so characterized would show diminished bone mass/volume elsewhere in the skeleton and biconcavities of the vertebrae and vertebral fractures to a greater degree. Conversely, one would expect older skeletalized adults with the characteristic radiographic manifestations of osteoporosis to show the cranial changes, if indeed the two are related. Such an association, if confirmed, might not validate the anemia hypothesis, but it would provide a clarification of terms.

Testing the anemia hypothesis will require much additional work, for we do not really know whether individuals with low or deficient Hgb and Hct levels are osteopoenic compared with their age peers.

Appendix I: Iron Content of Some Common Foods (mg/portion)

Food, as Served	Portion size [a]	Iron (mg)
Lamb's liver (broiled)	3½ oz	17.9
Calf's liver, fried	3½ oz	14.2
Beef kidneys, braised	3½ oz	13.1
Alligator meat	3½ oz	11.4
Armadillo meat	3½ oz	10.9
Chicken livers, simmered	3½ oz	8.5
Clams	5–10	7.5
Sunflower seeds	3½ oz	7.1
Beef heart, braised	3½ oz	5.9
Prune juice	1 cup	4.1
Roasted peanuts w/skin	2½ oz	3.4
Beef hamburger, cooked	1 patty	3.3
Beans, lima, cooked	⅔ cup	2.5
Spinach, cooked	3½ oz	2.0
Lettuce, raw	3 oz	2.0
Chicken, fried	¼	1.8
Peas, green, cooked	⅔ cup	1.8
Oatmeal, cooked	1 cup	1.7
Tomato juice	¾ cup	1.6
Rice, boiled	1 cup	1.2
Wheat, boiled	1 cup	1.2
Salmon, baked	Small serving	1.2
Bass, baked	1 serving	1.2
Potato, small baked	1	1.0
Chocolate bar	1 oz	1.0
Cod, baked	4 oz	0.9
Pine nuts (pinyon)	2 oz	0.7
Cornmeal, cooked	1 cup	0.5
Catfish	3½ oz	0.4
English walnuts	4–7	0.3
Corn grits, cooked	1 cup	0.2
Cow's milk	1 cup	< 0.1

[a] 3½ oz = 100 g.

Appendix II: Forms of Iron Used in Supplementation and Their Bioavailability

Reduced iron (elemental iron) may have high bioavailability if the particle size is small, being converted into the chloride ($FeCl_3$) by the action of gastric juice. Iron chloride is also now employed in fortification as is the sulfate $FeSO_4$, long used both for food fortification and in therapeutic doses. The sulfate, in fact, is the traditional iron salt for these purposes. Other iron salts include the gluconate, the carbonate ($FeCO_3$), the citrate, and also the lactate—the latter especially useful for milk fortification (cf. WHO technical Report 580, 1975).

Various studies have confirmed the bioavailability of iron from cooking vessels in which acidic foods are long simmered, spaghetti sauce being the type example. Iron salts in water supplies may be bioavailable, either through the action of gastric juice or in conjunction with acetic, citric, and (possibly) malic acid. The bioavailability of iron from foods depends both on the form of iron present and the presence of other foods.

Though the iron content of maize is low (ca. 0.4 mg per 6 oz serving) and a diet that is highly dependent on maize may therefore lead to iron-deficiency anemia, many American Indians did eat small animals whole, blood and all, thus providing a source of dietary iron with high bioavailability. However, recent paleoparasitological studies suggest a high degree of parasitization in the Anasazi, suggesting that they may have been increasingly anemic as irrigated africulture developed and as population densities soared.

References

Bazzano, G.S. (ed.). 1986. *Iron Fortification: Research on Iron Fortification and Iron Supplementation Conducted in the U.S.* New Orleans, LA: Touro Research Institute.

Control of Nutritional Anemia with Special Reference to Iron Deficiency: Report of an IASEA/USAID/WHO Joint Meeting 1975. Technical Report Series No. 580, Geneva World Health Organization.

Eads, M.G., O. Mickelsen, F.W. Morse, and H.R. Sandstead. 1949. The Nutritional Status of Negroes. *Journal of Negro Education* 18:291.

Garn, S.M. 1970. *The Earlier Gain and the Later Loss of Cortical Bone.* C.C Thomas. Springfield, IL.

Garn, S.M., and D.C. Clark. 1975. Hemoglobin and fatness. *Ecology of Food and Nutrition* 4:131–133.

Garn, S.M., and D.C. Clark. 1976. Problems in the nutritional assessment of Black individuals. *American Journal of Public Health* 66:262–267.

Garn, S.M., and W.R. Leonard. 1990. Reply to S. Boyd Eaton. *Nutrition Reviews* 48:229–230.

Garn, S.M., and A.S. Petzold. 1982. Fatness and hematologic levels during pregnancy. *American Journal of Clinical Nutrition* 36:129–130.

Garn, S.M., and A.S. Ryan. 1982. The effect of fatness on hemoglobin levels. *American Journal of Clinical Nutrition* 36:189–191.

Garn, S.M., and A.S. Ryan. 1983. Relationship between fatness and hemoglobin levels in the National Health and Nutrition Examination of the U.S.A. *Ecology of Food and Nutrition* 12:211–215.

Garn, S.M., N.J. Smith, and D.C. Clark. 1975. Lifelong differences in hemoglobin levels between blacks and whites. *Journal of the National Medical Association* 7:91–96.

Garn, S.M., D.C. Clark, and K.E. Guire. 1976a. Husband-wife similarities in hemoglobin levels. *Ecology of Food and Nutrition* 5:47–50.

Garn, S.M., H.A. Shaw, and K.D. McCabe. 1976b. Black-White hemoglobin differences during pregnancy. *Ecology of Food and Nutrition* 5:99–100.

Garn, S.M., S. Stinson, and G.H. Mayor. 1976c. The race difference in hemoglobin level in chronic renal failure patients. *American Journal of Clinical Nutrition* 29:240–241.

Garn, S.M., H.A. Shaw, K.E. Guire, and K.D. McCabe. 1977. Apportioning black-white hemoglobin and hematocrit differences during pregnancy. *American Journal of Clinical Nutrition* 30:461–462.

Garn, S.M., H.A. Shaw, and K.D. McCabe. 1978a. Effect of maternal smoking on hemoglobins and hematocrits of the newborn. *American Journal of Clinical Nutrition* 31:557.

Garn, S.M., H.A. Shaw, and K.D. McCabe. 1978b. Maternal smoking as a nutritional variable. *Ecology of Food and Nutrition* 7:143–145.

Garn, S.M., S.M. Bailey, and P.E. Cole. 1979. Biochemical resemblances among people living together. *Ecology of Food and Nutrition* 8:201–205.

Garn, S.M., S.A. Ridella, A.S. Petzold, and F. Falkner. 1981a. Maternal hematologic levels and pregnancy outcomes. *Seminars in Perinatology* 5:155–161.

Garn, S.M., A.S. Ryan, and S. Abraham. 1981b. New values defining "low" and "deficient" hemoglobin levels for white children and adults. *Ecology of Food and Nutrition* 11:71–74.

Garn, S.M., A.S. Ryan, G. Owen, and S. Abraham. 1981c. Income matched black-white hemoglobin differences after correction for low transferrin saturations. *American Journal of Clinical Nutrition* 34:1645–1647.

Garn, S.M., A.S. Ryan, G. Owen, and S. Abraham. 1981d. Suggested sex and age appropriate values for "low" and "deficient" hemoglobin levels. *American Journal of Clinical Nutrition* 34:1648–1651.

Health Services and Mental Health Administration. 1972. *Ten-State Nutrition Survey*. Washington DC: US Department of Health, Education and Welfare.

Interdepartmental Committee on Nutrition for National Defense. 1963. *Manual for Nutrition Surveys*. Washington DC: US Department of Health, Education and Welfare.

Jackson, R.T., and F.L.C. Jackson. 1991. Reassessing 'hereditary' interethnic differences in anemia status. *Ethnicity and Disease* 1:26–41.

Johnson, C.L., and S. Abraham. 1979. Hemoglobin and selected nonrelated findings of persons 1–74 years of age: United States, 1971–1974. *Advancedata* 46: 1–12.

Johnson, T.R., W.M. Moore, and J.E. Jeffries. 1978. *Children Are Different: Developmental Physiology*. Columbus, OH: Ross Laboratories.

Looker, A.C., C.M. Loria, M.A. McDowell and C.L. Johnson. 1990. Dietary Habits of Blacks and other Ethnic Minorities in the U.S. with Special References to Iron Status. In: *Functional Significance of Iron Deficiency*. Cyril O. Enwonwu (ed.) Meharry Medical College. Nashville, Tennessee.

Lowe, C.U., G. Forbes, S.M. Garn, G.M. Owen, N.J. Smith, W.B. Weil, Jr., and M.S. Nichaman. 1975. Reflections of dietary studies with children in the Ten-State Nutrition Survey of 1968–1970. *Pediatrics* 56:320–326.

Mayor, G.H., S.M. Garn, T.V. Sanchez, and H.A. Shaw. 1976. The need for differential bone mineral standards for Blacks. *The American Journal of Roentgenology, Radium Therapy and Nuclear Medicine* 126:1293–1294.

Milam, D.F., and J. Muench. 1946. Hemoglobin levels in specific race, age, and sex groups of a normal North Carolina population. *Journal of Laboratory and Clinical Medicine* 31:878.

Nelson, W.E., V.C. Vaughan III, and R.J. McKay. 1969. *Textbook of Pediatrics*. Philadelphia: W.B. Saunders.

Owen, G.M., A.H. Lubin, and P.J. Garry. 1973. Hemoglobin levels according to age, race, and transferrin saturation in preschool children of comparable socioeconomic status. *Journal of Pediatrics* 82:850–851.

Perry, G.S., T. Byers, R. Yip, and S. Margen. 1992. An examination of factors contributing to hemoglobin differences between blacks and whites, NHANES II, 1976–1980. *Journal of Nutrition* (in press).

Ronaghy, H., M.R. Spivey Fox, S.M. Garn, H. Israel, A. Harp, P.G. Moe, and J.A. Halsted. 1969. Controlled zinc supplementation for malnourished school boys: A pilot experiment. *American Journal of Clinical Nutrition* 22: 1279–1289.

Sinclair, H.M. 1948. The assessment of human nutrition. *Vitamins and Hormones* 4:101–162.

Tracer, D.P. 1991. *The interaction of nutrition and fertility among Au forager-horticulturalist of Papua New Guinea*. Ph.D. thesis. Ann Arbor: University of Michigan.

Wintrobe, M.M. 1974. *Clinical hematology*, 7th ed. Philadelphia: Lea & Febiger.

Chapter 3

Physiological, Pathological, and Dietary Influences on the Hemoglobin Level

G.R. Wadsworth

Introduction

The present chapter discusses normal variations in the hemoglobin level that are relevant in the diagnosis of anemia, the metabolism of iron in the body, the absorption of iron, and its presence and bioavailability in foods. The dietary intake of iron and possible causes of iron-deficiency anemia are also considered. These topics are appropriate in the general context of the book.

Physiological Significance of the Hemoglobin Level

Blood is often regarded as important primarily as a carrier of oxygen from the lungs to all the tissues of the body. Anemia is considered to be a condition associated with a decrease in this function, with the consequence that there is a lack of oxygen to fulfill metabolic needs. This does not always seem to be so because severe anemia can be associated with a marked increase over normal in the amount of oxygen being utilized by patients (T.S. Lee and G.R. Wadsworth 1968, unpublished observations). The body is able to adapt to the anemic state. One of the mechanisms of adaptation is an increase in the amount of dissociation of oxygen from oxyhemoglobin at the cellular level. But blood has important functions in addition to the transport of oxygen. One of these is the transport of heat from deeper to more superficial parts of the body, which promotes loss of excess heat from the skin and helps to maintain a body temperature within acceptable limits. Another function is the transport of nutrients to the tissues, of particular importance during the period of growth and during pregnancy. Any restriction to the flow of blood will inhibit normal growth, which, in the case of the placenta, might interfere with the growth and development of the fetus.

The viscosity of the blood has an important influence on the amount of nutrient material that reaches tissues. Blood of lower viscosity can flow more freely and thus convey oxygen and nutrients at a greater rate to the organs. The viscosity of blood varies both between and within individuals. It is a function of a number of interacting factors, including the deformability and degree of aggregation of erythrocytes, the nature of white blood cells, the composition of plasma, the diameter of the vessel through which blood is flowing, the speed of blood flow, the number of red cells, and hence the hemoglobin concentration, and others (Dormandy 1970; Dintenfass 1971). Despite this complexity the relative volume of erythrocytes to plasma (the packed red cell volume or PCV) and the hemoglobin level have consistently been found to correlate directly with overall viscosity of blood *in vivo*.

A decrease in the viscosity of blood can be achieved by reducing hemoglobin concentration through increasing the volume of plasma in the circulation. This form of hemodilution can be achieved experimentally or in clinical practice by intravenous infusion of a suitable fluid. Natural increases in plasma volume occur when a person moves from a cold to a hot environment (Barcroft et al. 1923). The corresponding degree of change in the concentration of hemoglobin can be demonstrated in the laboratory (Table 1), but can be greater in natural circumstances where temperature changes are greater.

Cooling either because of environmental conditions or in hibernation anesthesia is accompanied by a relatively high hemoglobin concen-

Table 1. The Effect of Environmental Temperature on the Hemoglobin Concentration

Subject in	Effective Temperature[a] (°F)	Hemoglobin Concentration (g/100 ml)
Cold room	61.5	16.1
Warm room	76.2	15.9
Warm room	77.0	15.5
Cold room	59.5	16.2

[a] Calculated from temperature, air movement, and relative humidity.
Source: Wadsworth (1952).

tration. This is associated with changes in blood viscosity and blood flow and with the control of heat exchange between the body and the environment.

Pregnancy and the period of growth are associated with relatively large volumes of circulating plasma. As a result these states are characterized by relatively low hemoglobin levels and blood viscosities. Despite this state of "physiological anemia" there is no decrease in the total amount of hemoglobin in the circulation—there is actually an increase in pregnancy—or in the supply of oxygen to the tissues (Mahomed and Hytten 1989). Hemodilution enhances the flow of blood through tissues without an increase in the amount of work done by the heart. Dormandy (1970) demonstrated with experimental animals that a 10% decrease in blood viscosity led to a 40% increase in cardiac output without any increase in heart rate, which is significant in relation to physical fitness in adults (Ernst et al. 1985) and in children (Brun et al. 1989).

Changes in blood viscosity, with associated changes in hemodynamics and hemoglobin levels, are of considerable importance. This is indicated by the relationships between the hemoglobin concentration and the course and outcome of pregnancy. Abernathy et al. (1966) identified a low hemoglobin level with the birth of a relatively large child, and a high hemoglobin level with prolongation of gestation, which is compatible with an inverse relationship between maternal PCV and the rate of premature birth observed by Lieberman et al. (1988). Garn et al. (1981) showed that within limits, perinatal death rates are inversely related to the maternal hemoglobin concentration. When the hemoglobin level rises during pregnancy preeclampsia tends to develop (Chesley 1972; Koller 1982). That these effects are the result of variations in the blood viscosity and blood flow to the uterus is indicated by the favorable results of hemodilution therapy in dealing with complications of pregnancy (Heilmann 1987). A relatively low blood viscosity may also be advantageous in regard to the development of cardiovascular disease (Dintenfass 1971). Vegetarians, who generally have less heart disease than others, have low blood viscosities and low hemoglobin levels (Ernst et al. 1986).

There is some evidence that in tropical conditions the hemodilution of pregnancy may be exaggerated. Lee and Wadsworth (1961) found, on measuring total plasma volume, that in Malaya some pregnant women with hemoglobin concentrations less than 10 g/100 ml had as much hemoglobin per unit fat-free body weight as normal men and women whose hemoglobin levels were as high as 16 g/100 ml. The frequency of hemoglobin levels down to less than 9 g/100 ml in pregnant women in the tropical environment of Singapore despite dietary supplements of iron is consistent with these observations (Kwa and Ko 1968).

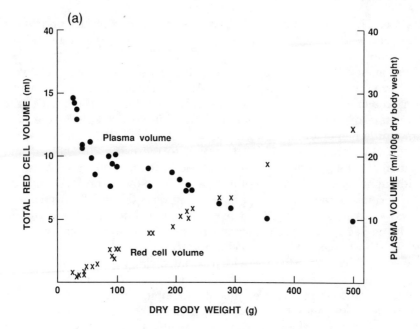

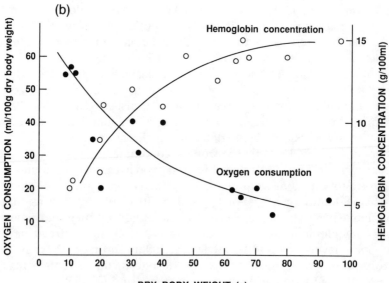

(c)

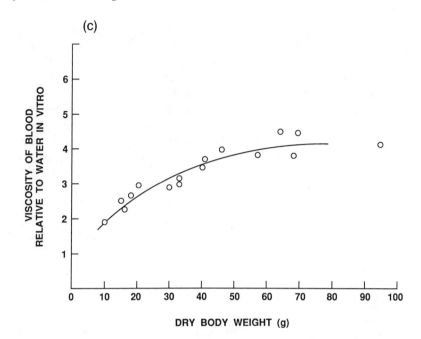

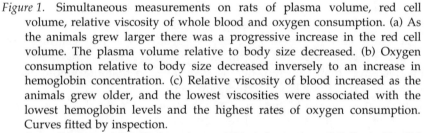

DRY BODY WEIGHT (g)

Figure 1. Simultaneous measurements on rats of plasma volume, red cell volume, relative viscosity of whole blood and oxygen consumption. (a) As the animals grew larger there was a progressive increase in the red cell volume. The plasma volume relative to body size decreased. (b) Oxygen consumption relative to body size decreased inversely to an increase in hemoglobin concentration. (c) Relative viscosity of blood increased as the animals grew older, and the lowest viscosities were associated with the lowest hemoglobin levels and the highest rates of oxygen consumption. Curves fitted by inspection.
Source: T.S. Lee and G.R. Wadsworth, unpublished observations, 1963. Drafted by Old Dominion U Graphics Department

Measurements in rats of the amount of metabolic tissue, oxygen consumption, hemoglobin level, total plasma volume, and *in vitro* relative viscosity of blood illustrated how these characteristics are interrelated as the body grows (T.S. Lee and G.R. Wadsworth 1963, unpublished observations). Metabolic activity, indicated by the rate of oxygen consumption in relation to body weight, decreased as the animals grew older and there was a concomitant increase in blood viscosity and the hemoglobin level. This was due partly to a progressive increase in the volume of circulating red cells, but more to a decrease in the plasma volume relative to body size (Figure 1).

When small rats were kept small by feeding them diets that contained little protein, low hemoglobin levels were maintained despite increasing age (G.R. Wadsworth 1968, unpublished observations). These low levels were due to relatively large plasma volumes, and the amount of hemodilution may have been an important factor in determining the rate of flow of blood consistent with cardiovascular characteristics and metabolic needs of animals of small size.

The absolute amounts of hemoglobin and plasma in the circulation in relation to the size and shape of the body do not seem to have been investigated in humans during the period of growth, although Palti (1983) found an association between stature and the hemoglobin level, and there seems to be an inverse relationship between rate of growth and hemoglobin level (Undritz 1964). In adults there are small degrees of correlation between various anthropometric characteristics and hematological indices (Micozzi et al. 1989). The relatively low hemoglobin level of women compared with that of men is accounted for by a larger plasma volume relative to fat-free body weight and a smaller number of red cells (Lee and Wadsworth 1961).

Hemoglobin concentrations are higher at the time of birth than later, partly because of the volume of blood transfused from the placenta into the child before the cord is tied. This should be associated with a high blood viscosity. However, infant plasma viscosity is relatively low (it is very low in preterm infants) because of a relatively low concentration of plasma proteins, especially fibrinogen. The low plasma viscosity has a greater effect than the high hemoglobin level so that the whole blood viscosity is relatively low (Linderkamp 1987).

There is evidence that the low hemoglobin levels in early childhood are temporary and physiological. Many surveys have shown that there is a spontaneous rise in these levels as children grow older. A study in Mexico reported by WHO (1972) found that anemia was of high prevalence among infants and young children in lower socioeconomic classes. When cereals to which iron had been added were given so as to provide 1.5 to 2.0 mg of iron per kg body weight a day anemia disappeared by the time the children reached the age of 2 to 3 years. However, the anemia also disappeared at this age among children who had not received the fortified cereal. These observations are compatible with those made by Burman (1972) in the United Kingdom and by Beal et al. (1962) in the United States.

The hemoglobin concentration of an individual does not remain constant from day to day, but fluctuates, sometimes appreciably. Variations over short periods are probably due to changes in the volume of plasma, although fluctuations in the reticulocyte count, also observed in healthy

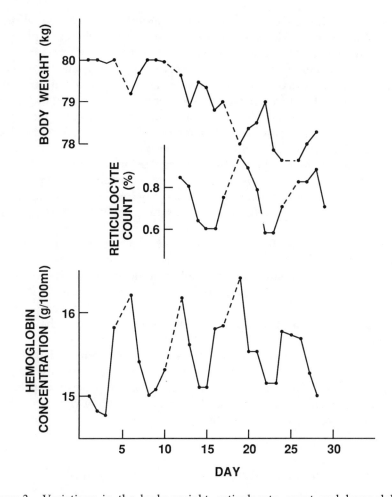

Figure 2. Variations in the body weight, reticulocyte count and hemoglobin concentration in a healthy young man. Measurements were made on successive days throughout a month.
Source: G.R. Wadsworth, unpublished observations, 1953. Drafted by Old Dominion U Graphics Department.

people, suggest that the volume of erythrocytes released into the circulation also varies from time to time. Changes in plasma volume may be due to movement of water between the extravascular fluid and blood, with no effect on body weight, or to hydration or dehydration, with corresponding changes in body weight. These associations are illustrated in Figure 2 and they are to be regarded as normal physiological phenomena.

In pathological states, changes in plasma volume may have appreciable effects on hemoglobin levels and blood viscosity. For example, plasma volume expands in congestive cardiac failure and contracts in severe diarrhea, especially in children. In polycythemia there is an abnormal increase in the production of erythrocytes and a large red cell volume in the circulation. However, in some cases there may be no obvious increase in the hemoglobin concentration because of a compensatory increase in the circulating plasma volume. In some patients with "apparent polycythemia" (Gaisbok's syndrome) chronic shrinkage of the plasma volume produces an increase in hemoglobin concentration even though the number of red blood cells does not increase. Correct diagnosis of these conditions requires measurements of the blood volume. Such determinations are also needed to evaluate the physiological significance of hemoglobin levels.

The above discussion shows that current accounts of the prevalence of anemia throughout the world, which are based on somewhat arbitrary criteria, may not recognize the physiological flexibility of the concentration of hemoglobin in the circulating blood. In most countries in which anemia has been found to be common fever, diarrheal diseases, limited rates of growth, and high environmental temperature may have effects on the hemoglobin level.

Physiological variations in hemoglobin concentration and those that are inherent in technical procedures may seem small, usually no more than 1 or 2 g/100 ml, but may often be sufficient to place an appreciable number of normal people in the "anemic" class when rigid criteria for lower levels of normal hemoglobin levels are applied.

Normal and Abnormal Metabolism of Iron

Approximately half of the total amount of iron in the body (about 3500 mg in the adult male) occurs in the circulating hemoglobin. Most of the rest, which constitutes "storage iron," is in various tissues, especially the liver, spleen, and bone marrow in association with the reticuloendothelial system of cells. The presence and amount of this iron do not seem to be of critical importance for adequate production of normal hemoglobinized erythrocytes (Brown et al. 1988). Storage iron may, therefore, consist of iron in excess of that needed for erythropoiesis. Each day about 21 mg of iron is released by the breakdown of effete red blood cells. This iron is a large proportion of the iron that circulates continually between different tissues in the body and is equal to the amount needed in the formation of new hemoglobin leaving the bone marrow. The inevitable, but very small, loss from the body is balanced by the absorption of 1 to 2 mg of iron from that sequestered from the diet in the mucosal cells of the intestine (Pollycove 1964). Thus, the daily requirement for iron is met almost entirely by sources inside the body.

Three "laws of erythrokinetics" have been discovered, largely through the use of radioactive materials (Pollycove 1964). The first is that the body conserves the iron that it contains; once in the body very little iron can get out under normal circumstances (McCance and Widdowson 1937). The second is that the amount of iron that enters from the intestine is inversely related to the amount of nonheme iron in storage in tissues. As these stores decrease, the amount absorbed by the intestine increases. The third law is that the amount of iron entering the body from the intestine is directly related to the rate of erythropoiesis; the greater the rate that red cells are being produced the greater the amount of iron absorbed.

The quantity of storage iron is indicated by the concentration of ferritin in plasma. Erythropoietic activity is indicated by the number of young erythrocytes (reticulocytes) in the circulation. Thus, according to the "laws" a low ferritin level and a high reticulocyte count should be associated with a high rate of absorption of iron from the diet. When results obtained by Taylor et al. (1986) are plotted on a graph an inverse relationship can indeed be seen between serum ferritin concentrations and the percentage absorption of radioactive iron although with a considerable degree of scatter of values. An absorption of almost 20% was associated with a serum ferritin level of less than 10 µg/liter and an absorption of less than 4% with ferritin levels in the region of 35 µg/liter. Baynes et al. (1987) found that the absorption of iron from ferrous sulfate taken by mouth was negatively correlated with the log serum ferritin concentration, with a coefficient of correlation of −0.54. This relatively low degree of association may be explained by influences on the serum ferritin level of factors other than the amount of storage iron (Jacobs and Worwood 1975). In the investigation of Baynes et al. (1987) a serum ferritin concentration of less than 20 µg/liter could be associated with absorption of up to 70% of the ingested iron. But the concentration of ferritin in plasma can itself be affected by the amount of iron that enters the body; the synthesis of ferritin is induced by the presence of iron (Harrison 1964) and serum levels are raised considerably by ingestion of large doses of the element. When a supplement of 60 mg of iron a day was given to preschool children the level of ferritin in serum rose from 20.6 to 59.3 ng/ml, a supplement of 120 mg led to a rise to 63.4 ng/ml, and one of 240 mg led to a rise to 79.7 ng/ml (Linpisarn et al. 1984). Conversely, serum ferritin levels quickly fall when the availability of iron is reduced (Milne et al. 1990). A rise in the concentration of ferritin in blood after administration of iron may not, therefore, be an indication of preexisting deficiency of iron. Furthermore, results of studies of the metabolism of intracellular iron (Bezkorovainy 1989a) indicate that the amount present as ferritin may not determine the amount of iron that is being utilized.

Although most of the iron in the body is conserved there are normally small losses, for example, in the urine and in cells that are desquamated from the skin surface. These small losses are balanced by corresponding gains from the intestine (Wadsworth 1969). According to the body's need for iron a variable amount that enters the intestinal mucosal cells passes either through the cells into the blood plasma or into ferritin within the cells (Bezkorovainy 1989b). In the latter event iron is lost when the mucosal cells are desquamated. When synthesis of mucosal intracellular ferritin reaches a maximum level iron may pass excessively into the bloodstream.

In iron deficiency or when a negative iron balance is caused by hemorrhage adaptive changes may occur. Thus, in patients with iron-deficiency anemia iron may be absent from the cells lost from the surface of the skin and there may be a reduction in menstrual loss of blood (Jacobs and Butler 1965; Pritchard 1966; Milne et al. 1990). A hazard as small as a single donation of blood is associated with a rise in the reticulocyte count, indicative of an increase in erythropoietic activity (Wadsworth 1955) and probably, therefore, an increase in the movement of iron into the body. This relationship is illustrated by the observations of Raja et al. (1988) on mice (Table 2).

Although the sensitivity of human responses according to the laws of

Table 2. Effect of Hypoxia on Intestinal Absorption of Iron in Mice

Group	No.	Hemoglobin Concentration (g/100 ml)	Reticulocytes Percent	Uptake (pmol/mg tissue/10 min)
Control	4	14.2 ± 0.7	1.5 ± 0.3	52.5 ± 7.0
Hypoxic (for 3 days)	5	16.3 ± 0.4	6.1 ± 0.6	140.0 ± 14.0

Source: Raja et al. (1988).

Table 3. Mean Percentage Absorption of Radioactive Iron
in Foods in Anemia

Food	Normal Controls	Iron-Deficient Patients
Oatcake	4.0	10.0
Eggs	2.2	5.6
Chicken meat	6.9	17.0

Source: Callender (1981).

ferrokinetics in the determination of how much iron is absorbed is not known precisely, those who have developed anemia in association with a depletion in iron stores have been found consistently to absorb more iron from iron salts and from foods than healthy subjects (Moore 1964). An illustration is given in Table 3.

According to the laws of ferrokinetics and observations such as those given in Table 3, there should be difficulty in the establishment of human anemia solely by dietary manipulation, as, indeed, is the case with rats and mice. Mechanisms for the conservation of iron and the increased absorption of iron according to need should redress an adverse balance. In addition, as the amount of iron in the diet decreases there is an increase in the proportion that is absorbed. Rodents are especially adaptable in this respect and enough iron can be obtained by the increase in the proportion absorbed, even from diets of natural foods of low iron content (Smith and Pannacculli 1958).

Foods that are used in tests on anemic patients cover a wide range and many people who do not have anemia probably live on the same foods. The question arises, why do some people with an apparent ability to absorb relatively large amounts of iron from food become iron deficient while the great majority of people who depend on the same foods remain normal? There seem to be two different types of people; one type requires relatively more iron and, despite adaptive mechanisms, is unable to meet these extra requirements by absorption from the diet. Unfortunately, inquiries by nutritionists into the natural history of iron deficiency have not been concerned very much with particular characteristics of individuals who become anemic, perhaps because undue attention is given to the nature of iron in foods. In the investigation of foods human subjects are, indeed, used, but only in place of experimental animals and not as important variables themselves in the relationship between dietary iron and blood formation.

Loss of storage iron as indicated by a decrease in the concentration of iron in the liver, and by a decrease in the level of ferritin in plasma, may not be due to a loss from the body but to deployment to another iron compartment within the body. Deployment of iron is controlled by transferrin, a protein in plasma to which iron is bound. Usually, the amount of transferrin is much in excess of the amount of iron available so that "transferrin saturation" with iron is normally less than 30%. When iron is being mobilized and in iron deficiency there is an increase in the concentration of transferrin in the blood and a decrease in its degree of saturation with iron. There is an appreciable increase in the transferrin level, even in the absence of iron deficiency, during pregnancy, and there is a relatively low transferrin iron saturation level during childhood (Milman and Cohn 1984). These changes do not seem to be consistently related to the amount of storage iron (King et al. 1987), and they may be controlled by particular patterns of endocrine activity. There is clinical evidence that hormones affect the concentration of transferrin in blood; men and women being treated with estrogens have an increased transferrin level (Laurell et al. 1969; Cartei et al. 1970). Oral contraceptives raise concentrations of transferrin in blood (Burton 1967; Jacobi et al. 1969; Horne et al. 1970) and also cause a marked increase in ferritin levels (Fressinelli-Gunderson et al. 1985). The influence of hormone balance on hematological characteristics is demonstrated by the fact that sex-related differences in these characteristics become apparent for the first time during puberty (Yip et al. 1984). When transferrin concentrations rise concurrently with an increase in the total plasma volume, as in pregnancy, the total amount of transferrin in the circulation is even greater than is at first apparent. The greater the amount of transferrin the greater the amount of iron drawn into the blood from the iron stores. Iron thus mobilized becomes available for the increased production of hemoglobin and myoglobin characteristic of pregnancy and growth. That iron is

Table 4. Concentrations of Iron in Liver at Different Stages of Life

Group	Iron in liver (μg/g wet wt.)
Neonates	342.5
Infants	107.8
Children	143.6
Men	233.0
Women (reproductive)	130.0
Women (postmenopausal)	302.6

Source: Chang (1973).

withdrawn from the tissues and prevented from accumulating in them during these phases of life is consistent with the observation that amounts of iron in liver decrease progressively during early childhood and remain small during the productive years of women. When women grow older iron becomes free to accumulate in storage, and the concentration in liver becomes high (Table 4).

During pregnancy removal of iron from storage is indicated by a decrease in the serum ferritin concentration, a decrease that is not prevented by the administration of iron (King et al. 1987). Serum ferritin levels are high at the time of birth, and fall to adult levels toward the end of the first year. These levels can be raised by ingestion of extra iron, but amounts in excess of those normally present in foods are required.

Each day about 35 mg of iron enters and leaves the circulating blood. Of this amount about 21 mg comes from the release of iron from effete erythrocytes and a further 7 mg or so from iron that entered the marrow but was not utilized in the synthesis of hemoglobin. All of this 28 mg of iron must pass through the reticuloendothelial system before reentering the plasma (Bezkroravainy 1989a). Thus about 80% of the total turnover of iron in the body depends on the integrity of the reticuloendothelial cells. This explains why iron-deficiency anemia may complicate malaria and other infections—in those conditions iron is sequestered in the reticuloendothelial cells. Iron sequestration also occurs when there is a deficiency of vitamin A (Mejia 1985) and dietary supplements of vitamin A enhance the utilization of iron (Bloem et al. 1990). The accumulation of iron outside the hematopoietic tissue is reflected in the relatively high level of plasma ferritin occurring in a number of chronic diseases (Brown et al. 1988). Iron-deficiency anemia that arises because of a disruption of the internal transfer of iron would develop more quickly than that caused primarily by dietary deficiency. A condition of "internal iron deficiency" persists in malaria after parasites disappear from the blood so that superficial inquires might lead to the false conclusion that an associated anemia was due to dietary causes.

Because malaria is highly prevalent in many parts of the world and is a potent cause of anemia, epidemiological and historical studies of anemia must take account of its occurrence and the age group that it affects. Malaria is particularly dangerous to the infant after the first few months of life, but as the child grows older an immunity to the parasite develops and malarial attacks diminish in intensity and frequency, although they may not disappear entirely. However, in places where malaria has been absent temporarily and is reintroduced older children may be severely affected. Variation in susceptibility to malaria, with associated anemia, might, by chance, be accompanied by variability in dietary patterns and difficulties could arise in the assignment of specific causes for the development of anemia. Malaria is relatively easily identifiable, but other infections that are recurrent and prolonged in many poorer communities cannot easily be identified without immunological tests. These infections, like malaria, can be important causes of anemia due to interference with the normal turnover of iron within the body.

Thus, the movement of iron between hematopoietic tissue and iron storage sites accounts for important physiological changes in the characteristics of the blood, and pathological changes that inhibit this movement are important causes of anemia.

Iron in Foods

Iron is abundant in the environment, being present in the earth's crust in the amount of 50,000 ppm, compared with only 57 ppm in the human body (Skoryna et al., 1980). Despite the abundance of iron in the environment anemia, due to lack of iron, is thought to be the most common deficiency disease in the world. The dramatic reduction in the amount of iron in the body compared with that in the environment is due to physiological control of the amount of the element that can pass through the wall of the intestine and to highly selective uptake of iron from the environment by materials that are consumed by man. Diets usually contain only from about 20 to 60 ppm of iron. The "anemogenic diet" has never been identified, first, because the dietary intake of individuals who are about to become anemic has never been measured with a sufficient degree of accuracy, if at all, and second, because no controlled tests have been made in which diets of varied and known composition have been fed to various kinds of people while their hemataological characteristics were being monitored. In any such attempts to determine the connection between the diet and iron deficiency the amounts of iron in different foods must be determined.

Iron is present in nearly all natural foods and is present in all known diets. Foods used traditionally in isolated communities may be important sources of iron. For example, the flesh of the mongongo fruit (*Ricinodendron rautanenii*) consumed by the !Kung contains 0.74 mg Fe/100 g, and the nut 2.3 mg Fe/100 g (Wehmeyer et al. 1969). These amounts are comparable with those in eggs (2.7 mg Fe/100 g), steak (2.5 mg Fe/100 g), and chicken (1.9 mg Fe/100g). Norton et al. (1984) were able to identify wild foods used by Native Americans in the Pacific Northwest for 12,000 years, some of which contain considerable amounts of iron (Table 5).

Table 5. Amounts of Iron in Some Foods Used Traditionally
by North American Indians

Local Name	Botanic Name	Iron (mg/100 g)
Bitterroot	*Lewisia rediviva*	33
Desert parsley	*Lomatium canbyi*	25
Wapatoo	*Sagittaria latifolia*	41
Fritillaria	*F. pudica*	88
Potato	*Solanum tuberosum*	3

Source: Norton et al. (1984).

Malaise and Parent (1985) listed 265 different plants growing wild in central Africa, and Ogle and Grivetti (1985) named 250 in Swaziland that can be used as foods. Many of these contain large amounts of iron (Table 6).

Considerable amounts of iron are added to a number of modern foods during their commercial preparation. Thus, many people, especially infants, ingest large amounts of iron. Babies in Britain fed from the breast get about 0.33 mg of iron a day, those fed on cow's milk about 0.74 mg a day, and those fed formula preparations up to 11.3 mg a day (Department of Health and Social Security 1974). Infants older than 4 months may be getting 16 mg of iron or even more a day because of the use of commercial foods fortified with iron (Rees et al. 1985; Penrod et al. 1990).

Contaminant iron can be appreciable in amount and may have been even more in the past than at present (Witts 1964). In some parts of Africa

Table 6. Some Wild Foods of Africa with a High
Content of Iron

Food	Iron (mg/100 g)
Balanities aegyptica (nut)	40
Sclerocarya birrea (nut)	60
Tylosema fassoglensis (seed)	40
Parkia fikicoidea (fruit pulp)	55
Pentanisia schweinfurthii (flower)	380
Cyperus esculentus (stem)	840
Dioscera praehensilis (rhizome)	150
Alternsethera sessilis (leaf)	400
Gynandropsis gynnandra (leaf)	3400
Solanum nigrum (leaf)	200

Source: Ogle and Grivetti (1985).

Table 7. Concentrations of Iron in Water
from Different Sources Used by Masai

Source	Iron (mg/100 ml)
Pipeline	0.65
Borehole	0.90
Rain pools	0.1 to 0.4

Source: Nestel and Geissler (1986).

cereals become heavily contaminated with iron-rich soil from the hooves of cattle used for threshing (Hercberg et al. 1987). Undritz (1964) stated that elephants in the wild depend on the high iron contents of soil and water for their existence. In captivity these animals often die unless given large supplements of iron. Water that is used to cleanse and cook foods often contains iron, which is consumed along with the foods, and iron from utensils can also enter the diet. The large amounts of iron in foods cooked in iron pots by the Bantu has often been cited in connection with the development of the pathological condition of iron overload. Possible contributions of iron from water are indicated in Table 7.

The iron in water may be an important source for infants. Traditional infant foods are commonly composed of the cooking water from the family pot and mashed starchy foods (Raphael 1984). These supplements to breast-feeding can be introduced soon after birth, although in small amounts.

Concentrations of iron given in standard tables of food composition are usually based on analyses of single foods. But, because of losses or gains of iron and alterations in the chemical nature and physical structure of foods during preparation and cooking, the amount and availability of iron may be quite different in foods consumed in meals from those processed in the laboratory. There may be differences in the amount of iron in the same kind of food derived from different sources. Thus, maize meal prepared commercially and used by Masai was found to contain 7.3 mg Fe/100 g; that from home grinding contained only 2.1 mg Fe/100 g (Nestel and Geissler 1986). According to tables of food composition, cassava root (*Manihot utilissima*) contains less than 1 mg Fe/100 g but Amorozo and Shrimpton (1984) found that this traditional food was the main source of iron for 40% of families who lived in a slum area of the Amazon, and the mean intake of iron was 19 mg/person/day. These authors quoted Maralhas (1964) who stated that cassava was a rich source of iron in South America, its region of origin. An explanation for the large amounts of iron in cassava prepared for cooking in rural households in Africa is probably contamination with rust from metal graters (Hegarty and Wadsworth 1968).

It appears that there are many dietary rich sources of iron available throughout the world. Traditional societies, both past and present, have probably consumed large amounts of iron because of its inadvertent addition to foods.

The Diet and Anemia

Discrepancies between the average intake of iron and average hemoglobin levels or the prevalence of anemia have been revealed. An example is provided by the results of an investigation made by Ong et al. (1983) in England (Table 8).

In Bangladesh, Hassan and Ahmad (1984) found, using the results of national surveys conducted on three occasions during the previous 20 years, that the mean intake of iron remained constant at about 23 mg/person/day, although 85% of the population is alleged to have anemia. In contrast, only 25% of Masai women and children with an average intake of iron of only 8 mg/day were found to be anemic by Nestel and Geissler (1986). The results of a number of other inquires provide evidence that low average hemoglobin levels occur over a wide range of average intakes of iron. The situation is confused by the employment of different methods of calculating the amount of iron ingested; those based on information contained in tables of food composition may provide values that are too low because they do not take into account the presence of contaminant iron. When samples of diets as consumed are analyzed chemically they often reveal the presence of relatively great amounts of iron. Other possible reasons for differing results in different inquires are variation in the amounts of iron released after digestion of

Table 8. Mean Intakes of Iron and Hemoglobin Levels of Pregnant Women of Different Ethnic Groups in England

	Indian	Bangladeshi	Pakistani
Number	19	10	17
Iron (mg/day)	11.8 ± 2.3	8.1 ± 2.3	16.3 ± 3.9
Hemoglobin (g/100 ml)	12.0 ± 1.12	12.6 ± 0.8	12.3 ± 1.13

Source: Ong et al. (1983).

foods and made available for absorption from the intestine, and inadequacy of the methods used to determine dietary intakes and incidence of anemia. Sanford (1960, 1961) showed that different amounts of iron in a soluble form are released when different foods are digested *in vitro* by pepsin in an acid medium, as is present in the stomach. The amounts of iron released in this way varied from about 2 to 85% according to the food. Jacobs and Greenman (1969) and Jacobs and Miles (1969) later made more extensive tests the results of which confirmed Sanford's observations that there is appreciable variation among foods in the amount of iron that passes from them into solution in the stomach.

Jacobs and Miles (1969) pointed out that although iron in some foods is soluble in an acid environment it becomes insoluble in the neutral to alkaline medium of the duodenum and ileum. However, precipitation from solution on this change of acidity is prevented when iron released in the stomach is combined with a mucopolysaccharide normally present in gastric juice. The iron–mucopolysaccharide complex remains in solution in an alkaline medium and contains iron available for absorption through the wall of the gut. Because of the large molecular size of the iron-mucopolysaccharide it is not itself absorbed; the iron moiety is first removed by chelating agents of small molecular size that can penetrate the intestinal mucosa. However, other substances present in gastric juice, one of which is gastrin, are capable of binding iron (Bella and Kim 1973; Baldwin et al. 1986).

Iron that passes through the intestinal wall to gain access to the body originates from various constituents of the chyme present in the lumen of the gastrointestinal canal. This chyme is a mixture of chemicals in solution, particulate matter, bacteria, viruses, and, very often, parasites of various kinds. Perhaps of great significance is the presence in chyme of lactoferrin and transferrin, conveyed by the bile, because of the involvement of these substances in the transfer of iron in biological systems. The living elements in the intestinal contents are themselves complex biochemical and physiological systems capable of consuming, synthesizing, and excreting many substances. The constituents of chyme have been acquired not only through ingestion, but also through the process of gastric digestion, and from gastric juice, bile, succus entericus, pancreatic juice, products of intestinal digestion, substances excreted by living organisms, and cells desquamated from the mucosal lining of the gastrointestinal canal. Within this mixture various chemical and physicochemical changes take place that probably vary both in extent and direction between individuals. The activities within chyme determine the amount of ionized iron and the extent of chelation of iron with small molecules able to pass through the wall of the small intestine. To now, no tests have been made in which samples of gut contents at various levels, at different times, in different types of consumer, and after the ingestion of different kinds of diet, have been analyzed. Thus, no direct evidence is available on the relative influences of chemical, physicochemical, physiological, pathological, and microbiological factors that ultimately determine how much iron moves into the body from the gut. Furthermore, there is a lack of understanding of how iron is actually transported from intestinal cells into the blood plasma and, hence, how this is regulated. Klausner (1988) has suggested that abnormalities in this transfer process could be a cause of hereditary hemochromatosis; could other abnormalities be a cause of iron-deficiency anemia? Balance studies in which comparison is made between the composition of the diet and that of the feces might seem to provide direct evidence on the amount of iron removed from foods that have been eaten. However, these studies are not satisfactory because the sensitivity of the methods for the quantitative analysis of iron in biological materials is often not great enough to detect the small differences between the amounts of dietary and fecal iron usually present. Furthermore, iron is contributed erratically to the feces from gastrointestinal secretions and also, perhaps to an appreciable extent, from desquamated mucosal cells. As already mentioned, iron that is absorbed from the lumen of the gut is first sequestered in these cells and may remain in them until they are detached. Although the life span of mucosal cells is only 1 to 2 days losses of sequestered iron takes several weeks (Schwartz 1986). Prolongation of balance studies long enough to take account of erratic fluctuations in the concentration of iron in the intestinal contents is not usually practicable. An indication of the variability under strict laboratory conditions encountered in such tests is given in Table 9.

Most of the information about the availability of iron in different foods is based on the use of radioactive preparations. As a result of such studies

Table 9. Apparent Retention of Iron by One Woman Determined from Analysis of Dietary and Fecal Iron[a]

Day of Experiment	Iron Intake (mg/day)	Fecal Iron (mg/day)	Retention (%)
1 (normal diet)	12.5	7.4	+ 41.1
3 (normal diet)	11.3	9.1	+ 19.4
5 (on experimental diet)	17.9	17.7	+ 1.6
12 (on experimental diet)	17.9	15.8	+ 11.9
13 (on experimental diet)	17.9	18.1	− 1.2

[a] The subject collected feces daily throughout the experiment and from day 4 onward remained on a constant diet. The figures in the table are selected examples of different days. *Source*: Narula (1968).

there is now a firm belief that iron in meat, contained in hemoglobin and myoglobin (heme-iron), is absorbed to a much greater extent than is iron contained in foods of vegetable origin. Iron in meat is absorbed without the need for any processing in the stomach, and products of the digestion of meat, probably amino acids, enhance the absorption of iron from the entire diet (Layrisse et al. 1984; Taylor et al. 1986). The superiority of meat in promoting regeneration of hemoglobin after severe hemorrhage in dogs was demonstrated long ago (Robscheit-Robbins and Whipple 1925). However, the availability of iron from meat is markedly reduced on prolonged heating during cooking (Martinez et al. 1986) and heme-iron is retained more firmly than non-heme-iron in the intestinal mucosal cells.

Classification of foods according to the extent to which radioactive iron

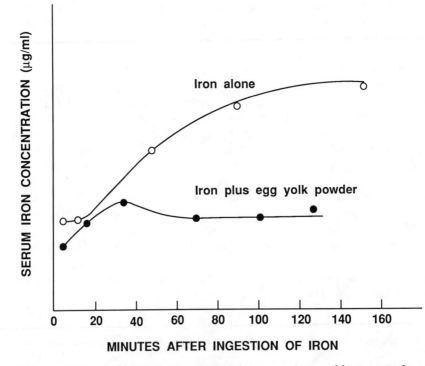

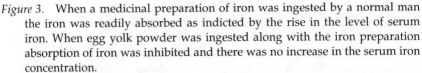

Figure 3.   When a medicinal preparation of iron was ingested by a normal man the iron was readily absorbed as indicted by the rise in the level of serum iron. When egg yolk powder was ingested along with the iron preparation absorption of iron was inhibited and there was no increase in the serum iron concentration.
Source: G.R. Wadsworth, unpublished observations, 1968. Drafted by Old Dominion U Graphics Department.

incorporated into or mixed with them is absorbed has become widely accepted and is used to assess the extent to which various diets provide iron to the body. There are, however, other factors apart from the bioavailability of iron in separate foods that influence the availability of iron from the whole diet. One is the presence of particular foods, of which beans, eggs, and cow's milk have been identified and studied. An illustration of the effect of powdered egg on the absorption of iron from ferrous sulfate is given in Figure 3.

Sadowitz and Oski (1983) observed that 30% of infants who had been given cow's milk before the age of 6 months and a hemoglobin concentration less than 11 g/100 ml and a serum ferritin level less than 12 μg/100 ml at the age of 9 to 12 months. These relatively low levels were present in only 17.4% of infants who had not been given cow's milk until after the age of 6 months. Similar observations were made by Reeves et al. (1984).

However, the most important dietary factor influencing iron absorption is the presence of a number of substances not routinely taken into account in surveys of dietary intakes and hemoglobin levels. Of these, vitamin C (ascorbic acid) has been investigated to the greatest extent, and it has been established that the presence of this vitamin may be the most critical factor determining the amount of iron obtained from many diets. Ascorbic acid is thought to chelate iron and carry it into the mucosal cells of the gut. Accordingly, recording intakes of vitamin C might be as important as recording intakes of iron. In this connection the relatively high concentration of vitamin C in human milk compared with cow's milk might be significant. The amount of vitamin C in traditional foods not included in most tables of food composition may be appreciable (Table 10).

Gillooly et al. (1983) made a detailed study of the effects on the absorption of iron of the presence of ascorbic acid and other organic molecules of small size. They demonstrated that citric, tartaric, and malic acids increased the amount of iron that passed into the body from a meal based on rice and was used in the formation of hemoglobin. They pointed out that these acids are normal components of a number of fruits and vegetables and are present in amounts comparable to those used in their tests. Accordingly, relatively large amounts of iron would be obtained by consumers from foods that contain them, such as, tomato, broccoli, cauliflower, cabbage, and sauerkraut. Lactic acid is also present in sauerkraut and may further enhance the availability of the dietary iron.

Citric acid is an essential constituent of the body and is involved in vital biochemical processes. It was first isolated, from lemon juice, by Scheele in 1784 (Partington 1962). Because of its chelating ability citric

Table 10. Ascorbic Acid Content of Some Leaf Vegetables Used
in Malaysia

Botanical Name	English Name	Ascorbic Acid (mg/100 g)	
		Mean	Range
Basella rubra	Ceylon spinach	88	47–131
Brassica juncea	Mustard green	82	59–100
Carica papaya	Papaya		
Light leaves		136	96–202
Dark leaves		197	147–241
Diplazium esculentum	Fern shoot	29	11–55
Manihot utilissima	Tapioca		
Light leaves		231	198–300
Dark leaves		482	401–567

Source: Caldwell (1972).

acid is widely used in food technology to remove traces of metals from
vegetable fats and other commodities liable to undergo rancidity. Wright
and Hughes (1975) found that a group of infants consumed 0.132 ± 0.0115
g/kg body weight of citric acid a day, 68% of which came from milk and
20% from canned foods. The mean intake by 20 nuns was 0.04 ± 0.0018
g/kg body weight, about one-third of which was from citrus fruits. Because citric acid is used in the food industry commercial products may

Table 11. Concentrations of Citric and Malic Acids
in Some Foods

Food	Citric Acid	Malic Acid
	(mg/100 g edible portion)	
Apple	64	270
Banana	320	500
Grapefruit	1720	—
Lemon juice	6200	300
Bread	37	—
Eggs	54	—
Human milk	150	—
Cherries	10	1250
Gooseberries	Trace	1400
Cauliflower	210	390

Sources: Diem (1962); Wright and Hughes (1975).

provide from 5 to 15% of the amount present in modern diets. The amounts of citric acid and malic acid present naturally in many foods indicate that they would be available to an appreciable extent from traditional diets (Table 11).

Some foods that lack one of the organic acids may have a large amount of another, so that in a mixed diet there may be a considerable additive effect.

In contrast to the enhancing effects of organic acids of small molecular size, other constituents of fruits and vegetables were found by Gillooly et al. (1983) to exert an inhibitory effect on the absorption of iron. They found, in particular, that sodium phytate, polyphenols, and large amounts of oxalate had this effect. Tannin is a polyphenol that is present in tea, many wines, and water used in arctic households (WHO 1982). Foods that contain a large amount of phosphate and probably, therefore, large amounts of phytate, are associated with low levels of absorption of dietary iron. These foods include rice bran, wheat germ, nuts, chocolate, and cheese. The effect of phytate on iron absorption may be counteracted by vitamin C (Hallberg et al. 1986), and calcium, which has an affinity for phytate, may reduce the amount available to combine with iron in the gut. The amount of phytate may also be reduced by certain methods of preparing and cooking foods. Absorption of iron from cereals is inhibited by lignins, some of which have a polyphenolic structure, and hemicellulose, both of which are components of dietary "fiber" (Gillooly et al. 1984). Some other natural constituents of plants, for example, hemaglutinins, also interfere with the availability of dietary iron. These substances are often destroyed during cooking, but there is variation in this respect depending on cooking practice in different households (Korte 1972).

Other, sometimes exotic, substances in foods affect the availability and utilization of iron; one example is lead.

Many children with high blood levels of lead have evidence of iron deficiency (Yip et al. 1981), although the anemia of lead poisoning is of the sideroblastic type in which there is a defect in the utilization of iron. Possibly 1.5% of children in metropolitan areas in the United States have blood levels of lead above 15 µg/dl (Mitchell and Baburich 1987). Lead poisoning has been known to occur in remote villages in the Middle East because stones that contain lead are used in grinding cereal grains.

Enhancement or inhibition of iron absorption by substances present in foods would affect not only the iron in those foods but iron from all sources.

There are, then, considerable variations in iron content among different samples of the same food, especially at the time of their consumption, differences in the availability of iron from different foods, and enhancing and inhibiting effects of various substances in the lumen of the gut on the extent to which iron is absorbed. Consequently, assessments of the amount of iron obtained by the consumer that depend on evaluation of the results of dietary studies in which use is made of standard tables of food composition are, in a functional sense, meaningless. Therefore, there is a need for accurate measurements of the actual amounts of iron which enter the systems of different people. Such measurements would indicate not only the net availability of dietary iron, but also the effects of intrinsic characteristics of the consumer, discussed below, which may influence absorption. So far, no such tests for field use have been proposed.

Serial determinations of the concentration of iron in serum show the extent to which iron is entering the blood stream from the gut (Figure 3), but repeated sampling of blood is not usually practicable. Man and Wadsworth (1969) observed that the total amount of iron excreted in the urine during 24 hours reflected the amount of iron in a mixed diet. For example, the average daily excretion of a man on a constant intake of 11.4 mg iron/day was 51.8 µg/day and on a constant intake of 35.7 mg iron/day the average excretion was 135.5 µg/day. Schultz-Lell et al. (1987) found that infants fed on breast milk which contained 440 µg of iron/liter excreted 0.005 ng/liter in their urine, while those fed a milk formula containing 1100 µg of iron/liter excreted 0.01 ng/liter. Man and Wadsworth (1969) supposed that a very small proportion of the iron that enters the blood from food is immediately diverted through the kidney, which, in this way, is taking continuous samples. The amount of iron excreted in 24 hours correlates closely with the amount in urine collected during the night or first thing in the morning. The urinary loss of iron by an individual, even on a constant intake, varies from day to day, especially in the case of women. Therefore, when urinary iron excretion is used as an indicator of the amount of iron being absorbed from the diet by an individual 24 hour or overnight samples of urine collected on a number of consecutive days should be analyzed. The average amount of iron lost in the urine by a group of people over a single period of 24 hours, by smoothing out individual variability, should indicate the average amount of iron being absorbed by that group. In this case the iron/creatinine ratio in casual samples of urine may be adequate because this mean ratio, for groups, is approximately the same whether determined on 24 hour, overnight, or casual samples (G.R. Wadsworth 1968, unpublished observation). However, the amounts of iron in urine are very small so that great care is needed to avoid contamination of specimens and the apparatus used in their analysis.

The above discussion leads to the conclusion that an important reason for discrepancies among the results of different investigations into the relationship between the diet and hemoglobin levels and the prevalence of anemia is a failure to take into account net biological availability of iron. There is a lack of appropriate methodology for determining how much iron is actually obtained from diets of various sorts, although measurement of iron in urine might be rewarding. Other possible reasons for discrepancies are failure to take into account the multifactorial etiology of iron-deficiency anemia, and failure to evaluate erratic and long-term variations in the dietary intakes of individuals and of groups. Such variations may be obscured when the results of inquiries are expressed only as averages.

All diseases are of multifactorial origin (Rothman 1976) and there may be variation in the relative importance of different causative factors among individuals or groups with a common disease. This variation is exaggerated when a condition is not a disease entity but a symptom common to a number of different pathological states. This is true of anemia, even when defined as "iron-deficiency anemia," as it is a symptom of a number of different pathological conditions, each of which may have multiple origins. Inquiries concerned with anemia and the diet must include observations not only on hemoglobin levels, but also on the presence or absence of hemorrhage, chronic disease, and other conditions.

Variations in the diet occur because of unpredictable fluctuations in the amounts and kinds of food eaten by individuals, established meal patterns within families according to the day of the week or season of the year, customary use or avoidance of some foods during pregnancy and lactation, seasonal changes in the availability or costs of particular foods, erratic use of some foods, and the use of unusual foods in times of shortage.

When food is scarce diets change in two ways: there is a reduction in the number of foods used and an increased use of unusual materials. In India and China important use of many wild foods has traditionally been made when necessary. Chou-Ting Wang, in about 1400 A.D., prepared a treatise describing 414 plants that could be used in times of famine (Read 1946). Some of these would have been useful sources of iron, for example, dandelion leaves, which contain about 3 mg of iron/100 g. The use of "famine foods" in Africa has already been mentioned.

The availability of traditional wild foods varies with the season (Ogle and Grivetti 1985). Seasonal shortages, which may amount to famine, are common in many communities and may distort apparent relationships between diet and anemia, especially when historical comparisons are made because any effect of a change of diet on the hemoglobin level would become obvious only after a considerable length of time. The extent of shortages is indicated by the observations of Pales (1954) in Sudan. In a particular year the intake of food, expressed as energy, was 800 kCal/head/day in July, but 3200 kCal/head/day in November. The intake of iron by Masai children ranged from 0.1 to 9.0 mg a day according to the month of the year (Nestel and Geissler 1986), but extra iron obtained and retained by the body during times of comparative plenty might be sufficient to prevent iron deficiency in times of famine.

Even in normal times occasional use may be made of unusual foods that would probably not be recorded in household dietary surveys. A great number of wild fauna may be eaten by those living in remote areas. Dwyer (1985) recorded the use in Papua New Guinea of lizards, spiders, frogs, beetle larvae, and others. Some of these "casual" foods may be rich in iron, for example, termites, which contain 52 mg Fe/100 g and snails, which contain 41 mg Fe/100 g (Hercberg et al. 1987).

Clearly, changes in the availability of foods and haphazard use of some foods would cause important variations in the dietary intake of individuals and groups living in more remote areas. Even in relatively prosperous and urban communities variations in the intake of nutrients can be considerable. Yudkin (1951) noted, for example, that over a period of 4 weeks the consumption of vitamin A could be as much as five times the amount in one week as in another week.

A considerable variation in the use of foods from time to time was found by Chapell (1955). This author carefully measured her own intake each day for a year. She calculated that the mean intake measured on different occasions separated by a week or two gave a closer estimate of the mean daily intake over a year than did measurements made on a few successive days, which is a common practice. Salvosa et al. (1979), found that when food was freely available to young children in an orphanage a stable mean food consumption by each individual could be obtained only by weighing all foods at the time of consumption on a randomly selected day once a week for at least 20 weeks. In this study very little correlation was found between the intake of food or different nutrients on different days.

Broad associations between a component of the diet and some pathological state may be revealed, or at least strongly suggested, when comparisons are made between average consumption and the known prevalence of a disease. In such cases even appreciable errors in the assessment of dietary intake may not be important (Block 1982). But in the case of anemia not even a broad association between the intake of iron and the prevalence of the condition has been established. Probably only by the study of individuals, who act as their own controls of nondietary influences on the hemoglobin level, and by measuring with precision the intake of iron over a long period is the extent to which the diet influences the hemoglobin level likely to be revealed. To the present, ideas about how much iron is consumed by various groups of people have been based on conventional dietary surveys. The majority of these employ a procedure in which individuals have to remember the kinds and quantities of foods that have been eaten during the previous 24 hours. Frequently the informant is a mother who has to recall not only her own intake, but also that of other members of her family. Despite the employment of expert interviewers and the use of aids such as household measures of known capacity, this source, according to the above discussion, is unlikely to provide information precise enough to reveal whether a relationship between dietary iron content and the hemoglobin concentration of the consumer actually exists.

Characteristics of the Consumer

In recent years the attention of researchers investigating the relationship between diet and iron-deficiency anemia has been confined largely to the availability of iron in foods. There is, however, marked and unexplained variation, revealed clearly in studies with radioactive iron, in the extent to which different individuals and the same individual from time to time, absorb iron from the same source. Results published by Baynes et al. (1987) showed that the range of an individual's absorption of radioactive iron in broccoli puree was from 4.4 to 30.3%, in cabbage puree from 8.7 to 62.5%, and in ferrous sulfate from 11.1 to 74.4%. So great is this variation that procedures have been adopted to reduce its effects on the results of dietary studies as far as possible. One way is to use large groups and to express results as averages. When individual values are not distributed along a Gaussian curve, but are markedly skewed, use has been made of the geometric mean instead of the arithmetic mean. A usual practice is to administer by mouth a standard dose of radioactive ferrous sulfate together with the food under test, which has been labeled with a different form of radioactive iron. Absorption of radioactivity from the food, and its subsequent appearance in circulating hemoglobin, is expressed as a proportion of that from the ferrous salt and this ratio is used to classify foods in terms of biological availability of iron. Such maneuvers are believed to compensate for interindividual variation in utilization of foods. In some tests radioactive iron has been incorporated biologically into foods. This seems to be satisfactory in the case of materials of animal origin. Incorporation of radioactive iron into plants, because they lack a rapid circulatory system, may not always be so satisfactory, and there is doubt as to whether the radioactive iron is in precisely the same compartments and in the same proportions as iron naturally present. Radioactive iron that is mixed with foods near to the time of consumption has been found to be absorbed to an extent comparable with radioactive iron incorporated biologically into foods. Most recent tests have used this procedure. However, it probably does not take account of differences between individuals in their ability to digest foods of various kinds and to release iron from them. Iron is present in foods of plant origin in the form of soluble substances, in the sap of xylem, phloem, and vacuoles, either as free ions or complexes of small molecular size, or as a component of structural and storage materials (Hazell 1985). When foods are analyzed for their content of iron they are first completely digested *in vitro*, which destroys the identity of the compounds originally present. Whether *in vivo* digestion of foods proceeds to a comparable extent in all individuals and in all circumstances is open to question. There is evidence that digestive ability can vary appreciably according to the type of food and the physical, and mental, state of the consumer (Beaumont 1833; Hirata et al. 1965). That variation in the secretion of gastric juice occurs among individuals is well established, but it has been gauged only in terms of the content of hydrochloric acid. The observations of Jacobs and Miles (1969) raises the question whether there is also variation in the secretion of the mucopolysaccharide needed to carry iron in a soluble form into the small intestine. The possibility of abnormality in gastric secretion as a cause of iron deficiency was at one time debated, but seems to have remained unconfirmed. Achlorhydria is a common feature of iron-deficiency anemia, although in many instances normal secretion is resumed after the anemia has been cured. There remain some cases, however, in which histamine-fast achlorhydria persists. The occurrence of an antibody to gastric mucosal cells in the blood of some people with achlorhydria and anemia (Wright 1974) raises the possibility of an autoimmune reaction, perhaps akin to that in pernicious anemia, which affects gastric function and the ability to obtain iron from foods of plant origin. In this case anemia would be revealed only when diets were grossly deficient in heme iron. However, the gastric mucosal antibody is not specific to iron-deficiency anemia and is present also in other chronic diseases. Tests for antibodies and gastric function of individuals have never been made in surveys of hemoglobin levels.

An important affliction of many people, especially adults, with iron-deficiency anemia is chronic hemorrhage, as in menorrhagia, peptic ulcer, gastric cancer, hemorrhoids, and other conditions. A particular form of loss of blood is the leakage of red cells from the circulatory system of a fetus into the mother's blood. Up to 50% of pregnancies exhibit this phenomenon, but only about 1% of fetuses so affected develop anemia from this cause (Bedrick and Williams 1983).

Blood loss from hookworm infestation varies according to the number and type of worm present. *Ankylostoma duodenale* may cause a loss of up to 0.26 ml/worm/day (Roche and Layrisse 1966). Schistsomiasis affecting the bladder is an important cause of chronic loss of blood and anemia. This form of parasitism was highly prevalent in Ancient Egypt and is still so in that region.

The most common form of excessive loss of blood is probably menorrhagia in women. Many anemic women are thought by medical practitioners to be suffering from menorrhagia on subjective evidence provided by the patient, but in the absence of the actual measurement of the amount of blood being lost the diagnosis may not always be accurate. In many communities in which anemia is relatively common menstrual characteristics have not been investigated in relation to hemoglobin levels. Suppression of menstruation for contraceptive purposes by the use of hormones does not affect average hemoglobin concentrations and, therefore, does not seem to reduce the prevalence of anemia (Burton 1967; Thein et al. 1969). Women, in any case, have a natural safeguard against becoming anemic in the form of a relatively great ability to absorb iron from the diet. Thus, Widdowson and McCance (1942) found that on an intake of iron of 15.3 mg/day a man absorbed 8.6% of the iron, and that a woman on about the same intake absorbed 13.8%. Man and Wadsworth (1969) found that one man on a standard diet excreted 52 μg of urinary iron in 24 hours on an intake of 11 mg, and one woman on about the same intake excreted 101 μg in 24 hours. These results are compatible with the proposal that women usually absorb about twice as much iron as do men on the same diet. This ability of women is increased up to 5-fold during pregnancy (King et al. 1987).

If anemia results from a loss of blood one must suppose that (1) enhanced absorption of iron fails to keep pace with the rate of loss through bleeding, or (2) that iron stores were depleted before the commencement of the bleeding, or (3) that the individual affected fails to "rise to the occasion" because of an inability to respond normally to a need for extra iron. An indication of such disability was given by Callender (1964), who observed that 10 of 27 patients with iron deficiency absorbed less heme iron than the mean absorption by normal subjects, although none of these patients had any other evidence of intestinal malabsorption.

Storage iron depletion has to be considerable before anemia develops. Thus, only a minority of those infested with hookworm become anemic and only when heavy parasite loads are indicated by the presence of 2000 eggs/g feces in women and children and 5000 eggs/g feces in men is there any relationship between ankylostomiasis and reduction in the hemoglobin level (Layrisse and Roche 1964). Hallberg et al. (1966) concluded on theoretical grounds that only when menstrual losses were of the order of 80 ml of blood at each menstruation would women be unable to maintain a normal iron balance. Conrad and Crosby (1962) showed that when blood was removed from healthy volunteers several times a week anemia did not develop until 1.5 g of iron had been removed. Clearly, the body normally has considerable ability to withstand a loss of iron and, therefore, reduced intakes or iron because of the nature of the diet would not normally be expected to be an acute cause of iron-deficiency anemia. A critical factor in the causation of such anemia, especially by the more acute forms of hemorrhage, is the amount of reserve iron in the stores. These stores are present from the earliest stages of life and accumulate to a maximum level by adulthood. Thereafter losses and gains of iron normally remain in equilibrium. Iron can be demonstrated in the fetus very early in its life and becomes measurable in amount by the fourth month (Table 12).

There is controversy about the influence of the iron status of the mother on the concentration of iron in the fetus, but probably only when maternal anemia is severe is the conceptus adversely affected. Krawinkel et al. (1990) found that the ferritin levels of cord blood of infants born to anemic mothers were well above 30 ng/ml. Usually, therefore, the newborn child begins life with an amount of iron adequate for its needs, and any deficiency of iron would be due to postnatal factors. At birth the

Table 12. Amounts of Iron in the Human Fetus[a]

Fetal age (weeks)	16	24	32	40
Weight (kg)	0.1	0.75	2.0	3.4
Total iron (mg)	5.0	45.9	141.0	278.0
Concentration of iron (mg/kg body weight)	50.0	61.2	70.5	81.8

[a] In the adult of average weight of 70 kg there is about 3500 mg of iron, giving a concentration of 50 mg/kg body weight.
Source: Widdowson (1980).

amount of storage iron is relatively great and there is a concentration of nonheme iron in the liver in the region of 300 µg/g, compared with about 200 µg/g in adult males (Chang 1973). During early infancy these stores are added to by a breakdown of surplus erythrocytes in the circulation, and at the same time, iron is being absorbed from milk. As indicated by serum ferritin levels, storage iron gradually decreases so that these levels fall from about 200 µg/100 ml during the first month to about 30 µg/100 ml at the age of 6 months, where they remain throughout life. However, because the liver is growing in size during childhood the total amount of iron being gained, despite the reduction in concentration in the liver, is increasing all the time, aided by the increase in the volume of red cells in the circulation.

During the entire history of man infants have been fed on human milk. This has been the main source of iron for the child during the first year of life. However, infants are commonly given supplementary foods from an early age, especially in western societies. In the United Kingdom Fox et al. (1984) found that up to 4.5% of infants were being given solid foods, mainly cereals, in the second week of life, and by 8 weeks up to about 35% were getting these foods. With the introduction of solid foods to the diet of children at an ever earlier age in recent times there has been an increase in the incidence of celiac disease due to adverse reactions to wheat gluten (Department of Health and Social Security 1974). Celiac disease is frequently associated with reduced levels of serum iron and serum ferritin (Bonamico et al. 1987). Under poor socioeconomic conditions supplementary foods can be a source of infection, which may affect the utilization of iron.

There is some difficulty today, especially in places where investigatory facilities are more available, in observing infants who get no other food than human milk. When this has been possible, evidence has been found that the breast-fed infant obtains enough iron during the first 6 months of life, or even longer. Thus, Siimes et al. (1984) found no difference between the iron status of solely breast-fed children and formula-fed children at the age of 6 months, although by the age of 9 months the breast-fed infants had lower concentrations of serum ferritin and lower iron saturation in serum transferrin. Similar results were obtained by Duncan et al. (1985). In their inquiry Siimes et al. (1984) found that between the ages of 7 and 8 months the hemoglobin level and the serum transferrin level were not affected by supplements of iron given to the mother. In another inquiry Iwai et al. (1986) found that infants of small birth weight, between 1.0 and 2.5 kg, who were fed only from the breast had hematological values at the age of 6 months comparable to those found by Siimes et al. (1984), but infants who had been fed on a formula that contained 8 mg Fe/liter had higher values.

The amount of iron in milk is of considerable interest because this milk is a "natural" diet and its study should provide invaluable information about the normal hematological state of the consumer. Millions of subjects are available on whom to study this natural relationship. Unfortunately, there is almost insuperable difficulty in measuring both the amount of milk ingested and its composition. In those communities most subject to anemia breast feeding is usually haphazard. Hamilton (1956) described the pattern in Papua New Guinea not so much as "demand feeding" but as "opportunity feeding," the child taking the breast whenever a suitable chance occurred, including times when the mother was at work and during the night. In such circumstances the measurement of the amount of milk imbibed does not seem possible. The composition of milk varies according to the period of lactation, and may vary from time to time during the day and even in the course of a single feeding. Thus, there is considerable difficulty in obtaining representative samples for analysis. For these reasons there are discrepancies among results reported by different investigators, and estimates of absorption of iron from human milk cannot be made with confidence. However, on the assumption that human milk is the natural food for the infant at an early stage of life and is of the right composition to meet physiological requirements, hematological studies on infants, such as those made by Iwai et al. (1986), indicate that many infants are getting too much iron because of being fed on artificial mixtures. In those studies infants who had been fed solely from the breast had an average serum ferritin level of 18 ng/ml at the age of 6 months and those who had been fed on a formula mix that contained 8 mg Fe/liter had an average level of 39.6 ng/ml. This indicates that the administration of extra iron early in life increases the amount of storage iron above what would have been acquired from human milk. Whether, in the long term, this increase is permanent and beneficial has not been investigated. Knowledge about variations in the amount of reserve iron in the body is far from complete, and the importance of changes during childhood in relation to the etiology of iron-deficiency anemia later on is not known. Present interest in the significance of "free radicals" and the influence of iron in their production (Halliwell, 1989), as a cause of disease, gives a new emphasis to the importance of determining the amounts of iron within the tissues, and the history of their accumulation. Sullivan (1989), for example, has assembled evidence that a critical factor in the development and out-

come of myocardial infarction is related directly to the amounts of iron
in cells.

Comments and Conclusions

Present ideas about the prevalence and causes of iron-deficiency
anemia are almost entirely based on somewhat arbitrary "normal"
hemoglobin levels, epidemiological studies of hemoglobin concentrations, and dietary patterns revealed by the 24-hour recall method of
determining the kinds and amounts of food consumed.

Concentrations of hemoglobin below which anemia is probably present
(WHO 1972) are well above those that lead to abnormal clinical signs and
symptoms and to disturbance of normal physiological functions (Brannon
et al. 1954; Lillie et al. 1954; Sharpey-Schafer 1944). Relatively low levels
that are interpreted as the presence of anemia may sometimes have normal physiological importance even in pathological conditions. Such low
levels are due to expansion of the volume of plasma in the circulation, and
not to a deficient production of hemoglobinised erythrocytes.

The interpretation of the results of hematological surveys is not
straightforward because of the influence on hemoglobin levels of numerous factors that may vary independently or in association with each
other. For example, the prevalence of malaria, which is commonly associated with relatively low hemoglobin concentrations, is determined by
aggregation of people, which first began in the past with the development of agriculture (Fiennes 1978), and altitude, terrain, and climate,
which determine the presence of the mosquito vector. The enzymology
(Targett 1983) and shape of erythrocytes and the chemical form of
hemoglobin in the human host, which are all genetically determined, and
which may lead independently to anemia, favor susceptibility or resistance to malarial infection. The prevalence of other infections and infestations that may affect the metabolism of iron, and hence lead to anemia,
is likewise determined by a number of factors, including household conditions and management, family size, the availability of water, climate,
terrain, and genetic traits. Some of these factors, for example, climate and
household management, also influence the availability and use of foods,
and hence the levels of intake of iron. The presence of chronic infection
may be unsuspected. In the case of malaria the absence of parasitemia
does not preclude the presence of malaria and the effects of this infection
on the blood can persist for many years after institution of antimalarial
projects (Crane and Kelly 1972). Scant attention has been given to this

complex situation by investigators into the possible effects of diet on the hemoglobin levels of different communities.

The significance of diet in the causation of iron-deficiency anemia is not certain because most of the available information about dietary intake of those who develop this deficiency is not sufficiently precise. An increase in the hemoglobin concentration after the administration of extra iron by mouth, although indicative of iron deficiency, is commonly accepted as proof that the diet was the cause, but is also effective in anemia associated with hemorrhage, cancer, and other conditions.

Whether iron-deficiency anemia develops at any particular time usually depends on the amount of storage iron that is present in the body at that time. This reserve iron is accumulated throughout the period of growth, commencing before birth. But there is as yet insufficient information of the natural history of the accumulation of iron in different types of individuals and, according to circumstances, to explain why some individuals develop anemia and others, seemingly exposed to the same hazards, do not.

If, as alleged, iron-deficiency anemia is a major health problem throughout the world at the present time, the prevalence of porotic hyperostosis might be expected to be high. But this condition is reported very rarely in modern literature, possibly because the presence of the abnormality, particularly in its minor forms, remains undetected. Radiography of the skull is seldom performed in clinical practice when anemia is present and is certainly not a routine procedure in field surveys. As well, all reports of cases of porotic hyperostosis indicate that it is likely to be present only in severe anemia, which is not nearly so common as minor deficiencies in hemoglobin levels. Finally, much of the anemia reported is in adults, who would not react by change in the structure of the skull. Much valuable information could be obtained by surveys in which skulls were routinely X-rayed at the time that hemoglobin levels were being determined; perhaps publication of this book will stimulate interest in the implementation of this procedure.

Witts (1964) said that, "It is a puzzle to me that 20–25% of women in the reproductive epoch in Great Britain should be anaemic despite the rise in the standard of living. It seems as if Nature has managed badly." He went on to suggest that an interval of 10,000 years was an inadequate time for man to adjust to a change of diet from one consisting of the products of hunting and gathering to one consisting largely of cereals which are cultivated. In view of the considerable ability of the living body to withstand large losses of blood, to adjust levels of absorption of iron from the diet, and to conserve iron in the body, Witts' suggestion does not seem tenable. An alternative explanation is that particular hematological characteristics designated as abnormal are not really so. Perhaps, as taught by Ryle (1947), we should judge normality according to features observed in people who are living their normal lives. If a large number of a population have relatively low hemoglobin levels, why is this not normal? An increase in these low levels sometimes observed after ingestion of large amounts of iron may be an adjustment to a new circumstance and not a sign of deficiency. A decision one way or the other will only be possible by ascertaining whether hemoglobin levels remain permanently raised and, more especially, whether they are ultimately associated with an increased level of health, as judged in terms of survival, efficiency, and subjective well-being (Wadsworth 1984).

References

Abernathy, J.R., G.B. Greenberg, H.B. Wells, and T.M. Frazier. 1966. Smoking as an independent variable in a multiple regression analysis upon birth weight and gestation. *American Journal of Public Health* 56:626.

Amorozo, M.C. De M., and R. Shrimpton. 1984. The effect of income and length of urban residence on food patterns, food intake and nutrient adequacy in an Amazonian peri-urban slum population. *Ecology of Food and Nutrition* 14:307.

Baldwin, G.S., R. Chandler, and J. Weinstock. 1986. Binding of Gastrin to Gastric Transferrin. *FEBS Letters* 205:147.

Barcroft, J., J.C. Meakins, H.W. Davies, J.M.D. Scott, and W.J. Fetter. 1923. On the relation of external temperature to blood volume. *Philosophical Transactions of the Royal Society Series B* 211:455.

Baynes, R.D., T.H. Bothwell, W.R. Bezwoda, A.P. MacPhail, and D.P. Derman. 1987. Relationship between absorption of inorganic and food iron in field studies. *Annals of Nutrition and Metabolism* 31:109.

Beal, V.A., A.J. Meyers, and R.W. McCammon. 1962. Iron intake, hemoglobin and physical growth during the first two years of life. *Pediatrics* 30:518.

Beaumont, W. 1833. Experiments and observations on the gastric juice and the physiology of digestion. Pittsburgh.

Bedrick, A.D., and M.L. Williams. 1983. Use of serum ferritin in evaluation of iron deficiency anemia in chronic fetal-maternal hemorrhage. *Clinical Pediatrics* Jan.:57.

Bella, A., Jr., and K.S. Kim. 1973. Iron binding of gastric mucins. *Biochimica Biophysica Act* 304:580.

Bezkorovainy, A. 1989a. Biochemistry of nonheme iron. I. Iron proteins and cellular iron metabolism. *Clinical Physiology and Biochemistry* 7:1.

Bezkorovainy, A. 1989b. Biochemistry of nonheme iron. II. Absorption of iron. *Clinical Physiology and Biochemistry* 7:53.

Block, G. 1982. A review of validations of dietary assessment methods. *American Journal of Epidemiology* 115, 492.

Bloem, M.W., M. Wedel, E.J. Van Altmaal, A.J. Speek, S. Saowakontha, and W.H.P. Schreurs. 1990. Vitamin A intervention: Short term effects of a single oral, massive dose on iron metabolism. *American Journal of Clinical Nutrition* 51:76.

Bonamico, M., A. Vania, S. Monti, G. Ballati, P. Mariani, G. Pitzalis, C. Benedetti, P. Falconieri, and A. Signoretti. 1987. Iron deficiency in children with celiac disease. *Journal of Pediatric Gastroenterology and Nutrition* 6:702.

Brannon, E.S., A.J. Merril, J.V. Warren, and E.A. Stead. 1954. The cardiac output in patients with chronic anemia as measured by the technique of right atrial catheterization. *Journal of Clinical Investigation* 24:332.

Brown, R.D., J. Benfatto, J. Gibson, and H. Kronenberg. 1988. Red cell ferritin and iron stores in patients with chronic disease. *European Journal of Haematology* 1989. 40:136.

Brun, J.F., M. Sekkat, C. Lagoueyte, C. Fedou, and A. Orsetti. 1989. Relationship between fitness and blood viscosity in untrained normal short children. *Clinical Hemorheology* 9:953.

Burman, D. 1972. Hemoglobin levels in normal infants aged 3 to 24 months and the effect of iron. *Archives of Disease in Childhood* 47:261.

Burton, J.L. 1967. Effect of oral contraceptives on hemoglobin, packed cell volume, serum iron and total iron-binding capacity in healthy women. *Lancet* i:978.

Caldwell, M.J. 1972. Ascorbic acid content of Malaysian leaf vegetables. *Ecology of Food and Nutrition* 1:313.

Callender, S.T. 1964. Digestive absorption of iron. In *Iron Metabolism*. F. Gross, S.R. Naegeli, and H.D. Philps, eds., p. 89. Berlin: Springer-Verlag.

Callender, S.T. 1981. Iron deficiency anaemia. In *Nutritional Problems in Modern Society*. A. Howard, ed., p. 1. London: John Libby.

Cartei, G., A. Meani, and D. Causarano. 1970. Rise of serum transferrin, serum iron and ceruloplasmin in men due to hexestrol and chlorotriannisene. *Nutrition Report International* 2:343.

Chang, L.L. 1973. Tissue storage iron in Singapore. *American Journal of Clinical Nutrition* 26:952.

Chapell, G.M. 1955. Long-term individual dietary surveys. *British Journal of Nutrition* 9:323.

Chesley, L.C. 1972. Plasma and red cell volumes during pregnancy. *American Journal of Obstetrics and Gynecology* 112:440.

Conrad, M., and W.H. Crosby. 1962. The natural history of iron deficiency induced by phlebotomy. *Blood* 20:173.

Crane, G.G., and A. Kelly. 1972. The effect of malaria control on haematological parameters in the Kaiapit Subdistrict, *Papua New Guinea Medical Journal* 15:38.

Department of Health and Social Security. 1974. *Present Day Practice in Infant Feeding*. London: Her Majesty's Stationary Office.

Diem, K. 1962. *Documenta Geigy, Scientific Tables*, 6th ed. Manchester: Geigy Pharmaceutical Company Limited.

Dintenfass, K. 1971. *Blood Microrheology—Viscosity Factors in Blood Flow, Ischaemia and Thrombosis*. London: Butterworths.

Dormandy, J.A. 1970. Clinical significance of blood viscosity. *Annals of the Royal College of Surgeons of England* 47:211.

Duncan, B., R.B. Schifman, J.J. Corrigan, Jr., and C. Schaefer. 1985. Iron and the exclusively breast fed infant from birth to six months. *Journal of Pediatric Gastroenterology and Nutrition* 4:421.

Dwyer, P.D. 1985. The contribution of non-domesticated animals to the diet of Etolo, Southern Highlands province, Papua New Guinea. *Ecology of Food and Nutrition* 17:101.

Ernst, E., A. Matrai, E. Aschbrenner, V. Will, and C. Schmidlechner. 1985. Relationship between fitness and blood fluidity. *Clinical Hemorheology* 5:507.

Ernst, E., L. Pietsch, A. Matrai, and J. Eisenberg. 1986. Blood rheology in vegetarians. *British Journal of Nutrition* 56:555.

Fiennes, R.N. 1978. *Zoonoses and the Origins and Ecology of Human Diseases*. New York: Academic Press.

Fox, P.T., M.D. Elston, S. Kerry, and E. Wheeler. 1984. How young English children were being fed in 1974: A report from the preschool child growth survey. *Ecology of Food and Nutrition* 14:129.

Frassinelli-Gunderson, E.P., S. Margen, and J.R. Brown. 1985. Iron stores in users of oral contraceptive agents. *American Journal of Clinical Nutrition* 41:703.

Garn, S.M., M.T. Keating, and F. Falkner. 1981. Hematological status and pregnancy outcomes. *American Journal of Clinical Nutrition* 34:115–117.

Gillooly, M., T.H. Bothwell, J.D. Torrance, A.P. McPhail, D.P. Derman, W.R. Bezwoda, W. Mills, R.W. Charlton, and F. Mayet. 1983. The effects of organic acids, phytates and polyphenols on the absorption of iron from vegetables. *British Journal of Nutrition* 49:331.

Gillooly, M., T.H Bothwell, R.W. Charlton, J.D. Torrance, W.R. Bezwoda, A.P. McPhail, D.P. Derman, L. Novegli, P. Morrall, and F. Mayet. 1984. Factors affecting the absorption of iron from cereals. *British Journal of Nutrition* 51:37.

Hallberg, L., A.N. Hogdahl, L. Nilsson, and G. Rybo. 1966. Menstrual blood loss—a population study. *Acta Obstetricia et Gynecolagica Scandinavica* 45:25.

Hallberg, L., M. Brune, and L. Rossander. 1986. Effects of ascorbic acid on iron absorption from different types of meals. *Human Nutrition Applied Nutrition* 40:97.

Halliwell, B. 1989. Tell me about free radicals, doctor: A review. *Journal of the Royal Society of Medicine* 32:747.

Hamilton, L. 1956. Nutrition survey, Sepik District, Department of Public Health, Port Moresby, Papua New Guinea, mimeo.

Hassan, N., and K. Ahmad. 1984. Studies on food and nutrient intake by rural population of Bangladesh: Comparison between intakes of 1962–64, 1975–76 and 1981–82. *Ecology of Food and Nutrition* 15:143.

Harrison, P.M. 1964. Ferritin and haemosiderin. In Iron *Metabolism*. F. Gross, S.R. Naegeli, and H.D. Philps, eds., p. 40. Berlin: Springer-Verlag.

Hazell, T. 1985. Minerals in foods: dietary sources, chemical forms, interactions, bioavailability. *World Review of Nutrition and Dietetics* 46:1.

Hegarty, P.V.J., and G.R. Wadsworth. 1968. The amount of iron in processed cassava (manihot utilissima). *Journal of Tropical Medicine and Hygiene* 71:51.

Heilmann, L. 1987. Blood rheology and pregnancy. *Balliere's Clinical Haematology* 1:777.

Hercberg, S., P. Galan, and N. Dupin. 1987. Iron deficiency in Africa. *World Review of Nutrition and Dietetics* 54:201.

Hirata, Y., T. Matsuo, and H. Kokubu. 1965. Digestion and absorption of milk protein in infant's intestine. *Kobe Journal of Medical Science* 11:103.

Horne, C.H.W., P.W. Howie, R.J. Weir, and R.B. Goodie. 1970. Effects of combined oestrogen-progestin and contraceptives on serum levels of alpha 2 macroglobulin, transferrin, albumin and Ig. *Lancet* i:49.

Iwai, Y., T. Takanashi, Y. Nakao, and H. Mikawa. 1966. Iron status in low birth weight infants on breast and formula feeding. *European Journal of Paediatrics* 145:63.

Jacobi, J.M., L.W. Powell, and T.J. Gaffney. 1969. Immunochemical quantitation of human transferrin in pregnancy and during the administration of oral contraceptives. *British Journal of Haematology* 17:503.

Jacobs, A., and E.B. Butler. 1965. Menstrual blood loss in iron deficiency anaemia. *Lancet* 2:407.

Jacobs, A., and D.A. Greenman. 1969. Availability of food iron. *British Medical Journal* i:673.

Jacobs, A., and P.M. Miles. 1969. Intestinal transport of iron from stomach to small-intestinal mucosa. *British Medical Journal* 4:778.

Jacobs, A., and M. Worwood. 1975. Ferritin in serum: Clinical and biochemical implications. *New England Journal of Medicine* 292:951.

Kwa, S.B., and M. Ko. 1968. Haemoglobin values in pregnancy—a survey of 1,000 consecutive normal mothers. *Singapore Medical Journal* 9:27.

King, J.C., M.N. Bronnstein, W.L. Fitch, and J. Weininger. 1987. Nutrient utilization during pregnancy. *World Review of Nutrition Dietetics* 52:71.

Klausner, R.D. 1988. From receptors to genes—insights from molecular iron metabolism. *Clinical Research* 36:494.

Koller, O. 1982. The clinical significance of hemodilution during pregnancy, *Obstetrical Gynecological Survey* 37:649.

Korte, R. 1972. Heat resistance of phytohemagglutinins in weaning food mixtures containing beans (*Phaseolus vulgaris*). *Ecology of Food and Nutrition* 1:303.

Krawinkel, M.B., M. Bethge, A.O. El Karib, H.M. Ahmet, and O.A. Mirghani. 1990. Maternal ferritin values and fetal iron status. *Acta Prediatrica Scandinavica* 79:467.

Laurell, C.B., S. Kullander, and J. Thorell. 1969. Plasma protein changes induced by sequential type of contraceptive steroid pills. *Clinical Chimica Act* 25:294.

Layrisse, M., and M. Roche. 1964. The relationship between anemia and hookworm infection; results of surveys of rural Venezuelan populations. *American Journal of Hygiene* 79:279.

Layrisse, M., C. Martinez-Torres, I. Leets, P. Taylor, and J. Ramirez. 1984. Effects of histidine, systeine, glutathione or beef on iron absorption in humans. *Journal of Nutrition* 114:217.

Lee, T.S., and G.R. Wadsworth. 1961. Assessment of anemia in clinical practice. *Clinical Science* 20:205.

Lieberman, E., K.J. Ryan, R.R. Monson, and S.C. Schoenbaum. 1988. Association of maternal hematocrit with premature labor. *American Journal of Obstetrics Gynecology* 159:107.

Lillie, E.W., P.B.B. Gatenby, and H.C. Moore. 1954. A survey of anemia in 4,314 cases of pregnancy. *Irish Journal of Medical Science* July:304.

Linderkamp, O. 1987. Blood rheology in the newborn infant. Balliere's *Clinical Haematology* 1:801.

Linpisarn, S., O. Thanangkul, C. Suwanraj, R. Kaewvichit, L.J. Kricka, and T.P. Whitehead. 1984. Iron deficiency in a Northern Thai population: The effects of iron supplements studied by means of plasma ferritin estimations. *Annals of Clinical Biochemistry* 21:268.

Malaise, F., and G. Parent. 1985. Edible wild vegetable products in the Zambian woodland area: A nutritional and ecological approach. *Ecology of Food and Nutrition* 18:43.

Man, Y.K., and G.R. Wadsworth. 1969. Urinary loss of iron and the influence on it of dietary levels of iron. *Clinical Science* 36:479.

Maralhas, N. 1964. Cinca estudos sobre a fairna de mandioca. *Publicacao de INPA, Serie Quimica* 6:1.

Martinez, C.T., I. Leets, P. Taylor, J. Ramirez, M. del V. Camacho, and M. Layrisse. 1986. Heme, ferritin, and vegetable iron absorption in humans from meals denatured of heme iron during the cooking of beef. *Journal of Nutrition* 116:1720.

Mahomed, K., and F. Hytten. 1989. Iron and folate supplementation in pregnancy. In *Effective Care in Pregnancy and Childbirth*. I. Chalmers, M. Ehkin, and M.J.N.C. Keirse, eds. p. 301. New York: Oxford University Press.

McCance, R.A., and E.M. Widdowson. 1937. Absorption and excretion of iron. *Lancet* 1:680.

Mejia, L.A. 1985. Vitamin A deficiency as a factor in nutritional anemia. *International Journal for Vitamin and Nutrition Research Symposium* 27:75.

Micozzi, M.S., D. Albanes, and R.G. Stevens. 1989. A Relation of body size and composition to clinical biochemical and hematolgic indeces in U.S. men and women. *American Journal of Clinical Nutrition* 50:1276.

Milman, N., and J. Cohn. 1984. Serum iron, serum transferrin, and transferrin saturation in healthy children without iron deficiency. *European Journal of Pediatrics* 143:96.

Milne, D.B., S.K. Gallagher, and F.H. Nielsen. 1990. Response of various indeces of iron status to acute iron depletion produced in menstruating women by low iron intake and phlebotomy. *Clinical Chemistry* 36:487.

Mitchell, F., and S. Baburich. 1987. The nature and extent of childhood lead poisoning in the United States. In *Trace Elements in Human Health and Disease*, p. 189. Copenhagen: WHO Regional Office for Europe.

Moore, C.V. 1964. Iron nutrition. In *Iron Metabolism*. G. Gross, S.R. Naegeli, and H.D. Philps, eds., p. 241. Berlin: Springer-Verlag.

Narula, K.K. 1968. Iron in foods, with special reference to their nutritional value, Ph.D. thesis, University of London.

Nestel, P. and C. Geissler, 1986. Potential deficiencies of a pastoral diet. *Ecology of Food and Nutrition* 19:1.

Norton, H.H., E.S. Hunn, C.S. Martinsen, and P.B. Keely. 1984. Vegetable food products of the foraging economies of the Pacific Northwest. *Ecology of Food and Nutrition* 14:219.

Ogle, B.M., and L.E. Grivetti. 1985. Legacy of the Cameleon: Edible wild plants of the Kingdom of Swaziland, Southern Africa. A cultural, ecological, nutritional study. Part II, Demographies, species availability and dietary use, analysis by ecological zone. Part IV, Nutritional analysis and conclusions. *Ecology of Food and Nutrition* 17:1 and 41.

Ong, S.P., J. Ryley, T. Bashir, and H.N. MacDonald. 1983. Nutrient intake and associated biochemical status of pregnant Asians in the United Kingdom. *Human Nutrition and Applied Nutrition* 37A:23.

Pales, L. 1954. L'alimentation en Afrique Française. *Organisme de Recherches sur l'Alimentation et la Nutrition Africaines*, Paris.

Palti, H., B. Pevsner, and B. Alder. 1983. Does anaemia in infancy effect achievement in developmental and intelligence tests? *Human Biology* 55:183.

Partington, J.R. 1962. *A History of Chemistry*, Vol. 3. New York: Macmillan.

Penrod, J.C., K. Anderson, and P.B. Acosta. 1990. Impact of iron status of introducing cow's milk in the second six months of life. *Journal of Pediatric Gastroenterology and Nutrition* 10:462.

Pollycove, M. 1964. Iron kinetics. In *Iron Metabolism*. G. Gross, S.R. Naegeli, and H.D. Philps, eds., p. 148. Berlin: Springer-Verlag.

Pritchard, J.A. 1966. Absence of menorrhagia in induced iron deficiency anaemia. *Obstetrics and Gynecology* 27:541.

Raja, K.B., R.J. Simpson, M.J. Pippard, and T.J. Peters. 1988. In vivo studies on the relationship between intestinal iron (Fe^{34}) absorption, hypoxia and erythropoiesis in the mouse. *British Journal of Haematology* 68:373.

Raphael, D. 1984. Weaning is always: The anthropology of breastfeeding behaviour. *Ecology of Food and Nutrition* 15:203.

Rothman, K.J. 1976. Causes. *American Journal of Epidemiology* 104:587.

Read, E.B. 1946. Famine foods listed in the Chiu Huang Pen Ts'Ao. *Henry Lester Institute of Medical Research*, Shanghai.

Rees, J.M., E.R. Monsen, and J.E. Merrill. 1985. Iron fortification of infant foods. *Clinical Pediatrics* 24:707.

Reeves, J.D., R. Yip, V.A. Kiley, and P.R. Dallman. 1984. Iron deficiency in infants: The influence of mild antecedent infection. *Journal of Pediatrics* 105:874.

Robscheit-Robbins, F.S., and G.H. Whipple. 1925. Blood regeneration in severe anaemia. II. Favourable influence of liver, heart and skeletal muscle. *American Journal of Physiology* 72:408.

Roche, M., and M. Layrisse. 1966. The nature and causes of "hookworm anaemia." *American Journal of Tropical Medicine and Hygiene* 15:1031.

Ryle, J.A. 1947. The meaning of normal. *Lancet* i:1.

Sadowitz, P.D., and F.A. Oski. 1983. Iron status and infant feeding practices in an urban ambulatory center. *Pediatrics* 72:33.

Salvosa, P.D., G.R. Wadsworth, and S.B. Bibera. 1979. The individual dietary intake of some children living in a childrens' home in Quezon City, Philippines. *Ecology of Food and Nutrition* 8:219.

Sanford, R. 1960. The release of iron from conjugates in food. *Nature (London)* 185:533.

Sanford, R. 1961. The effect of enzymic digestion of foods on the liberation of iron. *Australasian Annals of Medicine* 10:288.

Schwartz, R. 1986. Stable mineral isotopes in nutritional and related research. *World Review of Nutrition and Dietetics* 48:1.

Schultz-Lell, G., R. Buss, H-D. Oldigs, K. Dörner, and J. Schaub. 1987. Iron balances in infant nutrition. *Acta Paediatrica Scandinavica* 76:585.

Sharpey-Schafer, E.P. 1944. Cardiac output in severe anaemia. *Clinical Science* 5:125.

Siimes, M.A., L. Salmenpera, and J. Perheetupa. 1984. Exclusive breast-feeding for 9 months: Risk of iron deficiency. *Journal of Pediatrics* 104:196.

Skoryna, S.C., S. Inove, and M. Fuskova, 1980. Classification of biological effects of trace elements. In *Nutrition and Food Science*, Vol. 3. W. Santos, N. Lopes, J.J. Barbosa, D. Chaves, and J.C. Valente, eds., p. 105. New York: Plenum Press.

Smith, M.D., and I.M. Pannacculli. 1958. Absorption of inorganic iron from graded doses: Its significance in relation to iron absorption tests from the mucosal block theory. *British Journal of Haematology* 4:428.

Sullivan, J.L. 1989. The iron paradigm of ischemic heart disease. *American Heart Journal* 117:1172.

Targett, G.A.T. 1983. What determines the pathogenicity of parasites? *Journal of the Royal Society of Medicine* 76:888.

Taylor, P.G., C. Martinez-Torres, E.L. Romano, and M. Layrisse. 1986. The effect of cysteine-containing peptides released during meat digestion on iron absorption in humans. *American Journal of Clinical Nutrition* 43:68.

Thein, M., G.H. Beaton, H. Milne, and M.J. Veen. 1969. Oral contraceptive drugs: Some observations on their effect on menstrual loss and haematological indices. *Canadian Medical Association Journal* 101:679.

Undritz, E. 1964. Oral treatment of iron deficiency. In *Iron Metabolism*. F. Gross, S.R. Naegeli, and H.D. Philps, eds., p. 406. Berlin: Springer-Verlag.

Wadsworth, G.R. 1952. The effects of a tropical climate on the blood. M.D. thesis, University of Liverpool.

Wadsworth, G.R. 1955. Recovery from acute haemorrhage in normal men and women. *Journal of Physiology* 129:583.

Wadsworth, G.R. 1969. Losses of iron from the body as the basis for the determination of dietary iron requirements. *Singapore Medical Journal* 16:259.

Wadsworth, G.R. 1984. *The Diet and Health of Isolated Populations.* Boca Raton, FL: CRC Press.

Wehmeyer, A.S., R.B. Lee, and M.G. Whiting. 1969. The nutrient composition and dietary ingestion of some vegetable foods eaten by the !Kung Bushmen. *South African Medical Journal* 43:1529.

Widdowson, E.M. 1980. Chemical composition and nutritional needs of the fetus at different stages of gestation. In *Maternal Nutrition during Pregnancy and Lactation.* H. Aebi and G.R. Whitehead, eds., p. 39. Bern: Hans Huber Publishers.

Widdowson, E.M. and R.A. McCance. 1942. Iron exchanges of adults on white and brown bread diets. Lancet 1:588.

Witts, L.J. 1964. Summing up. In *Iron Metabolism.* G. Gross, S.R. Naegeli, and H.D. Philps, eds., p. 612. Berlin: Springer-Verlag.

World Health Organization (WHO). 1972. Nutritional anaemias. *World Health Organization Technical Report Series* 503, Geneva.

World Health Organization (WHO). 1982. *Environmental Health Problems in Arctic and Subarctic Areas,* Working Group Report, Copenhagen, 3–7 August 1981. Copenhagen: WHO Regional Office for Europe.

Wright, R. 1974. Immunological aspects of gastrointestinal disease. *Proceedings of the Royal Society of Medicine* 67:574.

Wright, E., and R.E. Hughes. 1975. Dietary citric acid. *Nutrition (London)* 29:367.

Yip, R., T.N. Norris, and A.S. Anderson. 1981. Iron status of children with elevated blood lead concentrations. *Journal of Pediatrics* 98:922.

Yip, R., C. Johnson, and P.R. Dallman. 1984. Age-related changes in laboratory values used in the diagnosis of anaemia and iron deficiency. *American Journal of Clinical Nutrition* 39:427.

Yudkin, J. 1951. Dietary surveys: Variation in the weekly intakes of nutrients. *British Journal of Nutrition* 5:177.

Chapter 4

Iron Withholding in Prevention of Disease

Eugene D. Weinberg

"In everything the middle road is the best; all things in excess bring trouble to me."

Plautus

"It is better to rise from life as from a banquet—neither thirsty nor drunken."

Aristotle

Introduction

During the past 60 years, much attention has been directed toward understanding the functions of iron in biological systems and the problems associated with iron deficiency. More recently, studies have begun to focus on the health hazards that result from iron overload and the mechanisms whereby cells and tissues attempt to protect themselves from this danger. Additionally, a great amount of clinical and laboratory research has been concerned with the ability of humans and other vertebrate animals to withhold iron from microbial and neoplastic cell invaders. This chapter describes the iron-withholding system, ways and consequences of its impairment, and possible methods and agents for its strengthening.

Cells of humans and other animals, as well as plants and most microorganisms, require well-defined amounts of iron for survival, replication, and expression of differentiated processes (Table 1). In contrast, excess iron is toxic.[1] These are inherently conflicting physiological and pathological roles of iron that raise a vexing dilemma for biological tissues. On

Table 1. Examples of Cellular Processes That Specifically Require
or are Modulated by Iron

Process	Site of Action of Iron
DNA synthesis	Ribonucleotide reductase (β_2 dimer)
RNA synthesis	RNA polymerase III
Electron transfer	Cytochromes, hydrogenase, ferredoxin, succinate dehydrogenase
Oxygen metabolism	Catalase, oxygenases, peroxidase, superoxide dismutase
Nitrogen fixation	Nitrogenase
Photosynthesis	Chlorophyll synthesis
Tricarboxylic acid cycle	Aconitase
Prokaryotic secondary metabolism	Repressor proteins
Myoblast and fungal differentiation	Unknown
Defense response by vertebrates	Neutrophil function, T lymphocyte activation, natural killer and B lymphocyte function

Source: Weinberg (1989).

the one hand, especially during multiplication, cells either must have a fairly constant and dependable source of available iron or have devised a method of internal storage of pools of the metal in an innocuous form. On the other hand, cells must take care not to acquire too much iron, particularly since most of them lack mechanisms of metal efflux. Iron stores can, indeed, be "an embarrassment to the body" (Wadsworth 1975).

Various forms of life have evolved a diversity of systems to regulate their acquisition and storage of iron (Weinberg 1984, 1989). In many cases, moreover, one kind of organism can prevent the growth of other kinds by restricting iron access of the latter. In some cases, a particular organism can utilize the iron-acquisition mechanism of neighboring organisms. In a few instances, organisms are known to employ excess iron to poison a neighboring form of life.

Our discussion will focus on the ability of humans to withhold iron from microbial pathogens and from neoplastic cells, while permitting our normal tissues to retain access to physiological levels of the growth-essential metal. We will review such pathological consequences of accumulation of excessive quantities of iron as infection, neoplasia, arthropathy, cardiomyopathy, and endocrine deficits. The chapter will conclude with a brief review of methods for preventing, and for minimizing the dangers of, iron overload.

The Iron-Withholding System

The presence of iron in human plasma was discovered in 1898. Three decades later, the metal was observed to be bound tightly to a plasma protein. The latter molecule was identified in 1946 by Schade and Caroline (1946). These microbiologists earlier had discovered that a related protein, conalbumin, is responsible for the powerful, broad-spectrum antimicrobial activity of egg white (Schade and Caroline 1944). They noted that conalbumin prevents microbial growth by withholding iron from potential bacterial and fungal invaders and they predicted that a similar protein would function in the same manner in plasma.

Schade and Caroline (1946) named the plasma protein that they had discovered "siderophilin." However, 1 year later, Holmberg and Laurell (1947) changed the name to "transferrin." The latter investigators altered the name because they had discovered that the protein has a second function, namely, that of transporting iron among the various tissues of the body. It is indeed intriguing that humans and other vertebrates employ the protein for dual purposes: that of withholding iron from microbial invaders and, at the same time, that of rendering the metal available to host cells for physiological use or for storage.

A third member of the transferrin class, termed lactoferrin, had been discovered in milk in 1939 but was not purified or clearly identified until 1960 (Groves 1960; Reiter 1978). In human milk, lactoferrin is an important constituent; it can represent as much as 20% of the protein content (Bezkorovainy 1980). Bovine milk contains only about one-tenth as much lactoferrin as does human milk. Lactoferrin is present also in such other exocrine fluids as bronchial mucous, nasal exudate, saliva, gastrointestinal fluid, hepatic bile, cervical mucous, seminal fluid, and tears.

Moreover, lactoferrin is a major component of the specific granules of polymorphonuclear leukocytes (Baggiolini et al. 1970). On migration of these defense cells to a septic site, degranulation occurs to cause release of the apoprotein. At the site of infection, apolactoferrin combines with iron derived from dying microbial invaders and injured defense cells. Iron-saturated lactoferrin molecules then are ingested by macrophages and assist these defense cells in killing pathogens (Lima and Kierszenbaum 1987). Ultimately, the resultant accumulation of iron suppresses further metabolic activity of the macrophages, thereby contributing to the down-regulation of the inflammatory process that occurs at the conclusion of the successful response to insult (Slater and Fletcher 1987).

Macrophages scavenge iron not only in septic sites but also in tissues threatened by neoplastic cell invasion. Various kinds of solid tumors, containing little iron, often are surrounded by macrophages replete with sequestered iron (Price and Greenfield 1958). Likewise, in Hodgkin's disease, heavy deposits of iron and its storage protein, ferritin, occur at the periphery of the tumor nodules (Smithyman et al. 1978).

Lactoferrin differs from transferrin and conalbumin in that it retains its avidity for iron as the pH declines below 4.0. Accordingly, it is an efficient scavenger of iron in septic areas in which the pH has been lowered by organic acids derived from the microbial invaders and immune defense cells. Not unexpectedly, humans deficient in lactoferrin-containing specific granules of polymorphonuclear leukocytes are at increased risk of gram-positive and gram-negative bacterial infections (Breton-Gorius et al. 1980).

The relatively large quantity of lactoferrin in human milk is an important contributor to the much lower incidence of infection in breast-fed infants as compared with the incidence in infants receiving milk formula or bovine milk (Bezkorovainy 1977). In addition to its ability to withhold iron from such potential infant intestinal pathogens as *Escherichia, Salmonella*, and *Clostridium*, the lactoferrin in human milk also may function to retard absorption of intestinal iron (derived from both bile and diet) in the human nursling (Brock 1980). During the first week of life, full-term healthy infants normally excrete 10 times more iron than they absorb (Cavell and Widdowson 1964). By 2 months, healthy infants have succeeded in decreasing the iron saturation level of their plasma transferrin from a mean of 69% (at birth) to 34% and, by 6 months, to 25%. Values less than ~30% are helpful in preventing infection (Weinberg 1984).

Transferrin, likewise, may serve in a protective manner to prevent excessive iron accumulation, especially in heart muscle (Hershko et al. 1987). The most important cause of death in hemosiderotic patients who have non-transferrin-bound (NTB) plasma iron is myocardial siderosis. Hershko et al. (1987) proposed that "the main physiological role of unsaturated transferrin may be protection of the myocardium from the harmful effects of NTB iron."

Despite the iron-expurgating efforts of lactoferrin and transferrin, humans and nearly all other forms of life inevitably acquire iron that is not immediately needed for metabolic use and that must be stored in a safe package. Early in evolution, in bacteria, plants, and animals, ferritin became available for this purpose. In animal cells, the iron-storage role is so important to continued viability that a special cytoplasmic control of ferritin messenger translation is employed (Bomford and Munro 1985).[2]

Each ferritin molecule can accommodate ≤ 4500 atoms of iron. The mass of the metal can be as much as 30–40% of the mass of the protein.

However, molecules with 1200–1400 atoms of iron are most efficient for short-term storage. When ferritin becomes highly satiated with the metal, partial degradation of the protein shell via lysosomal proteases may alter the molecule to the hemosiderin form (Theil 1987). Unlike ferritin, hemosiderin is water insoluble. The latter protein serves as a more durable iron sink (Deiss 1983). In liver biopsy specimens of iron-overloaded patients, the increase in ferritin over that in normal tissue was 10-fold whereas the increase in hemosiderin was 100-fold (Selden et al. 1980).

In the normal process of release of iron from ferritin storage, ferric ions are initially reduced by agents such as ascorbic acid in the case of macrophages, or reduced riboflavin or $FMNH^2$ in hepatic parenchymal cells (Frieden and Osaki 1974; Hershko 1977). The metal then must be reoxidized by ceruloplasmin or other ferroxidases to be acquired by transferrin for recycling to other tissues.

In addition to prior stationing of iron-binding proteins of the transferrin class at possible portals of invasion, it is important for potential hosts to be able to intensify the iron-withholding defense at the time of threatened invasion. It was noted above that extra lactoferrin is conveyed to the invasion site by the mobile polymorphonuclear leukocytes. However, it also would be useful to the host to be able to shut down dietary intake of iron and, as well, to lower the amount normally contained in transferrin. Humans and other vertebrate hosts promptly effect these measures.

In humans, intestinal absorption of iron compounds is reduced markedly during infection (Cartwright et al. 1946; Dubach et al. 1948). In a set of 19 children, for example, the mean absorption of an oral dose of ferrous ascorbate was 41.2% in health but only 15.1% during infection (Beresford et al. 1971). In a rodent model of inflammation, iron absorption was lowered by 74% (Hershko et al. 1974). Reduction of iron absorption begins at the time of initial microbial invasion and occurs well in advance of a generalized depression of intestinal absorption of other nutrients.

Evidence that humans develop a hypoferremic response to infection and chronic disorders (Table 2) began to accumulate six decades ago when Locke et al. (1932) observed that tubercular and cancerous patients lower their level of plasma iron. This consistent physiological response to insult is seen also in inflammatory conditions induced by collagen disease, cardiovascular accident, and endotoxin. Of course, if the pathological condition causes a release of storage iron (as in hepatitis) or a release of iron from erythrocytes (as in bartonellosis, malaria, or other hemolytic conditions), plasma iron levels will rise rather than fall. In the absence of

Eugene D. Weinberg

Table 2. Hypoferremic Response to Infection (Pekarek et al. 1969) and Neoplasia (Beamish et al. 1972)

	Day Postexposure to *Francisella tularensis*										
	0	1	2	3	4	5	6	7	8	9	10
Mean serum iron (μM)	22.3	18.0	15.5	11.2	10.0	6.4	7.3	12.3	13.0	13.2	15.3
Mean fever index (h × °F)	0	1	0	17	30	12	5	2	4	0	1

		Hodgkin's Disease				Non-Hodgkin's lymphoma
	Normal	Stage 1	Stage 2	Stage 3	Stage 4	
Number of persons	12	6	7	7	3	6
Serum iron (μM)	22.7 ± 1.8	16.4 ± 1.6	11.4 ± 1.5	8.6 ± 1.5	6.97 ± 0.61	10.7 ± 2.0
Fe saturation of Tf (%)	35 ± 3.7	27 ± 3.5	23 ± 2.6	18 ± 3.5	16 ± 1.2	17 ± 3.3

damage to parenchymal hepatocytes or to erythrocytes, plasma iron levels begin to decline early in the incubation phase of the disease. The extent of reduction often reaches 70%; on recovery, the level of plasma iron promptly returns to normal.

Plasma iron turns over about 10 times daily (Zschocke and Bezkorovainy 1974) and hypoferremia can be achieved quickly by suppression of the release of metal from splenic and hepatic macrophages that have processed decaying erythrocytes. In healthy hosts, the quantity of plasma iron is only 0.4% of the amount of storage iron; thus, withholding of ≤ 70% of the plasma iron by macrophages during the inflammatory response should present no logistical problem. Of course, synthesis of additional ferritin and hemosiderin, is required. The amino acids are most likely derived from catabolized muscle protein. When human monocytes differentiate into macrophages, their intracellular ferritin increases from 10 ng/10^6 cells to approximately 1000 ng/10^6 cells (Andreesen et al. 1984). In mature macrophages of noninflammed hosts, the ratio of hemosiderin iron to ferritin iron is 0.03/1 whereas in similar cells exposed to inflammatory agents, the ratio was observed to increase to 0.28/1 (Alvarez-Hernandez et al. 1986).

Retention of iron by macrophages during the inflammatory response apparently is induced by a monokine termed leukocytic endogenous mediator (LEM) (Weinberg 1984). This 13- to 16-kDa polypeptide is produced mainly by monocytes that have been derepressed by a variety of inflammatory agents, microbial invaders, and/or neoplastic cells. Another monokine, interleukin-1 (IL-1), described more recently, is considered by some investigators to have activities that include those ascribed to LEM (Dinarello 1984). However, careful monitoring of the acute phase response in a rodent model of human rheumatoid arthritis demonstrated that, at least in this system, the reduction in plasma iron of 58% developed 10 days prior to the appearance of splenic IL-1 (Connolly et al. 1988). In cultured hepatic macrophages, IL-1 could not substitute for the ability of rodent inflammed serum to prevent iron efflux (Kondo et al. 1988). Moreover, the infection resistance provided to neutropenic mice by a 17-kDa recombinant molecule, IL-1β, was considered to be unrelated to possible hypoferremic activity (van der Meer et al. 1988). In a different study, however, human recombinant IL-1 lowered plasma iron significantly in both normal and neutropenic mice (Gordeuk et al. 1988).

Another possible method of iron withholding that might be considered by invaded hosts would be that of increasing the normally small amount of iron (1 mg/day) excreted in either urine, sweat, and/or bile and feces. This method appears not to be employed. One reason for its undesirability is that, if it were to be utilized, severe iron deficiency might ensue, especially in a protracted infectious or other inflammation-induced episode. Moreover, during the process of augmented excretion of the metal, its presence might enhance microbial growth in the urinary tract, skin, or intestinal tract. Furthermore, expulsion of the metal presumably would require an organic carrier, thus resulting in the loss of useful nutrients. Nevertheless, urinary excretion of iron in humans is quite variable, ranging from ~0.2 to 200 μM (Bowering et al. 1976). Even in a given individual, considerable fluctuation occurs from day to day. Possible correlates of this large variation either with stages of specific infectious, neoplastic, or metabolic diseases and/or with excretion of low-molecular-weight iron carriers should be investigated.

Impairment of the Iron-Withholding System

Etiologies

The iron-withholding system can be compromised either by (1) the acquisition of an excessive amount of iron in particular body fluids, tissues, or cells, or (2) interference with the synthesis of the various iron-binding proteins (Table 3). In the first category, the source of the excess iron can be either exogenous or endogenous. If the former, the metal generally is acquired by ingestion, less commonly by injection or inhalation. If endogenous, the metal usually is derived from injured hepatocytes or ruptured erythrocytes. In women of child-bearing age, suppression of normal menstrual blood loss by use of high dose oral contraceptive agents or by hysterectomy also can contribute to excessive accumulation of endogenous iron. In the second category, the iron-withholding deficit can arise via a genetic defect or by a lack of dietary amino acids.

In regard to excessive intake of iron via dietary overload, one of the most thoroughly documented examples is that observed in adult males in Botswana, Kenya, Malawi, Mozambique, South Africa, Swaziland, Tanzania, Zambia, and Zimbabwe (Gordeuk et al. 1986; Hershko 1977; McLaren et al. 1983). Much of the excess metal is derived from iron cookware used to brew alcoholic beverages at acid pH values. The daily oral intake of nonheme iron in this population is estimated to be 50–100 mg, which results in a net tissue accumulation of 1–3 mg per day. Approximately 70% of the persons at risk have excessive tissue deposits of the metal at autopsy. Deposits of hemosiderin are unusually heavy in the spleen, bone marrow, and duodenal and jejunal villi. In the liver, hemosiderin accumulates first in the Kupffer phagocytic cells, and later in the parenchymal cells. In those patients who proceed to develop cirrhosis, iron is deposited in the myocardium, pancreas, adrenals, thyroid, and pituitary.

In populations that avoid use of iron cookware, ethanol itself can be a

Table 3. Conditions That Can Compromise the Iron-Withholding Defense System

---

I. Excessive intake of iron via intestinal absorption
   A. Excessive quantity of iron ingested
      1. Use of iron cookware
      2. Excessive consumption of red meats (heme iron)
      3. Excessive "fortification" of food with inorganic iron
      4. Accidental ingestion of iron tablets
   B. Enhanced iron absorption (normal quantity of iron in diet)
      1. Excessive consumption of alcohol
      2. Excessive consumption of ascorbic acid
      3. Pancreatic deficiency of bicarbonate ions
      4. Asplenia
      5. Excess erythropoietin from kidney graft
      6. Possible cell receptor defect in idiopathic hemochromatosis
      7. Erythropoietic defects due to
         a. Folic acid deficiency
         b. Porphyria cutanea tarda
         c. Various hemoglobinopathies
         d. Various anemias
II. Parenteral iron
   A. Intravenous multiple transfusions of whole blood or packed erythrocytes
   B. Intramuscular iron-dextran
III. Inhaled iron
   A. Mining iron ore, welding or grinding steel, cutting asbestos
   B. Painting with iron oxide powder
   C. Cigarette smoking
IV. Shifting of iron from body compartments into plasma
   A. Release of stored iron during hepatitis
   B. Release of erythrocyte iron during clinical episodes of hemolytic diseases
   C. Suppression of cellular iron assimilation from plasma by *Catharanthus* alkaloids
V. Reduction of normal excretion of iron in premenopausal women
   A. Hysterectomy
   B. Ingestion of high dose oral contraceptives
VI. Lack of transferrin
   A. Congenital defect in synthesis
   B. Lack of dietary amino acids for synthesis
      1. Kwashiorkor
      2. Jejunoileal bypass

---

salient factor in development of iron overload. In one study, for instance, a group of 20 alcohol abusers with no evidence of liver damage had a mean plasma iron concentration of 35 μM whereas a control group of 66 persons had a mean value of 18 μm (Rodriguez et al. 1986). In a different survey, a set of 35 noncirrhotic alcoholics had a mean hepatic iron concentration 3-fold higher than that of 16 normal persons ($p < 0.05$) (Chapman et al. 1982).

Ethanol enhances absorption of ferric iron from food by stimulation of secretion of HCl. The acid maintains the ferric ions in solution until they reach the absorbing area of the duodenum (Charlton et al. 1964; Jacobs et al. 1964). In achlorhydric patients, absorption of ferric ions is enhanced markedly by exogenous HCl. In normal persons who produce the acid, ethanol promotes excessive absorption (Table 4). In precirrhotic alcoholic patients, hepatic siderosis occurs frequently (Bomford and Williams 1976). Moreover, alcohol-induced liver disease results in an increase in transferrin saturation with iron that is even greater than the increase in iron stores (Milder et al. 1980). Furthermore, in 41 alcohol abusers, serum ferritin levels were elevated > 2-fold in 12 persons, > 5-fold in 11, and > 10-fold in 4 (Meyer et al. 1984).

In addition to ingestion of ethanol, several other conditions can enhance absorption of inorganic iron. For example, a 1/3 molar ratio of ascorbic acid to iron increased absorption of the metal from infant foods at least 6-fold (Morris 1983). In another study, absorption of iron from two wheat rolls and coffee was 2.5 times greater if orange juice that contained 70 mg ascorbic acid had been included in the meal (Lynch and Cook 1980).[3]

Augmented absorption of iron likewise occurs in persons with cystic fibrosis or chronic pancreatitis whose pancreatic tissues fail to secrete

Table 4. Enhancement of Intestinal Absorption of Inorganic Iron by Hydrochloric Acid and Ethanol

Form of Fe Ingested		Achlorhydric Patients			Normal Persons (N = 17)	
		H_2O	HCl	Ethanol	H_2O	Ethanol
Fe^{3+}	(N = 10)	2.2[a]	9.2	5.2 (N = 4)	4.1	22.6
Fe^{2+}	(N = 7)	10.9	19.3		18.8	17.5
Hb	(N = 7)	13.4	9.6		14.9	13.4

[a] Mean percentage of iron dose absorbed.
Source: Jacobs et al. (1964).

bicarbonate ions. In normal persons, the anion aids in preventing excessive uptake of the metal by forming insoluble iron complexes (Conrad and Barton 1981; Hershko 1977; Tonz et al. 1965). In a set of 14 normal children, the mean amount of an oral dose of ferric chloride absorbed was 6.8%. In 16 children of similar age to the controls but who had cystic fibrosis, a mean of 36.0% was absorbed (Tonz et al. 1965).

Increased iron accumulation occurs also in patients who have conditions of ineffective erythropoiesis due to folic acid deficiency, thalassemia, pernicious anemia, porphyria cutanea tarda, or such hemolytic anemias as hereditary spherocytosis (Hershko 1977; Milder et al. 1980). In these cases, erythroid hyperplasia and increased iron turnover stimulate above normal absorption of iron. Similarly, persons who have lost their spleen, whether through trauma or because removal was necessary for medical reasons, absorb elevated quantities of iron. In reports from three groups (Erlandson et al. 1962; Parkin et al. 1974; Pootrakul et al. 1980), the mean serum iron value for 75 normal persons was 20.16 μM; for 53 splenectomized persons it was 39.24 μM. In these studies, the latter had received minimal or no blood transfusions and none had ingested more than an occasional iron tablet. Absorption of an oral dose of the metal averaged 13.7% in 14 normal persons and 32.9% in 18 asplenic patients (Erlandson et al. 1962; Parkin et al. 1974).

In a series of 60 persons who had received renal transplants, 17 (28%) developed hemosiderosis (Rao and Anderson 1982). The condition could not be correlated either with splenectomy, blood transfusions, or parenteral iron preparations. Unfortunately, erythropoietin levels were not ascertained. Renal grafts supply this hormone to the recipients and, in some patients, abnormally high levels have been noted (Barber 1988).

Heme iron, chiefly derived from myoglobin and hemoglobin, is absorbed by a pathway distinct from nonheme (Wadsworth 1975; Conrad and Barton 1981; Morris 1983). Heme iron accounts for approximately 40% of the metal in animal tissue. Thus nonvegetarian Western diets contain about 10–15% of iron as heme. This value, of course, is much less in diets of the world population because of low meat consumption (Morris 1983). Unlike inorganic iron, heme is soluble at alkaline pH and insoluble in acid milieu. Accordingly, factors discussed above such as ethanol (Table 4), ascorbic acid (Lynch and Cook 1980), and bicarbonate ions that modulate absorption of inorganic ions have little or no influence on bioavailability of heme iron. For instance, 13 children with cystic fibrosis as well as 13 healthy children each absorbed a mean of 9.5–10% of a dose of hemoglobin iron (Tonz et al. 1965).

Persons who have idiopathic hemochromatosis maintain a positive iron balance of about 3 mg per day on normal diets. Such patients have diminished ability to excrete iron as well as to prevent excessive intestinal absorption.[4] Apparently they have a defect in expression of iron-regulated proteins in cells of the duodenal mucosa (Lombard et al. 1989). In contrast to that in persons with dietary iron overload, deposition of the metal is greater in parenchymal cells of the liver, heart, and endocrine glands than in the monocyte–macrophage cells of the liver, spleen, and bone marrow (Hershko 1977; Conrad and Barton 1981).

The clinical spectrum of hemochromatosis is wide. At one end, there are severely affected patients, usually males; at the other end are individuals with little or no clinical or biochemical evidence of iron overload. In between are the majority of persons who have varying degrees of excessive iron stores (Meyer et al. 1987). Possibly one or more of the enhancers of iron absorption listed in Table 3 function synergistically with the hemochromatosis defect to cause serious disease problems (Milder et al. 1980; McLaren et al. 1983; Irving et al. 1988).

As mentioned above, excessive exogenous iron also can enter the body via injection. In some patients, nonheme iron is injected intramuscularly. Usually, it is complexed with dextran to retard too rapid diffusion through the tissues. In most cases, the metal is contained in hemoglobin in intravenously transfused erythrocytes.[5] Quantities of the metal introduced intravenously first are stored in cells of the monocyte–macrophage system. At a later time, some of the surplus iron is recycled and stored in hepatic parenchymal cells (McLaren et al. 1983; Hershko 1988). Uniform distribution of stainable iron between monocyte–macrophage cells and parenchymal cells was observed in liver biopsy specimens of patients with transfusional iron overload (Schafer et al. 1981).

Inhalation of iron has been reported in such industrial workers as iron ore miners (Antoine et al. 1979), steel welders and grinders (Cordes et al. 1981), and children who applied iron oxide powder to clock faces assembled at home (Dreyfus 1936). Other children who swim in ponds contaminated by iron smelters have been found to be at risk of inhaling free-living protozoa that can traverse the nasal mucosa, penetrate the cribiform plate, and multiply in the gray matter of the brain (John 1982). The metal serves as a nutrient for the protozoa in the pond environment but also may be necessary for viability and virulence of the organism in the olfactory tract (Weinberg 1989). Note also that the silicates that comprise various forms of asbestos have a considerable amount of iron.[6]

The iron content of alveolar macrophages of cigarette smokers has been reported to be 3.7-fold higher than that of nonsmokers ($p < 0.02$) and the ferritin content 6.0-fold higher ($p < 0.01$) (McGowan and Henley

1988). The accumulation of iron by smokers' alveolar macrophages correlated with the quantity of cigarettes that had been smoked. The potential for iron toxicity in cigarette smokers is enhanced additionally by their lowered ceruloplasmin ferroxidase activity (Pacht and Davis 1988).[7]

Additional etiologies of iron overload are derived from destruction of compartments that normally contain the metal followed by its release into such body fluids as plasma. These endogenous sources of iron include that of the decaying parenchymal hepatocytes in hepatitis and of the ruptured erythrocytes in hemolytic episodes of such diseases as malaria, bartonellosis, sickling, leukemias, and lymphomas (Weinberg 1978).

Transient 2.5- to 4-fold elevation of plasma iron has been observed in cancer patients who are on *Catharanthus* alkaloid therapy. No appreciable changes occur in plasma levels of transferrin or ferritin, or in hematocrit or hemoglobin values. The cytotoxic alkaloids apparently are inhibiting the normal recycling of iron into the cellular compartment (Sethi et al. 1984).

A different etiology of endogenous iron overload is that in which normal excretion of the metal in menstruation is reduced in premenopausal women who use oral contraceptive agents or who have had a hysterectomy. Normally, the development of iron overload is retarded in premenopausal women by the release of 3–60 mg of the metal in each menstrual cycle and 500 mg in each pregnancy (Conrad and Barton 1981). In one survey, for example, serum ferritin in 30-year-old men was 4.5-fold higher than in 30-year-old women whereas it was only 1.5-fold higher in 60-year-old men as compared with 60-year-old women (Cook et al. 1976). In another study of 1472 women and 1270 men, serum ferritin in men in the 20- to 44-year-old age group was 2.7-fold higher than that of women. In the 45- to 64-year-old age group, the corresponding figure was only 1.7-fold (Gordeuk et al. 1986).

Unfortunately, about 60–80% of the estimated 150 million users of oral contraceptive agents have a reduction in menstrual blood release. In an early study, the median iron excretion in nonusers was 3.4-fold higher than that of users (Thein et al. 1969). A more recent study examined women who employed lower doses of oral contraceptive agents (mean of 400 μg progestin and 50 μg estrogen) (Frassinelli-Gunderson et al. 1985). Even with such moderate doses, the serum iron and ferritin values for 71 nonusers was, respectively, 78 and 64% of that of the 46 users ($p < 0.001$).

Manifestations of iron overload have been observed also in humans and other mammals in which normal amounts of the metal are ingested but in which synthesis of the iron-withholding proteins is prevented. Examples include (1) the autosomal recessively inherited disorder, congenital atransferrinemia (Hershko 1977; Bernstein 1987), and (2) lack of dietary amino acids for transferrin synthesis. Amino acid deprivation has been observed in children (McFarlane et al. 1970) and rats (Olusi and McFarlane 1978) on protein-deficient diets and in adults who have had a jejunoileal bypass (Pickleman et al. 1975). Because of their hypotransferrinemia, these various hosts are unable to withhold a sufficient amount of their iron from microbial invaders to preclude infection.

Clinical Consequences

Infection. During the past third of a century, the results of several hundred studies in animals and several score in humans have demonstrated clearly that hosts whose iron-withholding system is compromised are at increased risk of bacterial, fungal, and protozoan infection. Moreover, the corollary condition has been described in several dozen reports; that is, strengthening the iron-withholding system results in decreased risk of infection (Table 5). Representative studies have been cited in numerous reviews (Weinberg 1974, 1978, 1984, 1990, 1992).

Of course, some invaded hosts whose iron-withholding system is compromised may evade clinical disease by promptly mounting an effective antibody-mediated or cell-mediated immune defense. Furthermore, not every microbial strain can take advantage of the hyperferremic or hypotransferrinemic host (Kent et al. 1990). Microbial invaders attempt to obtain iron in diverse ways from hosts (Weinberg 1989). In many cases, novel cell surface proteins are produced in response to the iron limitation imposed by normal hosts. Not all of these proteins necessarily are in-

Table 5. Methods of Enhancement of the Iron-Withholding Defense System That Have been Shown to Decrease Risk of Bacterial Infection in Animal Models

1. Moderate restriction of iron in diet
2. Dietary restriction of copper (to lower ceruloplasmin level, thus preventing recycling of ferric iron to transferrin)
3. Hypoferremia induced by sham materials: endotoxin, bacterial cell walls, live attenuated bacteria
4. Hypoferremia induced by leukocytic endogenous mediator
5. Administration of an iron chelator that cannot be used by the bacteria
6. Administration of host iron-binding protein that cannot be used by the bacteria

Source: Weinberg (1984).

volved in iron uptake. Some may be needed in other ways for the establishment of the infection. Presumably, their formation, also, is triggered by iron limitation that serves as a signal to the microorganisms that they now may be invading host tissues.

Although the most obvious and most frequently demonstrated mechanism whereby excess iron enhances infection is that of serving as a nutrient for the invading microbial cells, the metal also can impair host defense cells (Weinberg 1984). Iron can suppress the phagocytosis-associated metabolic burst of macrophages. Chemotaxis, phagocytosis, and microbicidal action of both polymorphonuclear leukocytes and monocytes can be inhibited by excess iron (Van Asbeck et al. 1982; Ballart et al. 1986). Transferrin that is saturated $\geq 70\%$ with iron is much less effective in supplying the metal to lymphocytes for initiation of their DNA synthesis than is the protein saturated at values below 70% (Brock 1981). Moreover, iron overload reduces migration of B and T lymphocytes from the blood into the lymphatic system (de Sousa 1978) as well as the number of interleukin-2-secreting cells (Good et al. 1987), the number of T-helper cells (Pardalos et al. 1987), and the activity of natural killer cells (Kaplan et al. 1984; Akbar et al. 1986).

If human or animal hosts become markedly iron deficient (Hb < 10 g/dl) because of severe or prolonged blood loss or starvation, susceptibility to infection can increase presumably because the metal is needed to catalyze various components of the antibody- and cell-mediated immune defense systems (Gross and Newberne 1980; Weinberg 1978, 1984). A few animal studies are available on this topic in which appropriate controls and quantitative assays were employed (e.g., Hart et al. 1982). Studies on humans generally have reported anecdotal evidence with little or no microbiological data. Well-designed studies on iron deficiency are needed to determine the tissue concentrations of the metal at which risk of infection begins to occur as well as the precise intracellular deficits that are caused by iron famine. In such studies, the professional team should include not only a nutritionist, but, as important, a hematologist and a microbiologist.

Iron deficiency as determined by detection of abnormally low levels of serum ferritin, hemoglobin, and/or hematocrit is, of course, pathological (Dallman 1986; Sherman and Lockwood, 1987). In patients, it must not be confused with iron withholding, a normal physiological response to infection. The pathological deficiency should be managed by identification and correction of the blood loss and/or by the restoration of proper mineral nutrition. Iron withholding, on the other hand, should *not* be compromised by feeding or injecting excess iron. Rather, the underlying condition that has induced the hypoferremic response should be identified and, if possible, corrected.

Clinical reports of the association of iron overload with increased risk of infection continue to accumulate. The danger of injecting iron dextran into full-term, healthy young infants demonstrated clearly in the New Zealand studies (Barry and Reeve 1977; Becroft et al. 1977) has been confirmed in the New Guinea research (Oppenheimer et al. 1986a,b). It will be recalled that in the New Zealand project, a 7-fold increase in septicemias and meningitis caused by *E. coli* and other gram-negative bacteria occurred within 1 week of injection of 10–50 mg/kg iron (as dextran). Sera from infants who received the iron had a marked hyperferremia within 24 hours. In *in vitro* tests, these sera permitted a 5-fold increase in growth of *E. coli* in 5.5 hours as compared with sera obtained from the identical infants 1 hour prior to injection of iron. Moreover, the response of the infants' neutrophils to chemotactic stimuli was depressed by the iron overload. Control children of the same age who received no parenteral iron showed no increase in infection.

In the New Guinea study, 177 healthy 2-month-old infants, injected with 40 mg/kg iron (as dextran), developed more infections, needed more hospital admissions, and had longer hospital stays during the ensuing 10 months than did 190 normal, noninjected controls (Oppenheimer et al. 1986b). Malaria was especially troublesome; at 12 months of age, 58 iron-stressed infants had parasitemia as compared with 38 control children ($p < 0.01$) (Oppenheimer et al. 1986a). Splenomegaly was present in 81 of the experimental infants and in 66 of the controls ($p < 0.05$). Although it may be appropriate to give prophylactic intramuscular iron injections to *premature* infants to elevate their iron status to that of full-term children (Leikin 1960; Salmi et al. 1963), the New Zealand and the New Guinea research projects have shown unequivocally that it is no longer ethical to inject iron in healthy *full-term* infants.

Transfusional iron overload also can increase risk of infection. Older patients with cardiovascular problems and renal insufficiency are now routinely accepted for hemodialysis. Frequently, erythrocytes are administered to minimize angina pectoris and/or to improve the patients' level of activity. In one report, four patients who had each received approximately 20 units per year of packed red blood cells for 5–10 years and who now had hepatic siderosis and hyperferritinemia developed listeriosis (Mossey and Sondheimer 1985). None had an underlying malignancy nor were they receiving immunosuppressive medication or pregnant.

In a different study, 11 patients on hemodialysis for a mean of 6.4 years had received a mean of 24.9 g of iron in the form of either packed erythrocytes or iron-dextran and they had become hyperferritinemic (Boelaert et al. 1987). Each of these patients had episodes of generalized infection with *Yersinia enterocolitica*. In an earlier survey, five cases occurred among 539 dialysis patients who had iron overload (serum ferritin > 500 ng/ml); no cases occurred among 882 dialysis patients with lower serum ferritin values ($p < 0.05$) (Boelaert et al. 1987). Hemochromatotic patients also are at higher risk for *Yersinia* infections (Abbott et al. 1986; Hiesa et al. 1987).

In pediatric surveys (Butzler et al. 1978; Melby et al. 1982; Scharnetzky et al. 1984), 16 children with various etiologies of iron overload (accidental ingestion of iron tablets, aplastic anemia, thalassemia) or of hypotransferrinemia due to kwashiorkor were found to have septicemia caused by *Y. enterocolitica*. In four of the children, desferrioxamine had been given to relieve the iron intoxication.[8] In other reports, patients who received desferrioxamine for either iron or aluminum overload have developed infections due to *Vibrio vulnificus* (Mehtar 1988) and to *Mucor* sp. (Goodill and Abuelo 1987). In patients who present with gastrointestinal, pulmonary, or skin infections, use of the siderophore should be halted and appropriate antiinfective therapy should be employed until such time as the infection is cured (Boyce et al. 1985; Gallant et al. 1986).

Additional gram-negative bacteria that cause clinical disease, primarily in patients whose iron-withholding system is compromised, include dysgonic fermentor #2 (DF-2) (Weinberg 1987) and *Legionella pneumophila* (Quinn and Weinberg 1988). Each of these taxonomically dissimilar organisms requires specialized culture media to permit them to acquire iron in *in vitro* systems. DF-2 causes a septicemia mainly in alcoholic and/or asplenic persons who have had minor skin abrasions contaminated by saliva of healthy dogs, cats, or bears. *L. pneumophila* causes pneumonia by growing in alveolar macrophages of persons who generally are cigarette smokers. Although smokers attempt to render the excessive iron in their alveolar macrophages unavailable by incorporating it into insoluble hemosiderin, approximately 25% of the metal overload remains associated with ferritin (McGowan and Henley 1988) and thus potentially is accessible for growth of the bacteria.

Iron availability regulates the virulence of another gram-negative bacterium, *Pseudomonas aeruginosa*. Chronic obstructive pulmonary infection due to strains that produce iron-regulated factors of virulence[9] is the major cause of morbidity and mortality in patients with cystic fibrosis (Anwar et al. 1984). Although such patients absorb excess amounts of dietary iron (Tonz et al. 1965), the biochemical accessibility of the metal in pulmonary fluids might not be sufficiently high to repress synthesis of the virulence factors. For example, the iron might be sequestered by the 4-fold increase in lactoferrin that has been observed in saliva of cystic fibrosis patients (Smith et al. 1981).

Infectious diarrhea is one of the most prevalent causes of infant morbidity and mortality in developing parts of the world (Boesman-Finkelstein and Finkelstein 1985). Breast-fed infants fare far better than do their formula-fed counterparts largely because of lactoferrin and secretory immunoglobulin A (sIgA) in human milk. For instance, strains of *E. coli, S. typhimurium,* and *V. cholerae* grow very well in commercial infant formulas whereas human milk is bacteriostatic due to apolactoferrin and, as well, is bactericidal if sIgA also is present. The antibody without lactoferrin is inactive. Neither lysozyme nor complement is involved (Boesman-Finkelstein and Finkelstein 1985).

Iron-withholding defense has been observed often to be important in mycobacterial and systemic mycotic infections of animals and humans. In the 1970s, a surgical procedure for the correction of extreme obesity, jejunoileal bypass, was performed on several thousand patients. Unfortunately, kwashiorkor-like protein deficiency state associated with striking alterations in plasma amino acid levels developed in some of these individuals (Pickleman et al. 1975). Although the patients were able to maintain normal cell-mediated immunity (Tustin et al. 1980), during the postsurgical year some developed an increased susceptibility to mycobacterial and mycotic organisms present in their environment. The incidence of tuberculosis increased 60-fold (Bruce and Wise 1977; Pickleman et al. 1975) over that of the general population. The incidence of histoplasmosis and blastomycosis increased 31-fold as compared with that of persons who had been hospitalized for other reasons (Tustin et al. 1980).

Neoplasia.   Numerous cases of primary liver cancer as well as other neoplasms have occurred among persons who had become siderotic because of excessive ingested iron and/or inordinate intestinal absorption of the metal. In cancers that developed in young males recruited from several African nations for work in South African gold mines, 52% of 1694 neoplasms were primary hepatomas (Berman 1958; Robertson et al. 1971). In persons who have hemochromatosis, hepatoma and other kinds of neoplasms are common causes of death (Bomford and Williams 1976; Johnson et al. 1978; Milder et al. 1980; Niederau et al. 1985; Powell 1970; Purtillo and Gottleib 1973; Sherlock 1976). In one study, for example, liver cancer was 219 times more frequent among such patients than in the normal population (Niederau et al. 1985). Those who died of this malignancy had the highest amount of mobilizable iron, significantly higher than that of hemochromatotic patients who died from other causes. Cases have occurred even in patients who had not yet developed cirrhosis and who were being treated by phlebotomy (Fellows et al. 1988).

Ethanol consumption frequently has been linked to an increased incidence of various neoplasms. For instance, among 451 case-community-based control pairs of women, consumption of $\geq$ one glass of alcohol per day was associated with a 1.5-fold increase in risk of breast cancer ($p =$ 0.38) (Rohan and McMichael 1988). A quantitative review of 16 published studies noted that for women who consumed three glasses (36 g)/day of alcohol, the increase in risk of breast cancer over that in nondrinkers was 2-fold (Longnecker et al. 1988).

Of 47 male hepatitis B carriers who developed hepatocellular carcinoma, 40 drank alcohol and 7 abstained (Ohnishi et al. 1982). The average age of the former at the time of diagnosis of the neoplasia was 48.8 ± 8.1 years and of the latter, 61.4 ± 7.1 years ($p < 0.01$). In a set of 106,203 women and men, the relative risk for rectal cancer was 3.17-fold higher in persons with a daily intake of $\geq$ three drinks as compared with abstainers (Klatsky et al. 1988).

The remarkable geographic variation in the incidence of colonic cancer has been correlated with the amount of a dietary iron chelator, inositol hexaphosphate (phytic acid) (Graf and Eaton 1985). This compound is responsible for the ability of bran to inhibit intestinal absorption of inorganic iron (Hallberg et al. 1987). It occurs in substantial amount (1–5% by weight) in cereals but is present in negligible quantities in other high fiber foods such as fruits and vegetables. Thus, although the Danish population consumes twice as much dietary fiber as the Finnish people, the phytate intake of the latter is 20–40% higher because they consume more cereals. The Finns have a much lower incidence of colorectal cancer than do the Danes. Phytic acid is stable in the gut; by binding iron it inhibits the formation of hydroxyl radicals (Graf and Eaton 1985). The latter potentially are carcinogenic because of their ability to cause strand breakage and degradation of DNA (Halliwell and Gutteridge 1984).

Persons who have iron overload because of porphyria cutanea tarda are at increased risk for development of hepatocellular cancer. In a group of 342 patients followed for 15 years, 17 (5%) developed this malignancy (Bengtsson and Hardell 1986).

In May 1959, at a symposium on metals and disease, Arthur Furst stated: "One might worry about the iron-injectable compounds which are being tested and used. One could almost guess that someone is going to find iron dextran carcinogenic." That foreboding prediction was well founded; a few months after it was made, numerous reports (summarized in Weinberg 1981) began to appear that described the sarcomas that developed in rabbits and rodents at the sites of injection of iron-dextran. The percentage of cases and the time required for appearance of the neoplasia are dose dependent. The dextran component is not carcinogenic but serves merely to retard diffusion of the metal from the site of deposition. In humans, the time of development of the malignancy has ranged from a few months to 14 years (Robertson and Dick 1977; Weinbren et al. 1978).

As noted above, another portal for entry of excessive iron is inhalation by industrial workers and by cigarette smokers. The association of smoking with lung cancer is well established. Iron ore miners who smoked had an even higher incidence of lung cancer than nonminer smokers (Antoine et al. 1979). The genesis of these neoplasms in miners appears to derive from the combined action of tobacco smoke, various gases, and iron particles. Children, employed to polish clock screws with iron oxide, inhaled the powder; they developed lung cancer in young adulthood (Dreyfus 1936). Exposure to asbestos dust increases the incidence of malignant mesothelioma and bronchogenic carcinoma. This action of asbestos involves in part its high content of iron.[10]

In populations that have a high incidence of hepatitis B, long-term epidemiological studies have found that excess iron is associated with increased risk of general mortality and of cancer. For example, serum ferritin was higher and transferrin lower in Solomon Islanders who died during the subsequent decade (Stevens et al. 1983) and in Taiwanese government male workers who developed cancer (Stevens et al. 1986) as compared with appropriate controls. In the Taiwan investigation, the relative risk of cancer death for a man with 200 ng ferritin/ml and 200 mg transferrin/dl, as compared to a man with levels of 20 ng/ml and 400 mg/dl, respectively, was 2.9. In the Solomon Islands study, the correlation of elevated ferritin with mortality was more pronounced in women who were carriers of hepatitis B virus than in noncarriers.

Similarly, serum iron and transferrin saturation values are higher in patients with Down's syndrome or who are undergoing hemodialysis if they have become carriers of hepatitis B virus than if they do not become carriers (Lustbader et al. 1983). The excess iron is not caused by hepatocyte breakdown as determined by alanine-aminotransferase levels in the serum. The risk of persistent hepatitis B viral infection to development of primary hepatocellular carcinoma is nearly 100%. Survival and growth of the transformed liver cells may depend on a supply of iron from surrounding virus-infected nontransformed cells (Lustbader et al. 1983).

Additional associations of elevated iron burden with cancer morbidity and mortality continue to be recognized (Weinberg 1991). For example, in a set of 3355 men in the United States, 242 developed cancer. The mean total iron-binding capacity of the latter group was significantly lower (61.4 vs. 62.9 μM; $p = 0.01$) and transferrin saturation was significantly higher (33.1 vs. 30.7%; $p = 0.002$) than among the men who, during a 4-year period, remained free of cancer (Stevens et al. 1988). In 89 pediatric patients with acute lymphoblastic leukemia, transferrin iron saturation values of 43 were < 36% and of 46 were > 36%. Within the subsequent 2 years, five deaths occurred in the first set whereas 21 deaths occurred in the second set ($p < 0.001$) (Potaznik et al. 1987).

Of 103 children with neuroblastoma, 64 had serum ferritin values < 150 ng/ml and 39 had values > 150 ng/ml. In the subsequent 2 years, death occurred in 19% of the first set and in 83% of the second set ($p < 0.0001$) (Evans et al. 1987). Of 229 women presenting with early breast cancer, initial serum ferritin was ≤ 119 ng/ml in 172 and ≥ 201 ng/ml in 23 (Jacobs et al. 1976). The 3-year recurrence rate in the latter set was approximately 1.7-fold greater than in the former ($p < 0.04$). In a study of 94,500 women, the risk of developing lung cancer in the subsequent 7–16 years in persons whose hemoglobin value was > 13.8 g/dl was 2.3-fold greater than in those whose hemoglobin value was < 12.0 g/dl (Selby and Friedman 1988).

In a group of 122 adults who had undergone curative surgery for primary adenocarcinoma of the colon and rectum, the 5-year survival rate of those who had received perioperative blood transfusions was 50.86%; of those who had not been transfused it was 83.85% ($p < 0.005$) (Burrow and Tartter 1982). Of 156 patients with soft-tissue sarcomas of the extremities, 5-year survival also substantially was decreased in patients receiving perioperative transfusions (63% compared to 85%) ($p = 0.035$) (Rosenberg et al. 1985). Moreover, the greater the number of transfusions, the worse was the prognosis ($p = 0.0001$).

Arthropathy. About half of all patients with hemochromatosis have a fairly distinct arthropathy characterized by chronic symmetrical stiffening and swelling of the joints in the hands, wrists, and knees (Milder et al. 1980). The presence of iron in the joint synovium can act synergistically with other causes of joint disease to produce damage. In two groups totalling 197 hemochromatotic patients, joint pathology was present in 86 (43%) (Milder et al. 1980; Niederau et al. 1985).

In patients with rheumatoid arthritis, the level of ferritin in synovial fluid increases by 3- to 8-fold (Biemond et al. 1988). The protein tends to be satiated with iron and the metal is mobilized by superoxide. It is then free to catalyze production of hydroxyl radicals that proceed to destroy lipid membranes (Aust et al. 1985; Biemond et al. 1988). The inflammatory pathology in other autoimmune diseases such as lupus erythematosis may have the same etiology (Biemond et al. 1988). In hemophiliacs, the toxic iron is derived from blood that escapes into the joints (Biemond et al. 1988). The high incidence of polyarthritis that developed in patients following their jejunoileal bypass surgery (Shagrin et al. 1971) may have been a complication of their hypotransferrinemic condition.

Not surprisingly, intravenous injection of iron-dextran as well as feeding ferrous sulfate causes severe clinical exacerbation in patients with rheumatoid arthritis (Blake et al. 1981). Predictably, rheumatoid arthritis is more common in men than in women and, in the latter, its incidence increases rapidly after menopause (Blake et al. 1981). The disease is rare in underdeveloped rural populations presumably because parasitic infestations such as hookworm aid in preventing excessive accumulation of iron (Blake and Bacon 1982).[11]

Exacerbation of synovitis also has been reported in patients with ankylosing spondylitis or with spondylitis associated with Crohn's disease who are receiving injections of iron-dextran (reviewed in de Sousa et al. 1988). Circulating polymorphonuclear leukocytes and platelets of 29 patients with ankylosing spondylitis had, respectively, a 6-fold and a 2.4-fold increase in iron content over that of healthy controls ($p < 0.001$) (Feltelius et al. 1986).

Long-term functioning of the iron-withholding defense system in hosts invaded by microorganisms or cancer cells might contribute to arthropathy (Halliwell and Gutteridge 1984). Recall that a component of the normal inflammatory response to insult is the redistribution of iron from body fluids to storage in macrophages, a process that necessitates ferritin synthesis. If the inflammatory response is excessive or prolonged, some of the ferritin iron might be released into joints from decaying macrophages.

Moreover, iron-saturated ferritin can be metabolized into insoluble hemosiderin. Extensive accumulation of the latter protein can result in lysosome disruption and cell death (Selden et al. 1980; Alvarez-Hernandez et al. 1986). Additionally, lactoferrin, abundantly present in exudates of arthritic joints, has been suggested as being capable of providing iron to hydroxyl radical generating systems (Ambruso and Johnston 1981). Generally, however, lactoferrin is siderophraxic (Weinberg 1989), that is, the protein functions as an iron withholder rather than an iron supplier (e.g., Baldwin et al. 1984).

Cardiomyopathy. Cardiac muscle has a greater affinity for iron than does skeletal or smooth muscle. Unfortunately, "the iron heart is not a strong heart but a weak one" (Biya and Roberts 1971). Studies in animals have shown that excess iron in nurslings suppresses normal myocardial growth (Neffgen and Rakusan 1975). In isolated heart muscle strips (Artman et al. 1984) as well as in isolated baboon hearts (Wicomb et al. 1987), the metal impairs function by generating free radicals.[12] Similarly, iron contributes to the pathogenesis of reperfusion injury of ischemic myocardium (Ambrosio et al. 1987).

Iron overload has long been known to cause cardiac dysfunction. Accidental iron poisoning in children may result in cardiovascular collapse and death (Artman et al. 1984). In older individuals chronically stressed with excess iron, the most common cause of death is heart failure; autopsy reveals prominent myocardial deposits of the metal (Bothwell and Charlton 1979).

In a series of 34 hemochromatotic patients, 12 had developed congestive heart failure and eight additional patients had asymptomatic electrocardiographic abnormalities (Milder et al. 1980). In four of the severely affected persons, the cardiac dysfunction was rapidly progressive and fatal; alcoholism was present in each of these cases. Hemosiderin accumulates around the nuclear poles of myocardial fibers and in the conducting fibers of the atrioventricular node (Hershko 1977). Cardiomyopathy can be aggravated by administration of ascorbic acid to iron-overloaded patients (Henry 1979).

In a 24-year study of 2873 women (Gordon et al. 1978), a "sudden escalation in risk at the time of menopause" was observed in coronary heart disease. Likewise, in individuals who had had surgical menopause, *irrespective* of retention or removal of ovaries, the risk increased. In the age range 45–54 years, the subjects were 2.7-fold more likely to have coronary heart disease if they had had either surgical or natural menopause than if they were still premenopausal ($p < 0.01$). No association was found between incidence of coronary heart disease and either cigarette smoking or postmenopausal ingestion of estrogen. In a subsequent survey (Centerwall 1981), premenopausal hysterectomy was found to cause a 3-fold increase in cardiovascular disease during the patients' remaining premenopausal years.

Although Gordon et al. (1978) stated that men in the 45- 54-year-old age group were 15 times more likely to have coronary heart disease than premenopausal women of the same age, they failed inexplicably to mention the large difference in iron stores in the two groups as a possible contributing factor to the vast difference in risk. Finally, Sullivan (1981) called attention to the positive correlation of cardiovascular disease in men of increasing age from 35 to 59 years with their progressive accumulation of iron during this time span. He noted that women delay accumulation of iron until their menstrual flow begins to diminish.

As cited above, users of oral contraceptive agents generally have a lessened menstrual flow and consequently retain increased iron stores (Frassinelli-Gunderson et al. 1985). In a study of 556 women with myocardial infarction, aged 25–49 years, as compared with 2036 age-matched controls, the risk of development of the disease in oral contraceptive agent users was 3.5-fold higher than in nonusers (Slone et al. 1981). Even in women who had stopped use of oral contraceptives, the risk remained higher than in never-users, an observation that could be related to the level of iron stores in the various groups of subjects (Frassinelli-Gunderson et al. 1985). In the comparatively small number of women who develop hemochromatosis at an early age, amenorrhea due to hypogonadism is prominent; these patients have a high frequency of cardiomyopathy (Lamon et al. 1979).

Endocrine Deficits.   The most common endocrine dysfunctions caused by iron overload are hypogonadotrophic hypogonadism and insulin-dependent diabetes. The former condition usually results from iron-induced damage to pituitary and hypothalamic cells that normally synthesize, respectively, follicle-stimulating hormone and gonadotrophic- releasing hormone (Siemons and Mahler 1987). Often the anterior pituitary gland, especially the gonadotrophs, contains stainable iron, sometimes in massive amounts. The gonads generally have little or no excess deposits of the metal. In two studies that examined 144 hemochromatotic patients, 75 were hypogonadic (Milder et al. 1980; Niederau et al. 1985). In nonthalassemic patients with transfusional iron overload, gonadotropin was limited in 5 of 13 patients and pituitary ACTH reserve was limited in 10 of 12 patients (Schafer et al. 1981).

In the preinsulin era, type I diabetes was the most frequent cause of death in iron-overloaded patients (Milder et al. 1980). Hemosiderin deposits occur in pancreatic acinar tissue, islets, macrophages, and connective tissue of pancreatic ducts (McLaren et al. 1983). However, the development of the disease is not always directly correlated with the severity of iron overload. Factors in addition to iron deposits apparently contribute to development of the disease.[13] Nevertheless, in the group of 144 hemochromatotic patients cited above, 88 were diabetic. In a set of 15 nonthalassemic transfusional iron overload patients, all had glucose intolerance.

Miscellaneous Deficits. A cluster of neurologic complaints (e.g., fatigue, weakness, lethargy, apathy, disorientation) is associated with iron overload. Of the 144 hemochromatotic patients mentioned above, 93 had some type of neurologic symptom (Milder et al. 1980; Niederau et al. 1985). The globus pallidus and substantia nigra of the human brain normally contain approximately 50% more iron than does the liver. Excessive iron overload of these two brain regions is associated with tardive dyskinesia, Alzheimer's disease, and Huntington's chorea (Ashkenazi et al. 1982; Campbell et al. 1985).

In a different study of 10 patients on chronic maintenance hemodialysis who had developed severe iron overload because of prescribed oral and parenteral supplements, all developed proximal muscle weakness (Bregman et al. 1980). Muscle biopsy specimens revealed iron deposition in either macrophages and/or muscle fibers. Nine of the 10 myopathic patients had at least one of the so-called "hemochromatosis alleles" (i.e., HLA-A3, B7, or B14) whereas the expected frequency in the general population is only 25–33% ($p < 0.001$).

Osteoporosis is observed in patients with hemochromatosis, with nutritional iron overload, with thalassemia, and in those who are hemodialyzed (reviewed in de Vernejoul et al. 1984), but the mechanisms of iron toxicity is unclear. Three-month-old female pigs injected with 10.8 g of iron in 36 days (to simulate human hemochromatosis) developed iron deposits in both osteoclast and osteoblast cells as well as inside the bone matrix. The metal suppressed osteoblast recruitment and the rate of collagen synthesis but did not alter osteoclastic resorption (de Vernejoul et al. 1984).

Strengthening of the Iron-Withholding System

Prevention of Iron Overload

Intestinal barriers are in place to prevent assimilation of excessive amounts of iron (Wadsworth 1975). These include the barrier to entry at the surface of the mucosal cells, the ferritin within the cells, and the macrophages in the villous tips. As the mucosal cells and the macrophages become engorged with iron, they are shed into the lumen with consequent loss of the metal in the feces. However, these normal barriers cannot cope easily with such cultural practices as use of iron cookware; iron adulteration[14] of milk formula, of flour, and of cereals; consumption of ethanol; or of sugar-coating ferrous sulfate tablets that appear to small children to be candy.

Fortunately, there is increasing awareness that an effective way of strengthening the iron-withholding defense system is to avoid compromising it with these cultural practices. Mass medication of foodstuffs with the metal, for instance, should be replaced by administration of exogenous iron only to persons who truly are iron deficient.

In Sweden, food began to be adulterated with iron in 1948 (Olsson et al. 1978).Between 1962 and 1970, the amount of metal added to flour was increased 2.17-fold; by 1977, the incidence of primary liver cancer in Swedish women had increased by 3.5-fold (de Sousa and Potaznik 1984). At that time, the average daily intake of iron was 19 mg; 42% of this quantity was derived from the artificial incorporation of the metal into foodstuffs! A "surprisingly high incidence" (Olsson et al. 1978) of hemochromatosis began to be noticed in Sweden in 1975–1977. Therefore, a group of 347 persons, aged 30–39, from the general population were monitored for iron storage disease. The number of individuals affected was found to be 10-fold higher than would be expected in a normal population. Of the 197 men in the sample, four had early hemochromatosis; none of these persons was related. Five additional men consistently had high serum iron values but did not yet have sufficiently high stores to yield a positive desferrioxamine urinary iron excretion test. The 150 premenopausal women in the sample had not yet developed signs of iron overload.

Providentially, iron adulteration of foods in the United States is more restrained than in Sweden, although Crosby (1978) has estimated that 25% of our ingested iron is derived from this source. The combination of even this moderate overload with diets rich in red meats washed down with generous quantities of ethanol suggests obvious measures that could be adopted to strengthen our iron-withholding defense. In addition to freeing flour and cereals of added iron, we can recommend reduction in consumption of red meats and of ethanol. Several studies (reviewed in Sullivan 1983) have reported that mortality from ischemic heart disease is markedly lower in vegetarian than in nonvegetarian men. Moreover, if phytic acid in cereal fiber is indeed the salient factor in prevention of colonic cancer (Graf and Eaton 1985), we must be careful not to neutralize it by iron adulteration. Of course, other nutritional differences between vegetarian and nonvegetarian diets, such as cholesterol levels, might also play a role.

Although megadoses of ascorbic acid have not been found to lead to progressive iron accumulation in normal persons, those individuals who are at risk for hemochromatosis may be affected adversely (Cook et al. 1984). Persons already iron overloaded, for whatever reason, should reduce their intake of ascorbic acid to a minimum (Nienhuis 1981). The vitamin markedly increases the ability of the metal to catalyze lipid peroxidation (Hershko et al. 1987). Moreover, it enhances intestinal assimilation of iron as well as release of excess stores from monocyte–macrophages into the plasma. Synergism of iron and ascorbic acid has been observed in production of chromosome aberrations in cultured Chinese hamster ovary cells (Stich et al. 1979). Thus an ascorbic acid deficiency actually may be beneficial to patients who have iron overload (Nienhuis 1981).

Wadsworth (1975) has reminded us that "the human race has survived, and sometimes flourished, for hundreds of thousands of years without the purposeful addition to foods of inorganic forms of iron." He noted also that "extra iron given to the mother during pregnancy does not seem to benefit her offspring or herself. The increase in blood viscosity associated with an increase in hemoglobin concentration and hence an increase in blood pressure must be considered. . . . toxemia of pregnancy may be initiated by an interference, such as might follow an increase in blood viscosity, of the flow of blood through the placenta."

Indeed, in a study of pregnancies that had an unfavorable outcome, an increased incidence of prematurity and of fetal death was associated with maternal hematocrit values of >35% and hemoglobin values of > 11 g/dl in Blacks and > 12 g/dl in Whites (Garn et al. 1981). The results of six studies that comprised 3490 patients in which supplemental iron was compared with a placebo have been reviewed (Hemminki and Starfield 1978). In none of these studies did iron provide any beneficial effects on either infant or maternal morbidity or mortality. In pregnancy, iron is debited from the stores to increase the maternal red cell volume; the metal becomes available for return to storage after delivery (Hibbard 1988). Falsely boosting the red cell volume by iron supplementation is unnecessary and possibly undesirable (Hibbard 1988).

Accidental poisoning of young children who ingest maternal or pediatric iron tablets is relatively common and often fatal. These tablets are sold in the United States without prescription and their warning labels generally fail to mention potential lethality. In this country, iron is the fourth most common cause of poisoning in children ≤ 5 years (Murphy 1974).

A statement often heard in past decades is that "milk is a poor source of iron." This in spite of the fact that in all animals tested, the milk of the species allows an impressive accumulation of iron by the young during the time they feed solely on milk (Wadsworth 1975). Human breast milk contains about 14 μM iron; 50% of the metal can be absorbed by the infant (Oski 1976). Initial stores of iron in the full-term infant can sustain increase in red cell mass and tissue needs until birthweight has increased about 2.5 times, usually by 9 months or sometimes sooner (Oski 1976).

Accordingly, the combination of iron derived prenatally from placental sources and postnatally from maternal milk should preclude the need to supply supplemental iron to infants for 6 to 9 months. Two studies have validated this estimate. In one, 33 full-term, exclusively breast-fed infants were given no other source of iron for 6 months (Duncan et al. 1985). In the other study, 36 infants were tested in the same manner for 9 months (Siimes et al. 1984). None of the 69 infants developed an iron-deficiency anemia.

Other aspects of nutrition that can impact on iron metabolism in persons of all age groups include those of folic acid deficiency and of protein deficiency. In the former case, increased amounts of iron are assimilated in a vain attempt to compensate for the erythropoietic defect caused by the lack of the vitamin. In protein deficiency, the synthesis of transferrin is reduced by as much as 75% (Burger and Hogewind 1974). Thus even though a normal amount of iron is assimilated, the metal becomes freely available to potential microbial invaders. Accordingly, diets adequate in folic acid and in protein are essential for maintenance of a strong iron-withholding defense system.

Another method of prevention of iron overload is to minimize use of erythrocyte transfusions as much as possible. In end-stage renal disease, for example, recombinant human erythropoietin is now available (Eschbach et al. 1987). Of 18 patients who received effective doses of the hormone, 12 who had required transfusions no longer needed them. No organ dysfunction or other toxic effects were observed and no antibodies to the recombinant hormone were formed.

Additional methods of prevention of iron overload include minimizing inhalation of pollutants that contain iron. Another method, for premenopausal women, involves decreasing the dose level of oral contraceptive agents and, if menstrual flow continues to remain low, of shifting to a nonhormonal method of contraception.

Aspirin, even in low doses, can cause gastric irritation as well as inhibition of platelet function with increases in bleeding time (Sullivan 1982). This altered hemostasis can promote gastrointestinal blood loss even in the absence of an anatomic lesion. Loss of 1.5 ml/day would equal normal menstrual blood loss; thus, regular ingestion of aspirin would assist adult males and postmenopausal females to avoid iron deposition in cardiac tissue and so lower their risk of heart disease. An alternative procedure for prevention of iron cardiomyopathy would be the donation of three units of blood/year by adult males and postmenopausal females (Sullivan 1981). Multiple mechanisms whereby removal of excess iron might protect against coronary heart disease have been reviewed by Sullivan (1986). Therapeutic bloodletting is, of course, not novel. It has been used by healers in ancient China, India, Egypt, Israel, and Greece, by indigenous groups in North and South America, by Germanic tribes in Europe, and in Western medicine until the nineteenth century (Weinberg et al. 1986).

A different type of procedure to prevent iron overload is the immunization of children against hepatitis B in countries in which the disease is highly endemic. Reduction in prevalence of the acute illness will lessen the number of eventual carriers of the virus. The decrease in number of carriers will result in fewer hyperferremic individuals at increased risk of developing liver cancer. Another type of enhancement of the iron-withholding system, although not designed to prevent overload, is that of the possible development of immunizing agents against microbial cell surface receptor proteins that bind siderophores, transferrin, or lactoferrin. Immunization with epitopes of such products might interfere with the ability of pathogens to obtain iron from host tissues and fluids.

Management of Iron Overload

In conditions of iron overload in which phlebotomy can be utilized, the procedure may provide normal life expectancy if initiated prior to occurrence of such tissue damage as cirrhosis (Niederau et al. 1985). In contrast, cirrhotic hemochromatosis patients have a shortened life expectancy even when complete iron depletion has been achieved (Niederau et al. 1985). Unfortunately, patients who have hemoglobinopathies often require repeated blood transfusions; thus chelation rather than phlebotomy is required to elute the excess iron. Desferrioxamine, despite its difficulty of administration, remains the drug of choice. A few orally effective iron-chelating agents are being studied but none has been subjected to rigorous, expensive toxicity studies to allow their long-term use in humans (Hershko 1988). Given the extensive array of clinical conditions that are caused or exacerbated by iron overload, however, it is likely that the pharmaceutical industry may soon decide to invest in such studies.

Another medical use for novel iron chelators would be to serve as adjuncts to conventional antiinfective and antitumor chemotherapy. Of course, it would be essential to determine in pure culture that the microbial pathogen or tumor cell derived from the patient would be unable to use the chelator to obtain iron. Moreover, the chelator would need to bind selectively to the invading cells rather than to normal host cells. Even antiinfectives in present use might be functioning, in part, to deprive pathogens of iron. For instance, subinhibitory concentrations of some aminoglycosides suppress the formation of siderophores of *Pseudomonas aeruginosa* (Brown 1986; Morris and Brown 1988). The considerable array of antiinfectives with chelating potential has long been recognized (Weinberg 1957).

In cancer chemotherapy, powerful iron chelators such as parabactin and vibriobactin might be employed to synchronize growth of tumor cells and thus enhance the action of specific antitumor compounds (Bergeron et al. 1986). Chelating drugs that can withdraw iron selectively from tumor cells might also be developed. For example, leukemic blast cells from a 6-week-old infant were cultured and found to be suppressed by desferrioxamine (Estrov et al. 1987). Accordingly, the drug was administered intravenously and, in combination with low-dose cytosine arabinoside, caused a marked leukemic cytoreduction.

Alternatively, the introduction of toxic iron into neoplastic cells by compounds such as adriamycin (doxorubicin) or bleomycin, or into malarial-infected erythrocytes by lactoferrin (Fritsch et al. 1987), might be further explored. Monoclonal antibodies to receptor proteins on microbial cell surfaces or on tumor cells (cf. Taetle et al. 1986) are also candidates for possible development into medicinal agents.

Early Identification of Increased Risk
of Iron Overload

Since iron loading and organ damage can be prevented in hemochromatotic patients if prophylactic phlebotomy is performed *early* in the disease, it is important to detect the condition before onset of clinical symptoms. Edwards et al. (1988) have pointed out that if the estimate that five persons/1000 are homozygous for the hemochromatosis gene is correct, large scale screening of young adults may identify many at risk for organ damage in later life. These authors suggest measuring iron saturation of transferrin in the fasting state in women and men beginning in the 20- to 30-year-old age group during periodic health maintenance examinations.

Transferrin iron saturation values of $\geq 50\%$ in women and $\geq 62\%$ in men then would trigger an assay of their serum ferritin. If the latter is elevated, a liver biopsy would be indicated to confirm the diagnosis. Typing of histocompatability antigens is unnecessary. Transferrin iron saturation and ferritin values would be obtained for siblings and parents of the index patient, and all affected individuals would be urged to have periodic phlebotomy (Edwards et al. 1988).

As important as periodic phlebotomy is education of the individuals affected with hemochromatosis to be aware of and to avoid synergistic factors that might contribute to eventual organ deterioration. Outstanding among these is excessive consumption of alcohol. Other predisposing factors to avoid are megadoses of ascorbic acid, large quantities of red meats, use of iron cookware, and ingestion of cereals adulterated with iron.

Conclusions

Research and clinical observations during the past six decades have shown that humans and other vertebrates attempt to withhold growth-essential iron from bacterial, fungal, protozoan, and neoplastic cells. Powerful iron-binding proteins are stationed at potential sites of microbial cell invasion. Transferrin circulates in plasma and lactoferrin is contained in such exocrine secretions as tears, nasal exudate, saliva, bronchial mucus, gastrointestinal fluid, hepatic bile, cervical mucus, seminal fluid, and milk. Lactoferrin also is a constituent of the specific granules of circulating polymorphonuclear leukocytes. It is released on degranulation of these cells in septic areas. After combining with iron in the invaded sites, the metal-saturated protein is ingested by macrophages.

Macrophages attempt also to withhold iron from neoplastic cells and, as well, during inflammatory episodes, retain iron derived from decaying erythrocytes. Retention of the metal is induced by a hormone, leukocytic endogenous mediator, possibly a member of the interleukin-1 family. During the inflammatory episode, the macrophages synthesize increased amounts of the iron storage proteins, ferritin and hemosiderin. The iron-withholding process has been characterized as a "hypoferremic response to infection and chronic disorders."

The iron-withholding process includes also a suppression of intestinal cell absorption of dietary iron. If the response is prolonged, a low grade anemia may develop. Rarely is this anemia sufficiently severe to require blood transfusions. It is essential that physicians understand the distinction between iron deficiency, a pathological condition, and iron with-holding, a physiological response to insult. The pathological deficiency should be managed by identification and correction of the blood loss and/or by the restoration of proper mineral nutrition. Iron withholding, on the other hand, should *not* be compromised by feeding or injecting excess iron. Rather, the underlying condition that has induced the hypoferremic response should be identified and, if possible, corrected.

Unfortunately, numerous natural and iatrogenic factors can com-promise the iron-withholding defense system. These include (1) factors that promote excessive acquisition of iron via ingestion, injection, or in-halation, or by release of the metal from storage or from ruptured erythrocytes, and (2) factors that prevent adequate synthesis of iron bind-ing and iron storage proteins. Moreover, several cultural factors impair our ability to withhold iron from microbial and neoplastic cell invaders. Among these are use of iron cookware, excessive consumption of red meats, ethanol, and ascorbic acid, use of high dose oral contraceptive agents, and consumption of flour and cereals that have been adulterated with iron.

Excess iron is not readily excreted. Rather, it is stored in cells of the liver, joints, cardiac muscle, pancreas, and pituitary. Thus iron-over-loaded patients have greatly increased risk of hepatic neoplasia, arthro-pathy, cardiomyopathy, diabetes, and other endocrine disorders. Further-more, excess iron suppresses the metabolic functions of lymphocytes and macrophages so as to further impair our defense against infection and various kinds of neoplasia.

It is now possible to identify individuals who especially are predis-posed to iron loading and to communicate the dangers of excessive iron to these persons and their families. Methods for prevention of iron load-ing are self-evident and can be readily adopted. Methods for aiding iron-overloaded patients, however, are not always effective or available. Re-search and development of novel and improved methods and agents are sorely needed.

Notes

1. Superoxide-dependent formation of such reactive radicals as (*OH) is catalyzed by "free" ferric and ferrous ions (Neilands 1984). Hydroxyl radicals are prime candidates as the immediate cause of lipid peroxidation and of scission of DNA strands. Moreover, even the iron stored in intracellular ferritin may be

released *in vivo* to promote superoxide-dependent lipid peroxidation (Thomas et al. 1985).

2. The cytosol contains a large amount of inactive ferritin mRNA (Didsbury et al. 1986). Ferritin subunits possibly are attached to the initiation site. Entry of iron to the cytosol shifts the equilibrium toward assembly of completed ferritin shells so that the ferritin subunits are mobilized and the translatability of ferritin mRNA is increased sharply. Even in liver depleted of RNA by deprivation of protein, ferritin mRNA remains stable (Theil 1987).

3. Ascorbic acid, whether derived from bile, foodstuffs, or synthetic supplements, increases iron uptake by forming a chelate with ferric ions at acid pH that remains soluble at the alkaline pH of the duodenum (Lynch and Cook 1980; Nienhuis 1981).

4. Hemochromatosis, an autosomal recessive disease, formerly was believed to be rare. Presently, the frequency is estimated to be 3–8 homozygotic persons per thousand and 8–10 heterozygotic carriers per hundred (Cook et al. 1976; Edwards et al. 1988).

5. Each 500 ml of transfused whole blood contains approximately 200 mg of hemoglobin iron (Hershko 1988).

6. Chrysolite, crocidolite, and amosite, respectively, contain 3, 27, and 28% iron. The ability of asbestos to catalyze the generation of hydroxyl radicals from peroxide, as well as some of its carcinogenicity, has been attributed to its iron component (Weitzman and Graceffa 1984).

7. In smokers, 0.32 ± 0.009 units/mg; in nonsmokers, 0.42 ± 0.020 units/mg ($p < 0.005$).

8. Desferrioxamine, a siderophore produced by *Streptomyces griseus*, can assist some bacterial and fungal strains to obtain iron from hosts.

9. Low iron derepresses the synthesis by this organism of exotoxin A, elastase, and alkaline protease (Sokol and Woods 1984) as well as alginate (Boyce and Miller 1982).

10. In an *in vitro* study (Turver and Brown 1987), the ability of crocidolite to cause DNA strand breakage was almost completely prevented by desferrioxamine.

11. An intestinal burden of 100 hookworms, for example, can result in a daily loss of 1–5 mg iron (Roche et al. 1957).

12. The clinical use of an antitumor anthracycline, adriamycin, is limited by its dose-dependent cardiomyopathy, which leads to congestive heart failure (Aust et al. 1985). Manifestation of adriamycin cardiotoxicity requires iron and the damage is believed to result from generation of hydroxyl radicals with subsequent lipid peroxidation. Toxicity of the drug has been suppressed in animal heart tissue by superoxide dismutase, catalase, hydroxyl radical scavengers, and iron chelators (Aust et al. 1985).

13. The incidence of diabetes in families of hemochromatotic patients who themselves have the endocrine disease is 6-fold greater than in families of hemochromatotic patients who remain free of diabetes (Hershko 1977).

14. To emphasize the danger of the practice of adding iron to processed foods, "adulteration" rather than "addition" will be used in this chapter. Terms such as "enrichment" and "fortification" mask the injurious nature of iron addition and should be avoided.

References

Abbott, M., A. Galloway, and J.L. Cunningham. 1986. Haemochromatosis presenting with a double *Yersinia* infection. *Journal of Infection* 13:143–145.

Akbar, A.N., P.A. Fitzgerald-Bocarsly, M. de Sousa, P.J. Giardina, M.W. Hilgartner, and R.W. Grady. 1986. Decreased natural killer activity in thalassemia major: A possible consequence of iron overload. *Journal of Immunology* 136:1635–1640.

Alvarez-Hernandez, X., M.V. Felstein, and J.H. Brock. 1986. The relationship between iron release, ferritin synthesis and intracellular iron distribution in mouse peritoneal macrophages. *Biochimica Biophysica Acta* 886:214–222.

Ambrosio, G., J.L. Zweier, W.E. Jacobus, M.L. Weisfeldt, and J.T. Flaherty. 1987. Improvement of postischemic myocardial function and metabolism induced by administration of deferoxamine at the time of reflow: The role of iron in the pathogenesis of reperfusion injury. *Circulation* 76:906–915.

Ambruso, D.R., and R.B. Johnston, Jr. 1981. Lactoferrin enhances hydroxyl radical production by human neutrophils, neutrophil particulate fractions, and an enzyme generating system. *Journal of Clinical Investigation* 67:352–359.

Andreesen, R., J. Osterholz, H. Bodemann, K.J. Bross, U. Costabel, and G.W. Lohr. 1984. Expression of transferrin receptors and intracellular ferritin during terminal differentiation of human monocytes. *Blut* 49:195–202.

Antoine, D., P. Braun, P. Cervoni, P. Schwartz, and P. Lamy. 1979. Le cancer bronchique des mineurs de fer de Lorraine peut-il etre considere comme une maladie professionelle? *Revue French Maladie Respiratoire* 7:63–65.

Anwar, H., M.R.W. Brown, A. Day, and P.H. Weller. 1984. Outer membrane antigens of mucoid *Pseudomonas aeruginosa* isolated directly from the sputum of cystic fibrosis patient. *FEMS Microbiology Letters* 24:235–239.

Artman, M., R.D. Olson, R.J. Boucek, Jr., and R.C. Boerth. 1984. Depression of contractility in isolated rabbit myocardium following exposure to iron: Role of free radicals. *Toxicology and Applied Pharmacology* 72:324–332.

Ashkenazi, R., D. Ben-Schacar, and M.B.H. Youdim. 1982. Nutritional iron and dopamine binding sites in the rat brain. *Pharmacology and Biochemistry of Behavior* 17(Suppl. 1):43–47.

Aust, S.D., L.A. Morehouse, and C.E. Thomas. 1985. Roles of metals in oxygen radical reactions. *Journal of Free Radicals in Biology and Medicine* 1:3–25.

Baggiolini, M., C. DeDuve, P.I. Masson, and J.F. Heremans. 1970. Association of lactoferrin with specific granules in rabbit heterophil leukocytes. *Journal of Experimental Medicine* 131:559–570.

Baldwin, D.A., E.R. Jenny, and P. Aisen. 1984. The effect of human serum transferrin and milk lactoferrin on hydroxyl radical formation from superoxide and hydrogen peroxide. *Journal of Biological Chemistry* 259:13391–13394.

Ballart, I.J., M.E. Estevez, L. Sen, R.A. Diez, J. Giuntoli, S.A. deMiani, and J. Penalver. 1986. Progressive dysfunction of monocytes associated with iron overload and age in patients with thalassemia major. *Blood* 67:105–109.

Barber, W.H. 1988. Fetal hemoglobin and erythropoietin. *New England Journal of Medicine* 318:449.

Barry, D.M.J., and A.W. Reeve. 1977. Increased incidence of gram negative neonatal sepsis with intramuscular iron administration. *Pediatrics* 60:908–912.

Beamish, M.R., P.A. Jones, D. Trevett, I.H. Evans, and A. Jacobs. 1972. Iron metabolism in Hodgkin's disease. *British Journal of Cancer* 26:444–452.

Becroft, D.M.O., M.R. Dix, and K. Farmer. 1977. Intramuscular iron dextran and susceptibility of neonates to bacterial infection. *Archives of Diseases of Children* 52:778–781.

Bengtsson, N.O., and L. Hardell. 1986. Porphyrias, porphyrins, and hepatocellular cancer. *British Journal of Cancer* 54:115–117.

Beresford, C.H., R.J. Neale, and O.G. Brooks. 1971. Iron absorption and pyrexia. *Lancet* 1:568–572.

Bergeron, R.J. 1986. Iron: A controlling nutrient in proliferating processes. *Trends in Biochemical Science* 11:133–136.

Bergeron, R.J., P. Braylan, S. Goldey, and M. Ingeno. 1986. Effects of the *Vibrio cholerae* siderophore vibriobactin on the growth characteristics of L1210 cells. *Biochemical and Biophysical Research Communications* 136:273–280.

Berman, C. 1958. Primary carcinoma of the liver. *Advances in Cancer Research* 5:55–96.

Bernstein, S.E. 1987. Hereditary hypotransferrinemia with hemosiderosis, a murine disorder resembling human atransferrinemia. *Journal of Laboratory and Clinical Medicine* 110:690–705.

Bezkorovainy, A. 1977. Human milk and colostrum proteins: A review. *Journal of Diary Science* 60:1023–1037.

Bezkorovainy, A. 1980. *Biochemistry of Nonheme Iron,* pp. 127–206. New York: Plenum Press.

Biemond, P., A.J.G. Swaak, H.G. van Euk, and J.F. Koster. 1988. Superoxide dependent iron release from ferritin in inflammatory diseases. *Journal of Free Radicals in Biology and Medicine* 4:185–198.

Biya, L.M., and W.C. Roberts. 1971. Iron in the heart. *American Journal of Medicine* 51:202–221.

Blake, D.R., and P.A. Bacon. 1982. Iron and rheumatoid disease. *Lancet* 1:623.

Blake, D.R., N.D. Hall, P.A. Bacon, P.A. Dieppe, B. Halliwell, and J.M.C. Gutteridge. 1981. The importance of iron in rheumatoid disease. *Lancet* 2:1142–1143.

Boelaert, J.R., H.W. van Landuyt, Y.J. Valcke, B. Cantinieaux, W.F. Lornoy, J-L. Vanherweghem, P. Moreillon, and J.M. Vandepitte. 1987. The role of iron overload in *Yersinia enterocolitica* and *Yersinia pseudotuberculosis* bacteremia in hemodialysis patients. *Journal of Infectious Diseases* 156:384–387.

Boesman-Finkelstein, M., and R.A. Finkelstein. 1985. Antimicrobial effects of human milk: Inhibitory activity on enteric pathogens. *FEMS Microbiology Letters* 27:167–174.

Bomford, A.B., and H.N. Munro. 1985. Transferrin and its receptor: Their roles in cell function. *Hepatology* 5:870–875.

Bomford, A.B., and R. Williams. 1976. Long-term results of venesection therapy in idiopathic hemochromatosis. *Quarterly Journal of Medicine* 45:611–623.

Bothwell, T.H., and R.W. Charlton. 1979. Current problems of iron overload. *Recent Results in Cancer Research* 69:86–95.

Bowering, J., A.M. Sanchez, and M.I. Irwin. 1976. A conspectus of research on iron requirements in man. *Journal of Nutrition* 106:985–1074.

Boyce, J.R., and R.V. Miller. 1982. Selection of nonmucoid derivatives of mucoid *Pseudomonas aeruginosa* is strongly influenced by the level of iron in the culture medium. *Infection and Immunity* 37:695–701.

Boyce, N., N.M. Thomson, C. Wood, R.C. Atkins, and S. Holdsworth. 1985. Life-threatening sepsis complicating heavy metal chelation therapy with desferrioxamine. *Australia and New Zealand Journal of Medicine* 15:654–655.

Bregman, H., M.C. Gelfand, J.F. Winchester, H.J. Manz, J.H. Knepshield, and G.E. Schreiner. 1980. Iron-overload-associated myopathy in patients on maintenance haemodialysis: A histocompatability-linked disorder. *Lancet* 2:882–885.

Breton-Gorius, J., D.V. Mason, D. Buriot, J-L. Vilde, and C. Griscelli. 1980. Lactoferrin deficiency as a consequence of a lack of specific granules in neutrophils from a patient with recurrent infections. *American Journal of Pathology* 99:413–419.

Brock, J.H. 1980. Lactoferrin in human milk: its role in iron absorption and protection against enteric infection in the newborn infant. *Archives of Diseases in Children* 55:417–421.

Brock, J.H. 1981. The effect of iron and transferrin on the response of serum-free cultures of mouse lymphocytes to concanavalin A and lipopolysaccharide. *Immunology* 43:387–392.

Brown, A.E. 1986. Ferrous complexes and chelating compounds in suppression of fungal diseases of cereals. In *Iron, Siderophores, and Plant Diseases.* T.R. Swinburne, ed., pp. 233–242. New York: Plenum Press.

Bruce, R.M., and L. Wise. 1977. Tuberculosis after jejunoileal bypass. *Annals of Internal Medicine* 87:574–576.

Burger, F.J., and Z.A. Hogwind. 1974. Changes in trace elements in kwashiorkor. *South African Medical Journal* 48:502–504.

Burrow, L., and P. Tartter. 1982. Effect of blood transfusions on colonic malignancy recurrence rate. *Lancet* 2:662.

Butzler, J.P., M. Alexander, A. Segers, N. Cremer, and D. Blum. 1978. Enteritis, abscess, and septicemia due to *Yesinia enterocolitica* in a child with thalassemia. *Journal of Pediatrics* 93:619–621.

Campbell,W.G., M.A. Raskind, T. Gordon, and M. Shaw. 1985. Iron pigment in the brain of man with tardive dyskinesia. *American Journal of Psychiatry* 142:364–365.

Cartwright, G.E., M.A. Lauritzen, P.J. Jones, I.M. Merrill, and M.M. Wintrobe. 1946. The anemia of infection. I. Hypoferremia, hypercupremia, and alterations in porphyrin metabolism in patients. *Journal of Clinical Investigation* 25:65–80.

Cavell, P.A., and E.M. Widdowson. 1964. Intakes and excretions of iron, copper, and zinc in the postnatal period. *Archives of Diseases in Children* 39:496–501.

Centerwall, B.S. 1981. Premenopausal hysterectomy and cardiovascular disease. *American Journal of Obstetrics and Gynecology* 139:58–61.

Chapman, R.W., M.Y. Morgan, M. Laulicht, A.V. Hoffbrand, and S. Sherlock. 1982. Hepatic iron stores and markers of iron overload in alcoholics and patients with idiopathic hemochromatosis. *Digestive Disease Science* 27: 909–916.

Charlton, R.W., P. Jacobs, H. Seftel, and T.H. Bothwell. 1964. Effect of alcohol on iron absorption. *British Medical Journal* 2:1427–1429.

Chiesa, C., L. Pacifico, F. Renzulli, M. Midulla, and L. Garlaschi. 1987. *Yersinia* hepatic abscesses and iron overload. *Journal of the American Medical Association* 257:3230–3231.

Connolly, K.M., V.J. Stecher, and L. Kent. 1988. Examination of interleukin-l activity, the acute phase response, and leukocyte subpopulations in rats with adjuvant-induced arthritis. *Journal of Laboratory and Clinical Medicine* 111: 341–347.

Conrad, M.E., and J.C. Barton. 1981. Factors affecting iron balance. *American Journal of Hematology* 10:199–225.

Cook, J.D., C.A. Finch, and N.J. Smith. 1976. Evaluation of the iron status of a population. *Blood* 48:449–454.

Cook, J.D., S.S. Watson, K.M. Simpson, D.A. Lipschitz, and B.S. Skikne. 1984. The effect of high ascorbic acid supplementation on body iron stores. *Blood* 64:721–726.

Cordes, L.C., E.W. Brink, P.J. Checko, A. Lentner, R.W. Lyons, P.S. Hayes, T.C. Wu, D.G. Tharr, and D.W. Fraser. 1981. A cluster of *Acinetobacter* pneumonia in foundry workers. *Annals of Internal Medicine* 95:688–693.

Crosby, W.H. 1978. The safety of iron-fortified food. *Journal of the American Medical Association* 239:2026–2027.

Dallman, P.R. 1986. Biochemical basis for the manifestations of iron deficiency. *Annual Review of Nutrition* 6:13–40.

Deiss, A. 1983. Iron metabolism in reticuloendothelial cells. *Seminars in Hematology* 20:81–90.

de Sousa, M. 1978. Lymphoid cell positioning: A new proposal for the mechanism of control of lymphoid cell migration. *Symposia of the Society of Experimental Biology* 32:393–409.

de Sousa, M., and D. Potaznik. 1984. Proteins of the metabolism of iron, cells of the immune system, and malignancy. In *Vitamins, Nutrition, and Cancer*. D. Prasad, ed., pp. 231–239. Basel: Karger.

de Sousa, M., R. Dynesius-Trentham, F. Mota-Garcia, M.T. da Silva, and D.E. Trentham. 1988. Activation of rat synovium by iron. *Arthritis and Rheumatism* 31:653–661.

de Vernejoul, A. Pointillart, C. Cywiner-Golenzer, C. Morieux, J. Bielakoff, D. Modrowski, and L. Miravet. 1984. Effects of iron overload on bone remodeling in pigs. *American Journal of Pathology* 116:377–384.

Didsbury, J.R., E.C. Theil, R.E. Kaufman, and L.F. Dickey. 1986. Multiple red cell ferritin mRNAs, which code for an abundant protein in the embryonic cell type, analyzed by cDNA sequence and by primer extension of the 5'-untranslated regions. *Journal of Biological Chemistry* 261:949–955.

Dinarello, C.A. 1984. Interleukin-1 and the pathogenesis of the acute phase response. *New England Journal of Medicine* 311:1413–1418.

Dreyfus, J.R. 1936. Lungencarcinom bei Geschwistern nach Inhalation von eisenoxyhaltigem Staub der Jugend. *Zeitschrift für Klinische Medizin* 130: 256–260.

Dubach, R., S.T.E. Callender, and C.V. Moore. 1948. Studies in iron transportation and metabolism. VI. Absorption of radioactive iron in patients with fever and with anemias of varied etiology. *Blood* 3:526–542.

Duncan, B., R.B. Schifman, J.J. Corrigan, Jr., and C. Schaefer. 1985. Iron and the exclusively breast-fed infant from birth to six months. *Journal of Pediatric Gastroenterology and Nutrition* 4:421–425.

Edwards, C.Q., L.M., Griffen, D. Goldgar, C. Drummond, M.H. Skolnick, and J.P. Kushner. 1988. Prevalence of hemochromatosis among 11,065 presumably healthy blood donors. *New England Journal of Medicine* 318:1355–1362.

Erlandson, M.E., B. Walden, G. Stern, M.W. Hilgartner, J. Wehman, and C.H. Smith. 1962. Studies on congenital hemolytic syndrome. IV. Gastrointestinal absorption of iron. *Blood* 19:359–369.

Eschbach, J.W., J.C. Egrie, M.R. Downing, J.K. Browne, and J.W. Adamson. 1987. Correction of the anemia of end-stage renal disease with recombinant human erythropoietin. *New England Journal of Medicine* 316:73–78.

Estrov, Z., A. Tawa, X-H. Wang, I.D. Dube, H. Sulh, A. Cohen, E.W. Gelfand, and M.H. Freedman. 1987. In vitro and in vivo effects of deferoxamine in neonatal acute leukemia. *Blood* 69:757–761.

Evans, A.E., G.J. D'angio, K. Propert, J. Anderson, and H-W. L. Hann. 1987. Prognostic factors in neuroblastoma. *Cancer* 59:1853–1859.

Fellows, I.W., M. Stewart, W.J. Jeffcoate, P.G. Smith, and P.J. Toghill. 1988. Hepatocellular carcinoma in primary hemochromatosis. *Gut* 29:1603–1606.

Feltelius, N., U. Lindh, P. Venge, and R. Hallgren. 1986. Ankylosing spondylitis: a chronic inflammatory disease with iron overload in granulocytes and platelets. *Annals of the Rheumatic Diseases* 45:827–831.

Frassinelli-Gunderson, E.P., S. Margen, and J.R. Brown. 1985. Iron stores in users of oral contraceptive agents. *American Journal of Clinical Nutrition* 41: 703–712.

Frieden, E., and S. Osaki. 1974. Ferroxidases and ferrireductases: their role in iron metabolism. *Advances in Experimental Medicine and Biology* 48:235–265.

Fritsch, G., G. Sawatzki, J. Treumer, A. Jung, and D.T. Spira. 1987. *Plasmodium falciparum*: inhibition *in vitro* with lactoferrin, desferriferrithiocin, and desferricrocin. *Experimental Parasitology* 63:1–9.

Furst, A. 1960. Chelation and cancer: discussion. In *Metal-Binding in Medicine*. M.J. Seven and L.A. Johnson, eds., p. 346. Philadelphia: J.B. Lippincott.

Gallant, T., M.H. Freedman, H. Velland, and W.H. Francombe. 1986. *Yersinia* sepsis in patients with iron overload treated with deferoxamine. *New England Journal of Medicine* 314:1643.

Garn, S.M., M.T. Keating, and F. Falkner. 1981. Hematological status and pregnancy outcomes. *American Journal of Clinical Nutrition* 34:115–117.

Good, M.F., D.E. Chapman, L.W. Powell, and J.W. Halliday. 1987. The effect of experimental iron-overload on splenic T cell function: Analysis using clonal techniques. *Clinical Experimental Immunology* 68:375–383.

Goodill, J.J., and J.G. Abuelo. 1987. Mucormycosis—a new risk of deferoxamine therapy in dialysis patients with aluminum or iron overload. *New England Journal of Medicine* 317:54.

Gordeuk, V.R., R.D. Boyd, and G.M. Brittenham. 1986. Dietary iron overload persists in rural sub-Saharan Africa. *Lancet* 1:1310–1313.

Gordeuk, V.R., P. Prithviraj, T. Dolinar, and G.M. Brittenham. 1988. Interleukin-l administration in mice produces hypoferremia despite neutropenia. *Journal of Clinical Investigation* 82:1934–1938.

Gordon, T., W.B. Kannel, M.C. Hjortland, and P.M. McNamara. 1978. Menopause and coronary heart disease. *Annals of Internal Medicine* 89:157–161.

Graf, E., and J.W. Eaton. 1985. Dietary suppression of colonic cancer. *Cancer* 56:717–718.

Gross, R.L., and P.M. Newberne. 1980. Role of nutrition in immunologic function. *Physiological Reviews* 60:188–302.

Groves, M.I. 1960. The isolation of a red protein from milk. *Journal of the American Chemical Society* 82:3345–3350.

Hallberg, L., L. Rossander, and A.-B. Skanberg. 1987. Phytates and the inhibitory effect of bran on iron absorption in man. *American Journal of Clinical Nutrition* 45:988–996.

Halliwell, B., and J.M.C. Gutteridge. 1984. Oxygen toxicity, oxygen radicals, transition metals and disease. *Biochemical Journal* 219:1–14.

Hart, R.C., S. Kadis, and W.L. Chapman. 1982. Relationship of nutritional iron deficiency to susceptibility to *Proteus mirabilis* pyelonephritis in the rat. *Canadian Journal of Microbiology* 28:713–717.

Hemminki, E., and B. Starfield. 1978. Routine administration of iron and vitamins during pregnancy: review of controlled clinical trials. *British Journal of Obstetrics and Gynaecology* 85:404–410.

Henry, W. 1979. Echocardiographic evaluation of the heart in thalassemia major. *Annals of Internal Medicine* 91:892–894.

Hershko, C. 1977. Storage iron regulation. *Progress in Hematology* 10:105–147.

Hershko, C. 1988. Oral chelating drugs: coming but not yet ready for clinical use. *British Medical Journal* 296:1081–1082.

Hershko, C., J.D. Cook, and C.A. Finch. 1974. Storage iron kinetics. VI. The effect of inflammation on iron exchange in the rat. *British Journal of Haematology* 28:67–75.

Hershko, C., G. Link, and A. Pinson. 1987. Modification of iron uptake by hypoxia, ascorbic acid, and α-tocopherol in iron-loaded rat myocardial cell cultures. *Journal of Laboratory and Clinical Medicine* 110:355–361.

Hibbard, B.M. 1988. Iron and folate supplements during pregnancy: Supplementation is valuable only in selected patients. *British Medical Journal* 297:1324–1326.

Holmberg, C.G., and C-B. Laurell. 1947. Investigations in serum copper. I. Nature of serum copper and its relation to the iron-binding protein in human serum. *Acta Chemica Scandinavia* 1:944–950.

Irving, M.G., J.W. Halliday, and L.W. Powell. 1988. Association between alcoholism and increased hepatic iron stores. *Alcoholism: Clinical and Experimental Research* 12:7–13.

Jackson,A.M., and M.H.N. Golden. 1978. The human rumen. *Lancet* 2:764–766.

Jacobs, A., B. Jones, C. Ricketts, R.D. Bulbrook, and D.Y. Wang. 1976. Serum ferritin concentration in early breast cancer. *British Journal of Cancer* 34:286–290.

Jacobs, P., T.H. Bothwell, and R.W. Charlton. 1964. Role of hydrochloric acid in iron absorption. *Journal of Applied Physiology* 19:187–188.

John, D.T. 1982. Primary amebic meningoencephalitis and the biology of *Naegleria fowleri*. *Annual Review of Microbiology* 36:101–123.

Johnson, P.J., N. Krasner, B. Portmann, A.L.W.F. Eddleston, and R. Williams. 1978. Hepatocellular carcinoma in Great Britain: Influence of age, sex, Hb$_s$Ag status, and aetiology of underlying cirrhosis. *Gut* 19:1022–1026.

Kaplan, J., S. Sarnaik, J. Gitlin, and J. Lusher. 1984. Diminished helper/suppressor lymphocyte ratios and natural killer activity in recipients of repeated blood transfusions. *Blood* 64:308–310.

Kent, S., E.D. Weinberg, and P. Stuart-Macadam. 1990. Dietary and medical prophylactic iron supplements: Helpful or harmful? *Human Nature* 1:53–79.

Klatsky, A.L., M.A. Armstrong, G.D. Friedman, and R.A. Hiatt. 1988. The relations of alcoholic beverage use to colon and rectal cancer. *American Journal of Epidemiology* 128:1007–1015.

Kondo, H., K. Saito, J.P. Grasso, and P. Aisen. 1988. Iron metabolism in the erythrophagocytosing Kupffer cell. *Hepatology* 8:32–38.

Lamon, J.M., S. Marynick, R. Rosenblatt, and S. Donnelly. 1979. Idiopathic hemochromatosis in a young female. *Gastroenterology* 76:178–183.

Leikin, S.L. 1960. The use of intramuscular iron in the prophylaxis of iron deficiency anemia of prematurity. *American Journal of Diseases of Children* 99:739–745.

Lima, M.F., and F. Kierszenbaum. 1987. Lactoferrin effects on phagocytic cell function. *Journal of Immunology* 139:1647–1651.

Locke, A., E.R. Main, and D.O. Rosbach. 1932. The copper and non-hemoglobinous iron content of the blood serum in disease. *Journal of Clinical Investigation* 11:527–542.

Lombard, M., A. Bomford, M. Hynes, N.V. Naoumov, S. Roberts, J. Crowe, and R. Williams. 1989. Regulation of the hepatic transferrin receptor in hereditary hemochromatosis. *Hepatology* 9:1–5.

Longnecker, M.P., J.A. Berlin, M.J. Orza, and T.C. Chalmers. 1988. A meta-analysis of alcohol consumption in relation to risk of breast cancer. *Journal of the American Medical Association* 260:652–656.

Lustbader, E.D., H-W. L. Hann, and B.S. Blumberg. 1983. Serum ferritin as a predictor of host response to hepatitis B virus infection. *Science* 220:423–425.

Lynch, S.R., and J.D. Cook. 1980. Interaction of vitamin C and iron. *Annals of the New York Academy of Sciences* 355:32–44.

McFarlane, H., S. Reddy, K.J. Adcock, H. Adeshima, A.R. Cooke, and J. Akene. 1970. Immunity, transferrin, and survival in kwashiorkor. *British Medical Journal* 4:268–270.

McGowan, S.E., and S.A. Henley. 1988. Iron and ferritin contents and distribution in human alveolar macrophages. *Journal of Laboratory and Clinical Medicine* 111:611–617.

McLaren, G.D., W.A. Muir, and R.W. Kellerman. 1983. Iron overload disorders: Natural history, pathogenesis, diagnosis, and therapy. *CRC Clinical Reviews of Laboratory Sciences* 19:205–266.

Mehtar, S. 1988. Adult epiglottitis due to *Vibrio vulnificus*. *British Medical Journal* 296:827–828.

Melby, K., S. Slordahl, T.J. Gutteberg, and S.A. Nordbro. 1982. Septicaemia due to *Yersinia enterocolitica* after oral overdoses of iron. *British Medical Journal* 285:467–468.

Meyer, T.E., C. Kassianides, T.H. Bothwell, and A. Green. 1984. Effects of heavy alcohol consumption on serum ferritin concentrations. *South African Medical Journal* 66:573–575.

Meyer, T.E., D. Ballot, T.H. Bothwell, A. Green, D.P. Derman, R.D. Baynes, T. Jenkins, P.L. Jooste, E.D. Du Toit, and P. Jacobs. 1987. The HLA linked iron loading gene in an Afrikaner population. *Journal of Medical Genetics* 24:348–356.

Milder, M.S., J.D. Cook, S. Stray, and C.A. Finch. 1980. Idiopathic hemochromatosis, an interim report. *Medicine* 59:34–49.

Morris, E.R. 1983. An overview of current information on bioavailability of dietary iron to humans. *Federation Proceedings* 42:1716–1720.

Morris, G., and M.R.W. Brown. 1988. Novel modes of action of aminoglycoside antibiotics against *Pseudomonas aeruginosa*. *Lancet* 1:1359–1360.

Mossey, R.T., and J. Sondheimer. 1985. Listeriosis in patients with long-term hemodialysis and transfusional iron overload. *American Journal of Medicine* 79:397–400.

Murphy, B.F. 1974. Hazards of children's vitamin preparations containing iron. *Journal of American Medical Association* 229:324.

Neffgen, J.F., and K. Rakusan. 1975. Iron supplementation in suckling rats: its effect on the heart. *Recent Advances in Study of Cardiac Structure and Metabolism* 10:707–716.

Neilands, J.B. 1981. Iron absorption and transport in microorganisms. *Annual Review of Nutrition* 1:27–45.

Neilands, J.B. 1984. Methodology of siderophores. *Structure and Bonding* 58:1–24.

Niederau, C., R. Fischer, A. Sonnenberg, W. Stremmel, H.J. Trampisch, and G. Strohmeyer. 1985. Survival and causes of death in cirrhotic and in noncirrhotic patients with primary hemochromatosis. *New England Journal of Medicine* 313:1256–1262.

Nienhuis, A.W. 1981. Vitamin C and iron. *New England Journal of Medicine* 304:170–171.

Ohnishi, K., S. Iida, S. Iwama, N. Goto, F. Nomura, M. Takashi, A. Mishima, K. Kono, K. Kimura, H. Musha, K. Kototo, and K. Okuda. 1982. The effect of chronic habitual alcohol intake on the development of liver cirrhosis and hepatocellular carcinoma. *Cancer* 49:672–677.

Olsson, K.S., P.A. Heedman, and F. Staugard. 1978. Preclinical hemochromatosis in a population on a high-iron-fortified diet. *Journal of American Medical Association* 239:1999–2000.

Olusi, S.O., and H. McFarlane. 1978. Iron therapy and refeeding in experimentally malnourished rats. *Pediatric Research* 12:625–630.

Oppenheimer, S.J., F.D. Gibson, S.B. MacFarlane, J.B. Moody, C. Harrison, A. Spencer, and O. Bunari. 1986a. Iron supplementation increases prevalence and effects of malaria: Report on clinical studies in Papua New Guinea. *Transactions of Royal Society of Tropical Medicine and Hygiene* 80:603–612.

Oppenheimer, S.J., S.B.J. MacFarlane, J.B. Moody, O. Bunari, and R.G. Henrickse. 1986b. Effect of iron prophylaxis on morbidity due to infectious disease: Report on clinical studies in Papua New Guinea. *Transactions of Royal Society of Tropical Medicine and Hygiene* 80:596–602.

Oski, F.A. 1976. Anemia in children. *Hospital Practice* 63–72.

Pacht, E.R., and W.B. Davis. 1988. Decreased ceruloplasmin ferroxidase activity in cigarette smokers. *Journal of Laboratory and Clinical Medicine* 111:661–668.

Pardolos, G., F. Kanakoudi-Tsakalidis, M. Malaka-Zafiriu, H. Tsantali, M. Athanasiou-Metaxa, G. Kallinikos, and G. Papaevangelou. 1987. Iron-related disturbances in multitransfused children. *Clinical Experimental Immunology* 68:138–143.

Parkin, J.D., B. Rush, R.J. DeGroot, and R.S. Budd. 1974. Iron absorption after splenectomy in hereditary spherocytosis. *Australia and New Zealand Journal of Medicine* 4:58–61.

Pekarek, R.S., K.A. Bostian, P.J. Bartelloni, F.M. Calia, and W.R. Beisel. 1969. The effects of *Francisella tularensis* infection on iron metabolism in man. *American Journal of Medical Sciences* 258:14–25.

Pickleman, J.R., L.S. Evans, J.K. Kane, and R.J. Freeark. 1975. Tuberculosis after jejunoileal bypass for obesity. *Journal of American Medical Association* 234:744

Pootrakul, P., R. Rugiatsakul, and P. Wasi. 1980. Increased transferrin iron saturation in splenectomized thalassemic patients. *British Journal of haematology* 46:143–145.

Potaznik, D., S. Groshen, D. Miller, R. Bagin, R. Bhalla, M. Schwartz, and M. de Sousa. 1987. Association of serum iron, serum transferrin saturation, and serum ferritin with survival in acute lymphocytic leukemia. *The American Journal of Pediatric Hematology/Oncology* 9:350–355.

Powell, L.W. 1970. Tissue damage in haemochromatosis. An analysis of the roles of iron and alcoholism. *Gut* 11:980.

Price, V.E., and R.E. Greenfield. 1958. Anemia in cancer. *Advances in Cancer Research* 5:199–284.

Purtillo, D.T., and L.S. Gottlieb. 1973. Cirrhosis and hepatoma occurring at Boston City Hospital (1917–1968). *Cancer* 32:458–462.

Quinn, F.D., and E.D. Weinberg. 1988. Killing of *Legionella pneumophila* by human serum and iron-binding agents. *Current Microbiology* 17:111–116.

Rao, K.V., and W.R. Anderson. 1982. Hemosiderosis: an unrecognized complication in renal allograft recipients. *Transplantation* 33:115–117.

Reiter, B. 1978. Review of the progress of dairy science: antimicrobial systems in milk. *Journal of Dairy Research* 45:131–147.

Robertson, A.G., and W.C. Dick. 1977. Intramuscular iron and local oncogenesis. *British Medical Journal* 1:946.

Robertson, M.A., J.S. Harrington, and E. Bradshaw. 1971. The cancer pattern in African Gold mines. *British Journal of Cancer* 25:395–402.

Roche, M., M.E. Perez-Gimenez, M. Layrisse, and E. Di Prisco. 1957. Study of urinary and fecal excretion of radioactive chromium Cr^{51} in man. Its use in the measurement of intestinal blood loss associated with hookworm infection. *Journal of Clinical Investigation* 36:1183–1192.

Rodriguez, M.C.N., M.S. Henriquez, A.F.D. Turon, F.J. Novoa, J.G. Diaz, and P.B. Leon. 1986. Trace elements in chronic alcoholism. *Trace Elements in Medicine* 3:164–167.

Rohan, T.E., and A.J. McMichael. 1988. Alcohol consumption and risk of breast cancer. *International Journal of Cancer* 41:695–699.

Rosenberg, S.A., C.A. Seipp, D.E. White, and R. Wesley. 1985. Perioperative blood transfusions are associated with increased rates of recurrence and decreased survival in patients with high-grade soft-tissue sarcomas of the extremities. *Journal of Clinical Oncology* 3:698–709.

Salmi, T., P. Hanninen, and T. Peltonen. 1963. Applicability of chelated iron in the care of prematures. *Acta Paediatrica Scandinavia* 140:114–115.

Schade, A.L., and L. Caroline. 1944. Raw hen egg white and the role of iron in growth inhibition of *Shigella dysenteriae, Staphylococcus aureus, Escherichia coli,* and *Saccharomyces cerevisiae. Science* 100:14–15.

Schade, A.L., and L. Caroline. 1946. An iron-binding component in human blood plasma. *Science* 104:340–341.

Schafer, A.I., R.G. Cheron, R. Dluhy, B. Cooper, R.E. Gleason, J.S. Soeldner, and H.F. Bunn. 1981. Clinical pathological consequences of acquired transfusional overload in adults. *New England Journal of Medicine* 304:319–324.

Scharnetzky, M., R. König, M. Lakomek, W. Tillman, and W. Schröter. 1984. Prophylaxis of systemic yersiniosis in thalassemia major. *Lancet* 1:791–792.

Selby, J.V., and G.D. Friedman. 1988. Epidemiologic evidence of an association between body iron stores and risk of cancer. *International Journal of Cancer* 41:677–682.

Selden, C., M. Owen, J.M.P. Hopkinds, and T.J. Peters. 1980. Studies on the concentration and intracellular localization of iron proteins in liver biopsy specimens from patients with iron overload with special reference to their role in lysosomal disruption. *British Journal of Haematology* 44:593–603.

Sethi, V.S., Z. Shihabi, and C.L. Spurr. 1984. Increase of serum iron concentrations in Rhesus monkeys and humans on administration of vincristine, vinblastine, or vindesine. *Cancer Treatment Reports* 68:933–936.

Shagrin, J.W., B. Frame, and H. Duncan. 1971. Polyarthritis in obese patients with intestinal bypass. *Annals of Internal Medicine* 75:377–380.

Sherlock, S. 1976. Hemochromatosis: Course and treatment. *Annual Review of Medicine* 27:143–149.

Sherman, A.R., and J.F. Lockwood. 1987. Impaired natural killer cell activity in iron-deficient rat pups. *Journal of Nutrition* 117:567–571.

Shoji, A., and E. Ozawa. 1986. Necessity of transferrin for RNA synthesis in chick myotubules. *Journal of Cellular Physiology* 127:349–356.

Siemons, L.J., and C. Mahler. 1987. Hypogonadotropic hypogonadism in hemochromatosis: Recovery of reproductive function after iron depletion. *Journal of Clinical Endocrinology and Metabolism* 65:585–587.

Siimes, M.A., L. Salmenpera, and J. Perheentopa. 1984. Exclusive breast feeding for 9 months: Risk of iron deficiency. *Journal of Pediatrics* 104:196–199.

Slater, K., and J. Fletcher. 1987. Lactoferrin derived from neutrophils inhibits the mixed lymphocyte reaction. *Blood* 69:1328–1333.

Slone, D., S. Shapiro, D. Kaufman, L. Rosenberg, O.S. Miettinen, and P.D. Stolley. 1981. Risk of myocardial infarction in relation to current and discontinued use of oral contraceptives. *New England Journal of Medicine* 305:420–424.

Smith, Q.T., M. Krupp, and M.J. Hamilton. 1981. Salivary lactoferrin in cystic fibrosis. *IRCS Medical Science: Biochemistry* 9:1040–1041.

Smithyman, A.M., G. Munn, B. Koznier, C.T.C. Tan, and M. de Sousa. 1978. Spleen cell populations in Hodgkin's disease. *Advances in Experimental Medicine and Biology* 114:585–588.

Sokol, P.A., and D.E. Woods. 1984. Relationship of iron and extracellular virulence factors to *Pseudomonas aeruginosa* lung infections. *Journal of Medical Microbiology* 18:125–133.

Stevens, R.G., S. Kuvibidila, M. Kapps, J.S. Friedlaender, and B.S. Blumberg. 1983. Iron-binding proteins, hepatitis B virus, and mortality in the Solomon Islands. *American Journal of Epidemiology* 118:550–561.

Stevens, R.G., R.P. Beasley, and B.S. Blumberg. 1986. Iron-binding proteins and risk of cancer in Taiwan. *Journal of National Cancer Institute* 76:605–610.

Stevens, R.G., D.Y. Jones, M.S. Micozzi, and P.R. Taylor. 1988. Body iron stores and the risk of cancer. *New England Journal of Medicine* 319:1047–1052.

Stich, H.F., L. Wei, and R.F. Whiting. 1979. Enhancement of the chromosome-damaging action o f ascorbate by transition metals. *Cancer Research* 39: 4145–4151.

Sullivan, J.L. 1981. Iron and the sex difference in heart disease risk. *Lancet* 1: 1293–1294.

Sullivan, J.L. 1982. Iron, aspirin, and heart disease risk. *Journal of American Medical Association* 247:751.

Sullivan, J.L. 1983. Vegetarianism, ischemic heart disease, and iron. *American Journal of Clinical Nutrition* 37:882–883.

Sullivan, J.L. 1986. Sex, iron, and heart disease. *Lancet* 2:1162.

Taetle, R., J. Castagnola, and J. Mendelsohn. 1986. Mechanisms of growth inhibition by anti-transferrin receptor monoclonal antibodies. *Cancer Research* 46:1759–1763.

Theil, E.C. 1987. Ferritin: Structure, gene regulation, and cellular function in animals, plants, and microorganisms. *Annual Review of Biochemistry* 56:289–315.

Thein, M., G.H. Beaton, H. Milne, and M.J. Veen. 1969. Oral contraceptive drugs: some observations on their effect on menstrual loss and hematological indices. *Canadian Medical Association Journal* 101:73–76.

Thomas, C.E., L.A. Morehouse, and S.D. Aust. 1985. Ferritin and superoxide-dependent lipid peroxidation. *Journal of Biological Chemistry* 260:3275–3280.

Tonz, O., S. Weiss, H.W. Strahm, and E. Rossi. 1965. Iron absorption in cystic fibrosis. *Lancet* 2:1096–1099.

Turver, C.J., and R.C. Brown. 1987. The role of catalytic iron in asbestos induced lipid peroxidation and DNA-strand breakage in C3H10T$\frac{1}{2}$ cells. *British Journal of Cancer* 56:133–136.

Tustin, A.W., A.B. Kaiser, R.W. Bradsher, and J.L. Herrington. 1980. Unusual fungal infections following jejunoileal bypass surgery. *Archives of Internal Medicine* 140:643–645.

Van Asbeck, B.S., J.J.M. Marx, A. Struyvenberg, and J. Verhoeff. 1982. Defects of phagocytic cells in patients with iron overload. *Antonie van Leeuwenhoek Journal of Microbiology and Serology* 48:192–194.

van der Meer, J.W.M., M. Barza, S.M. Wolff, and C.A. Dinarello. 1988. A low dose of recombinant interleukin 1 protects granulocytopenic mice from lethal gram-negative infection. *Proceedings of the National Academy of Sciences U.S.A.* 85:1620–1624.

Wadsworth, G.R. 1975. Nutritional factors in anaemia. *World Review of Nutrition and Dietetics* 21:75–150.

Weinberg, E.D. 1957. The mutual effects of antimicrobial compounds and metallic cations. *Bacteriological Reviews* 21:46–68.

Weinberg, E.D. 1974. Iron and susceptibility to infectious disease. *Science* 184:952–956.

Weinberg, E.D. 1978. Iron and infection. *Microbiological Reviews* 42:45–66.

Weinberg, E.D. 1981. Iron and neoplasia. *Biological Trace Element Research* 3:55–80.

Weinberg, E.D. 1984. Iron withholding: A defense against infection and neoplasia. *Physiological Reviews* 64:65–102.

Weinberg, E.D. 1986. Regulation of secondary metabolism by trace metals. In *Cell Metabolism: Growth and Environment*. T.A.V. Subramanian, ed., pp. 151–160. Boca Raton: Chemical Rubber Corporation Press.

Weinberg, E.D. 1987. DF-2 sepsis: A sequela of sideremia? *Medical Hypotheses* 24:287–289.

Weinberg, E.D. 1989. Cellular regulation of iron assimilation. *Quarterly Review of Biology* 64:261–290.

Weinberg, E.D. 1990. Cellular iron metabolism in health and disease. *Drug Metabolism Reviews* 22:531–579.

Weinberg, E.D., 1992. Roles of iron in neoplasia: Promotion, prevention, and therapy. *Biological Trace Element Research*, 34:in press.

Weinberg, E.D. 1992. Roles of iron in functions of activated macrophages. *Journal of Nutritional Immunity* 1:41–63.

Weinberg, R.J., S.R. Ell, and E.D. Weinberg. 1986. Blood-letting, iron homeostasis, and human health. *Medical Hypotheses* 21:441–443.

Weinbren, K., R. Salm, and G. Greenberg. 1978. Intramuscular injections of iron compounds and oncogenesis in man. *British Medical Journal* 1:683–685.

Weitzman, S.A., and P. Graceffa. 1984. Asbestos catalyzes hydroxyl and superoxide radical generation from hydrogen peroxide. *Archives of Biochemistry and Biophysics* 228:373–376.

Wicomb, W.N., D.K.C. Cooper, and D. Novitzky. 1987. Loss of myocardial viability following hypothermic perfusion storage from contaminating trace elements in the perfusate. *Transplantation* 43:23–28.

Zschocke, R.H., and A. Bezkorovainy. 1974. Structure and function of the transferrins. II. Transferrin and iron metabolism. *Arzneimittel Forschung* 24: 726–737.

Chapter 5

Anemia in Past Human Populations

Patricia Stuart-Macadam

Introduction

Evidence for anemia in prehistoric populations can be inferred by the presence of a paleopathologic condition of bone known as porotic hyperostosis. Porotic hyperostosis is a term introduced by Angel (1966) to describe characteristic bone lesions of the skull affecting the outer compact layer of bone and the middle layer, or diploë. The normally smooth, dense compact bone is pierced by small holes of varying size and frequency, and the diploë is increased in thickness. The lesions are usually symmetrical in distribution and occur mainly on the orbital roof (cribra orbitalia) and skull vault, particularly the frontal, parietal, and occipital bone (Figures 1 and 2). Orbital and vault lesions of porotic hyperostosis can occur concurrently or independently. Although orbital lesions often occur without vault lesions, vault lesions rarely occur without associated orbital lesions; in a large Romano-British skeletal sample of 752 individuals, vault lesions were associated with orbital lesions in 88% (45/51) of cases. The more severe vault lesions were associated with orbital lesions in every case (Stuart-Macadam 1982, 1987a). There has been some question as to whether a relationship between lesions on the orbit and skull vault actually exists, but research utilizing a number of criteria has confirmed the relationship and strongly supports a common etiology (Stuart-Macadam 1982, 1987b, 1989).

There is a long history of interest in and speculation about this paleopathology, going back at least 100 years. Vault lesions have been described since the mid-nineteenth century (Rokitansky 1848; Virchow

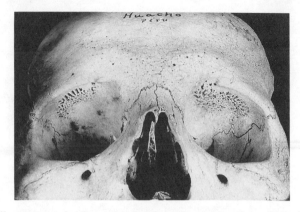

Figure 1.   Illustration of cribra orbitalia (San Diego Museum of Man).

1848; Owen 1859). Welcker (1885, 1888) was the first to fully describe what he termed a "conglomeration of small apertures in the roof of the orbits or 'cribra orbitalia.'" Shortly afterward Toldt (1886), Adachi (1904), Ahrens (1904), and Oetteking (1909) produced papers on the same subject. Since the incidence of lesions appeared to vary among different populations and geographic areas sampled, cribra orbitalia was thought to be a racial trait or geographic characteristic. Soon other etiologies and terminologies became associated with the lesions. Wood-

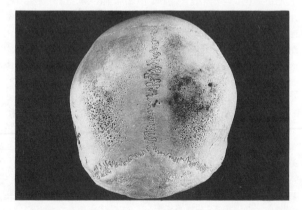

Figure 2.   Illustration of vault lesions of porotic hyperostosis (San Diego Museum of Man).

Jones (1910) thought that the condition might have been caused by the carrying of water jugs on the head. Toldt (1886) suggested that cribra orbitalia was a normal developmental phenomenon rather than a pathology. Koganei (1912) renamed the pathology "external cribra cranii" and suggested that irritation or inflammation of the periosteum produced by mechanical factors, such as compression by tumors of the lacrimal glands, might explain the development of cribra orbitalia. Hrdlička (1914) included the orbital lesions in the broader classification of "symmetrical osteoporosis," many cases of which he found in Peruvian coastal groups. He felt that the vault lesions indicated a systemic disorder, probably of toxic rather than nutritive or degenerative nature. Research in Denmark by Møller-Christensen in 1953 showed that geography was not such an important factor as had previously been thought. Introducing the term "usura orbitae," he showed that the prevalence in two populations from the same geographic region could be quite different. He attributed the development of lesions to the pressure of an enlarged lacrimal gland associated with certain diseases including leprosy and some blood disorders.

In 1961 Henschen suggested that nutritional causes may contribute to the development of both orbital and vault lesions, which he termed "cribra cranii." Nathan and Haas (1966) suggested that periosteal inflammation due to local eye infections such as trachoma or acute or chronic conjunctivitis might be a contributing factor. Since the severe lesions appear to be associated with hypertrophy of the diploic bone layer, Hamperl and Weiss (1955, after Müller 1935) and Angel (1966) suggested that the condition be called "spongy hyperostosis" and "porotic hyperostosis," respectively. They applied these terms to both orbital and vault lesions. Angel's term "porotic hyperostosis" came into popular usage and replaced previous terms for the lesions, although the earlier "cribra orbitalia" continues to be used to refer to the orbital lesions.

The first researchers to link porotic hyperostosis with anemia were Moore and Williams, who in 1929 independently suggested that anemia was responsible for the development of porotic hyperostosis. Williams also put forward dietary deficiencies as a possible causative factor. This idea was mentioned again in 1961 by Henschen, who stressed the possibility that nutritional conditions, and possibly chronic infectious diseases, might produce orbital as well as vault lesions. Nathan and Haas (1966) concurred, noting that nutritional factors would explain the wide distribution of cribra orbitalia in time and space, as well as its occurrence in both human and nonhuman primates. They found that in cave sites in Israel where the inhabitants were thought to have died from starvation there was a much greater prevalence of cribra orbitalia than in relatively well-nourished groups from other cave sites.

However, the anemia theory gradually gained popularity and acceptance. Moore (1929), Williams (1929), and Hooton (1930) had noticed the similarity between radiographs of ancient skulls with lesions and those of clinical cases of various hemolytic anemias. A number of researchers since that time have attributed porotic hyperostosis to anemia of one type or other (Angel 1964, 1966, 1967; Zaino 1964; Moseley 1961, 1966; Hengen 1971; Carlson et al. 1974; El-Najjar et al. 1975, 1976; Lallo et al. 1977; Mensforth et al. 1978, etc.)

Stuart-Macadam (1982, 1985, 1987a,b) provided empirical evidence to support the anemia hypothesis by completing a study that compared skull radiographs of patients with various types of anemia and radiographs of archaeological skulls with porotic hyperostosis. A number of bone changes including "hair-on-end" trabeculation, outer table thinning, texture changes, diploic thickening, orbital roof thickening, and orbital rim changes were observed on both types of radiographs. A consideration of these and other aspects of porotic hyperostosis, including macroscopic and microscopic appearance, distribution by age and sex, and other demographic factors, also supports the anemia hypothesis (Stuart-Macadam 1982, 1987b).

The evidence clearly shows that porotic hyperostosis is indicative of an anemic condition that affected some prehistoric populations. However, there are many different kinds of anemia; the question remains as to which type affected populations in the past? Some researchers (Angel 1964, 1966, 1967; Zaino 1964, 1967) suggested that porotic hyperostosis was the result of a genetic anemia, such as thalassemia or sickle cell anemia. This was partly due to the fact that it has only been appreciated in the last 35 years that acquired anemia, such as iron-deficiency anemia, could also be associated with bone changes. Angel was quite justified in supposing that the anemic changes he saw in skeletal collections from Greece may be associated with thalassemia, as this is an inherited disorder that is found today in that area. Mosely (1961) was the first researcher to suggest that an acquired iron-deficiency anemia could be responsible for porotic hyperostosis. This hypothesis was reiterated by many later researchers (Hengen 1971; Carlson et al. 1974; El-Najjar et al. 1976; Lallo et al. 1977; Mensforth et al. 1978) and has now gained wide popularity in the anthropological literature.

It is very possible that in some cases of porotic hyperostosis the anemia was a genetic type, particularly in areas of the world where malaria was common and balanced polymorphisms evolved as an adaptive mechanism. However, it is likely that most cases of porotic hyperostosis reflect an acquired anemia, such as iron-deficiency anemia. Three lines of evidence support this hypothesis:

1.   Calculations based on the very highest gene frequencies for genetic anemias seen today show that the probability of finding individuals from archaeological collections with skeletal changes due to genetic anemia is quite low (Stuart-Macadam 1982).
2.   There are high levels of porotic hyperostosis in groups from northern Europe and North America, where genetic anemias are not known to have existed in the past.
3.   The severe bone changes that are associated with the genetic anemias, particularly as they affect the postcranial skeleton, have rarely been found in archaeological collections (see Hershkovitz et al. 1991).

Given that porotic hyperostosis is most probably representative of an acquired iron-deficiency anemia, what factors could have been operative in the past that would have led to the development of this condition? Today iron-deficiency anemia (or low hemoglobin/hematocrit) is said to be caused by a number of factors, including blood loss, deficiency in the diet during periods of accelerated growth, inadequate absorption of iron, general nutritional deficiencies, and others (Robinson 1972). Speculation by anthropologists regarding which factors are responsible for porotic hyperostosis has focused on two hypotheses:

1.   dietary deficiency and inadequate absorption of iron, particularly related to high maize consumption; and
2.   a combination of factors, including infection and diet.

The dietary deficiency hypothesis was put forward as early as 1929 when Williams suggested that nutritional deficiencies may be responsible for porotic hyperostosis. This idea was reiterated by Henschen (1961), Nathan and Haas (1966), and El-Najjar et al. (1975, 1976). El-Najjar et al. suggested that the phytates in a predominantly maize diet would inhibit the absorption of iron and lead to high levels of porotic hyperostosis. Other researchers have adopted this theory, even to the extent of suggesting that high levels of porotic hyperostosis in a population indicate a high reliance on maize.

The second hypothesis supports the idea that the interaction of a number of factors, including diet, parasitic infection, and infectious disease, is critical in the production of porotic hyperostosis. Hengen (1971) was the first to suggest this approach. He said:

Changes in the hygienic conditions and of the incidence of iron deficiency
anemias in former times depended without doubt largely on deviations of
the climate, differences in the habits of daily life, procuring and preparation
of food, types of housing, keeping of domestic animals, disposal of excre-
ment and so on.

Carlson et al. (1974) followed this approach when they speculated that
poor diet, parasitic infection, and weanling diarrhea contributed to the
development of iron-deficiency anemia in Nubian populations. Lallo et
al. (1977) suggested that there was a synergistic relationship between
microbial infection, malabsorption due to weanling diarrhea, and the
nutrient depletion that occurs with rapid growth in the etiology of
porotic hyperostosis at a site in Libben, Ohio. Walker (1986) considered
that the high prevalence of porotic hyperostosis on one of the Santa Barbara Channel Islands could be explained by the interaction between diet
and diarrheal infections.

Both of these hypotheses incorporate the assumption that diet plays a
significant role in the etiology of iron-deficiency anemia. Certainly, in
discussions of porotic hyperostosis, diet is almost always invoked as an
explanation for iron-deficiency anemia (an exception is Kent 1986). In
fact, some anthropologists consider porotic hyperostosis to be a good indicator of nutritional stress in prehistoric populations. Is it valid to consider porotic hyperostosis in this way? A review of the physiology and
metabolism of iron, together with data from clinical and anthropological
studies, suggests that it is not. There may be other, more compelling, explanations for the development of iron-deficiency anemia, and hence
porotic hyperostosis, in prehistoric populations.

The physiology and metabolism of iron, one of the most important
body nutrients, has evolved to ensure that there is always an adequate
supply for the body. Iron is absorbed by the duodenum of the small intestine; the factors that control absorption are not fully understood, but
the absorption is efficient and adaptable. Absorption of iron from a given
diet can vary enormously, from 0 to 50%, depending on age, sex, physiological state, iron status, condition of health, and other factors. For example, because of greater physiological needs, women and children absorb more iron than men from the same diet. Women in the last trimester
of pregnancy absorb even greater amounts of iron than average women.
Individuals of both sexes who are iron deficient also increase their absorption of iron. One study of iron-depleted men showed that they consistently absorbed iron at a rate that was up to seven times that shown
by iron-loaded men (Wadsworth 1975). When the body becomes overloaded with iron absorption decreases. As the level of iron in the diet is

increased, the proportion absorbed decreases. The body actually seems as much concerned with too much iron in the system as too little.

Human iron metabolism is based on conservation, hence it is almost a closed system; as much as 90% of the iron in the body is recycled. About 90% of the iron needed by the bone marrow each day to manufacture new red blood cells is obtained from the destruction of old red blood cells and the consequent liberation of iron. The remaining 10% is derived from release of storage iron and absorption from the diet by the intestine (Hoffbrand and Lewis 1981). The body successfully conserves most of its iron, and under normal conditions losses are miminal.

As a result of the conservative nature of iron metabolism only a small amount of iron is needed from the diet to compensate for losses and dietary lack of iron is of minor importance in most cases of iron deficiency. Crosby (1974) states that unless there is blood loss it is difficult to contrive a diet so poor in iron as to cause iron-deficiency anemia. It has been estimated that it would take 6 to 8 years for an adult male to deplete body iron stores and develop iron-deficiency anemia solely as the result of dietary lack (Hoffbrand and Lewis 1981). Arthur and Isbister (1987) say that "even if iron intake was reduced to nil, which is virtually impossible even with the most frugal diets, it would still take at least two to three years to develop iron deficiency anemia, and probably even longer because losses would decline as levels declined." A study of 1205 men, women, and children from the Aberdeen area in Scotland showed that those people who developed iron-deficiency anemia consumed no less iron than others (Davidson et al. 1933). Observations extending over many years showed a wide variation in hematological levels among children on similar intakes of iron, and supplementation with iron did not increase the levels (Wadsworth 1975). In a study of 272 infants with iron-deficiency anemia, Woodruff (1958) found that low birth weight as the result of prematurity or twinning was the most common predisposing factor. He noted that the poor diets of the severely anemic infants were similar to those of a much larger number of infants who did not develop anemia of the same degree of severity, and concluded that factors other than diet are important in the etiology of severe iron-deficiency anemia in infancy. A study by Picciano and Deering (1980) reported that in 96 healthy infants fed diets consisting of mother's milk or milk formula fortified with differing amounts of iron, dietary intakes did not correlate with hemoglobin, hematocrit, serum iron, or percentage saturation of transferrin. The results of many surveys conducted in different countries showed that there was no relationship between hemoglobin levels and mean intake of iron, and were unsuccessful in explaining the absence of anemia in the face of low dietary intake (Wadsworth 1975).

There is an increasing body of evidence that supports the concept that iron deficiency is associated with the development of the body's defense system (Weinberg 1974, 1978, 1984, and this volume Chapter 4). With chronic infections and inflammatory conditions, the body's natural response is to decrease intestinal absorption of iron, prevent the release of iron into the blood from the reticuloendothelial system, and increase the amount of iron stored in the liver. This state of hypoferremia may be a natural protective response to render blood less suitable for bacterial growth. Apparently the assimilation of iron is a necessity for microbial growth—in fact microbes synthesize substances that bind iron. This may explain the prompt and consistent response of the body to bacterial invasion by reducing the amount of iron in the blood plasma. This is effected by simultaneously decreasing the amount of iron absorbed by the intestine and increasing the amount of iron stored in the liver (Weinberg 1974). Studies have shown that if iron is deleted from the blood, the host's defense is strengthened, and if iron is added, microbial growth is enhanced. It is definitely to the advantage of the host to be transiently hypoferremic in the situation of microbial invasion. A number of *in vivo*, *in vitro*, and clinical studies lend support to the concept that iron deficiency is not always detrimental, but may increase the body's defense against infections.

It follows that a child deficient in iron should have an advantage over the child who is replete, at least in areas where there are high levels of pathogenicity. It could be that the so called "physiological iron lack" that occurs in children between the ages of 6 and 18 months is actually an evolutionary adaptation (Stuart-Macadam 1988). It is interesting that this iron lack occurs in all infants, regardless of the amount of iron supplementation in their diet, and in animals during comparable periods of their lives. This is the time of immunological vulnerability when the passive immunity conferred by the mother is being lost, while at the same time exposure to pathogens increases. A similar evolutionary adaptation may apply to women during pregnancy (Stuart-Macadam 1988). Apparently, during the first 3 months of pregnancy absorption of iron from the diet decreases.This is the period when the fetus is most vulnerable to environmental insults because of rapid growth and development and the incomplete development of the placenta. As a defense against pathogens, it would be advantageous for a pregnant woman to have a lowered iron status during the pregnancy, and particularly during the first trimester. Perhaps the consistently low mean hemoglobin levels seen in many populations in tropical countries reflect adaptation to chronic and/or extremely high pathogen loads, rather than a consequence of iron-poor diets. Certainly, in areas of the world where groups are faced with overwhelming malnutrition and/or undernutrition, with a corresponding lack of many essential body nutrients, diet is going to play an important role in the development of iron-deficiency anemia. However in groups not having severe nutritional deprivation, pathogen load could be a more critical factor in the etiology of iron-deficiency anemia. Problems could result as the body tries to maintain a balance between lowered iron absorption as a defense against pathogens, and the need for iron, especially in women and children, who have greater physiological requirements for iron.

The flexibility of iron metabolism, the factors known to be responsible for iron-deficiency anemia in clinical studies, and the role of iron in the defense against pathogens all suggest a third hypothesis to explain the presence of porotic hyperostosis in archaeological populations, namely, that porotic hyperostosis is related to the total pathogen load of a population. A heavy pathogen load will increase the incidence of parasitic, infectious, viral, and fungal diseases, many of which have the effect of reducing the iron status of individuals. Some diseases such as malaria have a direct effect on blood cells, causing hemolysis and sometimes severe anemia (Davidson et al. 1975). Parasitic infestation, such as hookworm (*Ancylostoma duodenale* and *Necator americanus*), can result in anemia by producing chronic blood loss. Today hookworm anemia affects some 20% of the world's population and is endemic in a zone extending from the southern United States to northern Argentina in the Western Hemisphere, and in the Mediterranean countries, South Asia, and Africa (Wintrobe 1974). Other diseases do not have a direct effect on the blood, but do produce anemia associated with acute or chronic infections; this is said to be the second most common form of anemia after iron-deficiency anemia (Zucker 1980). Such diseases include a number that are known to have affected past populations, including chronic mycotic infections, tuberculosis, and osteomyelitis. The anemia is, in effect, the body's attempt to withhold iron from the invading microorganisms.

Arthur and Isbister (1987) state that iron deficiency is commonly misdiagnosed, with the usual error being confusion with the anemia of chronic disease. This is not surprising, since both anemias share some of the same features, including low serum iron. It is very likely that anemia of chronic disease was also common in the past and that it contributed to a generally lowered iron status among individuals in populations exposed to high and/or chronic pathogen loads.

On the basis of this theory it is postulated that porotic hyperostosis will occur more frequently in populations with greater pathogen loads, for whatever reason. The total pathogen load could be a function of many

factors, such as climate (tropical or temperate), geography (closer or farther from the equator), topography (lowland or highland), aggregation
(crowded city or village), hygiene, food resources, seasonality, customs,
period in history (effects of modern medicine, for example), economy
(hunter, gatherer, or agriculturalist), etc. In areas or periods of higher
pathogen load the population as a whole may have a lower mean iron
status and the threshold between iron deficiency and anemia is more
easily crossed.

What is the archaeological picture of porotic hyperostosis and how
does it fit with the hypotheses that have been generated? Does diet seem
to be a major contributing factor?

There appear to be three major trends in the occurrence of porotic hyperostosis:

1. Temporal: porotic hyperostosis increased through the Neolithic
   period and then decreased toward the twentieth century.
2. Geographic: porotic hyperostosis increased in frequency the
   nearer the country of origin is to the equator.
3. Ecological: porotic hyperostosis occurred more frequently in lowland or coastal sites than in highland sites.

Within these broad trends the picture is not clear, with many variations
in frequency among sites and through time. As a result, porotic hyperostosis can occur with different frequencies in the same time period and
geographic area but within differing microenvironments. Examination of
the broad trends and the exceptions to the trends should provide clues to
the occurrence of porotic hyperostosis, and hence of iron-deficiency
anemia.

Temporal

Porotic hyperostosis first appears at the transition from Upper
Paleolithic to Mesolithic periods in Africa and the Mediterranean (Angel
1978). However, at that time it was an extremely rare occurrence. Meik-
lejohn (1984) found very little cribra orbitalia from the Neolithic and
Mesolithic periods in western Europe. Kennedy (1984) found that with a
single exception, preagricultural remains that he examined in India and
Sri Lanka did not exhibit porotic hyperostosis. The frequency increased
in the Neolithic period in many areas of the world. Lallo et al. (1977)
studied material from an area in Illinois and found that cribra orbitalia
was much more prevalent after agriculture appeared than in the preced-

ing hunting and gathering period. Angel (1978) found that porotic hyperostosis increased in the Mesolithic in Greece and reached high frequencies in the Neolithic to Middle Bronze Age times.

During and after the Neolithic the picture becomes very complex, with prevalences varying greatly among groups from differing ecological niches, geographic areas, and time periods. However, the prevalence does seem to decrease steadily toward the twentieth century. Angel (1978) found a nearly straight-line reduction in adult frequency from 21 to 2% in Greece over the 4000 years from late Neolithic to classical times. Hengen (1971) found that there was a statistically significant decrease in prevalence of cribra orbitalia in skeletal remains from an area in Germany (Wurtemberg) from the twelfth century to the late nineteenth and early twentieth century. In a study of Swedish skulls, Henschen (1961) found cribra orbitalia to be present in mid-nineteenth century skulls, but absent in 2000 skulls collected since 1939.

Exceptions

Although there was a steady decrease in porotic hyperostosis in Greece from Neolithic to classical times, during the postclassical period porotic hyperostosis showed great increases (Angel 1978). Brothwell reports a 15% frequency of porotic hyperostosis in seventeenth-century London, but at the eighteenth- to nineteenth-century Spitalfields Church site in London the frequency is 34% (Cox 1988).

Geography

Porotic hyperostosis has been found to occur in skeletal collections from every country and continent. However, Hengen (1971) observed that the closer the country of origin is to the equator, the more common it is to see cribra orbitalia. His conclusion was based on the analysis of 5698 skulls, mainly from the nineteenth and twentieth centuries.

Ecology

Hrdlička found porotic hyperostosis to be much more common in individuals from coastal areas of Peru than in highland areas. El-Najjar et al. (1976) studied a series of 539 crania from a 120 mile radius repre-

Geographic Latitude (degrees) (Northern or Southern)	Frequency of Cribra Orbitalia (%)
90–71	1.28
70–61	3.24
60–51	3.64
50–41	4.13
40–31	6.92
30–21	8.23
20–11	12.66
10–0	13.19

(Taken from Hengen, 1971)

senting Anasazi Indian sites from the American Southwest. They found that cribra orbitalia was more common at canyon bottom sites than higher altitude sage plain sites. In Ecuador, Ubelaker (1984) found that porotic hyperostosis was rare in highland sites and more common in lowland sites. Angel studied 1750 adult and 584 juvenile skeletons from Greece and Turkey. He found that in Anatolia, Greece, and Cyprus from the seventh to second millennia B.C., porotic hyperostosis occurred frequently in farming populations living in marshy areas, but rarely in those people inhabiting dry or rocky areas (Angel 1972). Angel also found differences in prevalence of porotic hyperostosis between highland and lowland areas, with highland coastal sites having much lower prevalences than lowland coastal sites. He studied 10 samples including Catal Huyak, situated in an inland drainy marshy plateau region, Nea Nikomedeia, on the marshy Macedonian plain, Kephala, on a rocky headland, and Karatas, in the Lycian mountains, Khirokitia, a dry valley in the hills of Cyprus, and Bamboula, close to large salt marshes. Five prehistoric populations living close to "permanent" marshes had fairly high frequencies of severe porotic hyperostosis, while five groups in dry environments had lower frequencies of porotic hyperostosis. He later studied a number of Neolithic and Bronze Age populations and found a similar pattern.

Exceptions

Angel discovered that during the Bronze Age in Greece the differences in prevalence of porotic hyperostosis between highland and lowland sites were not present. At Lerna, a coastal lowland site, 6.4% of the Bronze Age population had porotic hyperostosis, whereas at similar sites in the

Neolithic there were frequencies up to 67%. Møller-Christensen (1953) observed that individuals from a medieval leper hospital at Naestved, Denmark had twice as many orbital lesions as those from a monastery located on the same island during the same time period. Nathan and Haas (1966) found a statistically significant difference in the frequency of cribra orbitalia between children from ordinary burial places in Israel and those from caves used for refuge, which had a much higher frequency. Walker (1986) found that a group from the Santa Barbara Channel Islands showed higher frequencies of porotic hyperostosis than mainland groups from the same time period.

Discussion

Are the data consistent with the dietary hypothesis, or one in which diet plays a major role? The overall frequency of porotic hyperostosis does increase during the Neolithic period, suggesting that the appearance of iron-deficiency anemia is associated with the development of agriculture. It has been suggested that increasing reliance on maize or grain, which is an inferior source of iron, was responsible for iron-deficiency anemia. However, as Kent has argued, (1986) this association could be seen as correlation, which does not necessarily imply a cause and effect relationship. It can be seen from the data that groups with a heavy reliance on agriculture have varying prevalences of porotic hyperostosis, some low and some high, as do groups that are known to rely more heavily on animal protein food sources. For example, Ubelaker (1984) found little porotic hyperostosis in an Ecuador highland site where there was intensive agriculture. In some other areas in North America where maize and cereal grains were known to have been important dietary sources, porotic hyperostosis has been found in only a few individuals (Larsen 1987). Conversely, Walker (1986) found that a group from the Santa Barbara Channel Islands showed a high frequency of porotic hyperostosis even with an iron-rich diet from marine sources. Cybulski (1977, 1985) has shown that in a number of areas inhabited by hunters and gatherers, there were high prevalences of porotic hyperostosis. He found that postcontact human remains from the British Columbia coast had a widespread distribution of porotic hyperostosis. El-Najjar et al. (1976) found differences between canyon bottom and sage plain sites that they attributed to differences in maize consumption, but Reinhard's studies (1987, and this volume, Chapter 8) have shown that the proportion of maize in the diet was the same. Although factors that arise in the Neolithic do appear to be associated with iron-deficiency anemia these studies show that there is no consistent pattern associated with agriculture per se. The dietary hypothesis also fails to explain the general trend of increasing porotic hyperostosis with increasing proximity to the equator.

Does the hypothesis that an interaction of diet, intestinal parasites, and disease fit the pattern of porotic hyperostosis? This explanation goes much further, but it does not really explain why there has been a general decrease in prevalence from the Neolithic through to modern times. This would infer that diet has improved and/or that intestinal parasites and diseases have decreased steadily from the Neolithic. There is no evidence to support this happening simultaneously in areas as diverse as Greece or Germany.

Does the hypothesis of pathogen load fit the observed patterns? Variations in pathogen load satisfactorily explain both the broad trends and the exceptions to the trends. Pathogen load, by contributing to increased incidences of infection and chronic disease, and thereby stimulating the defense system into maintaining a lowered iron status, is a critical factor in the development of iron-deficiency anemia. With the advent of agriculture, populations and population density increased, and diseases that are population dependent for their transmission became more prevalent. This meant that individuals were exposed to greater numbers of disease organisms. The rise of towns and cities meant that people were living in close proximity, and hygiene must have suffered, again increasing exposure to disease organisms. Deforestation associated with clearing of agricultural land led to an enormous change in ecology and a subsequent increase in numbers of mosquitos in many areas of the world. This must have been associated with a great increase in malaria, which could explain why porotic hyperostosis became more common during the Neolithic period. Improvements in hygiene and sanitation in the last 100 years could explain why porotic hyperotosis decreased during that time, especially in Europe.

This hypothesis could explain why Angel (1972) found a dramatic rise in porotic hyperostosis in the postclassical period. During this time in Greece there was a slight warming trend, the sea level rose, expanding marshy areas. The rise in porotic hyperostosis occurs concurrently with the known increase and spread of the malarias that accompanied these changes. Malaria, of course, is directly associated with iron-deficiency anemia.

Why was there a higher prevalence of porotic hyperostosis in London (Spitalfields) in the eighteenth to nineteenth century than in the seventeenth century? The environment of eighteenth- and nineteenth-century

London was far less wholesome than it had been in the seventeenth century. There were huge increases in population accompanied by problems in housing, water supply, and sanitation (Cox 1988). All these factors increased the exposure of the population to pathogens and the possibility of acquired anemia. Why did Cybulski find high levels of porotic hyperostosis in hunters and gatherers from the British Columbia coast? Cybulski (1977) suggests that European-induced infectious diseases may have contributed.

The increase of porotic hyperostosis with closer proximity to the equator can also be explained by the hypothesis. In temperate climates, with cold winters, pathogen survival is inhibited compared with areas that are warm year round. Consequently, there are far fewer pathogens in areas with temperate climates than in areas with subtropical or tropical climates. The pathogen load in countries closer to the equator would therefore be much higher than in cooler countries farther away from the equator. According to Masawe et al. (1974), up to 80% of children, young adult women, and pregnant mothers in the tropics have anemia. The commonest types are iron-deficiency anemia and anemia of chronic disorders. Their results show that although some types of anemia are associated with a high frequency of infections, patients with negative iron stores have significantly less bacterial infections than patients with positive iron stores. Masawe and Nsanzumhire (1973) reported that growth of bacteria *in vitro* in blood from patients with iron-deficiency anemia was considerably less than growth in blood from people with normal hemoglobin values.

Normally there are greater numbers of pathogens in lowland, or coastal areas than at higher altitudes. This may explain why Hrdlička (1914), Angel (1972, 1978), and Ubelaker (1984) found more porotic hyperostosis in lowland sites than highland sites, and why El-Najjar et al. (1976) found less in sage plain sites than canyon bottom sites. In fact, a study by Reinhard (1987) plus this volume, Chapter 8, shows that although the proportion of maize in the diet was probably the same in both areas, canyon bottom sites showed significantly higher levels of parasites. Walker (1986) suggests that higher levels of porotic hyperostosis in Santa Barbara Channel island groups than in contemporaneous mainland groups may be related to the contamination of water sources as a result of increased population density. Settlement of people around a limited number of water sources may have resulted in contamination by enteric bacteria.

Angel found that by the end of the Bronze Age differences in prevalence of porotic hyperostosis between highland and lowland sites had disappeared. Why? At this time there was climatic change that resulted in a decrease in the sea level of about 2 m, shrinking marshland areas and reducing malaria mosquito habitat. Improved technology resulted in the development of irrigation, which further decreased swamp areas thus effectively reducing the breeding grounds for parasite-carrying mosquitos. Again, on the basis of the pathogen load hypothesis it is not surprising that Møller-Christensen (1953) found that individuals living in a leper hospital had higher levels of anemia than individuals living in a monastery on the same island. Surely general conditions, including hygiene, would have been much better in the monastery. The same holds true for the differences between children from ordinary burial places in Israel and those from caves used for refuge. Conditions must have been much worse in caves of refuge, with diseases, perhaps undernutrition, and poor hygiene all contributing to anemia.

Anthropologists have become increasingly aware of the complexity of the story of porotic hyperostosis and the multifactorial nature of its etiology. The simplistic view that diet is the major factor in its etiology or that porotic hyperostosis is a "nutritional stress" indicator needs to be replaced by a greater understanding of iron metabolism and an awareness of the interaction between specific populations and their environment. It has become apparent that factors such as ecology, hygiene, aggregation, disease, and the role of iron in the body's defense system are of far greater importance than diet in producing iron-deficiency anemia and porotic hyperostosis. All these factors ultimately affect the total pathogen load of a population, which is the key to the occurrence of iron-deficiency anemia in past human populations.

References

Adachi, B. 1904. Die porositat des schadels. *Zeitshrift für Morphologie und Anthropologie* 7:373.

Ahrens, E. 1904. Cited in Nathan and Haas (1966).

Angel, J.L. 1964. Osteoporosis: Thalassemia? *American Journal of Physical Anthropology* 22:369–374.

Angel, J.L. 1966. Porotic hyperostosis, anemias, malarias and the marshes in prehistoric Eastern Mediterranean. *Science* 153:760–762.

Angel, J.L. 1967. Porotic hyperostosis or osteoporosis symmetrica. In *Diseases in Antiquity*. D. Brothwell and A.T. Sandison, eds., Springfield, IL: Charles C Thomas.

Angel, J.L. 1972. Ecology and population in the Eastern Mediterranean. *World Archaeology* 4(1):88–105.

Angel, J.L. 1978. Porotic hyperostosis in the Eastern Mediterranean. *Medical College of Virginia Quarterly* 14(1):10–16.

Arthur, C.K., and J.P. Isbister. 1987. Iron deficiency: Misunderstood, misdiagnosed and mistreated. *Drugs* 33:171–182.

Carlson, D., G. Armelagos, and D. van Gerven. 1974. Factors influencing the etiology of cribra orbitalia in prehistoric Nubia. *Journal of Human Evolution* 3:405–410.

Crosby, W.H. 1984. The rationale for treating iron deficiency anemia. *Archives of Internal Medicine* 144:471.

Cox, M. 1988. Personal communication.

Cybulski, J.S. 1977. Cribra orbitalia, a possible sign of anemia in early historic native populations of the British Columbia Coast. *American Journal of Physical Anthropology* 47:31–40.

Cybulski, J.S. 1985. Further observations on cribra orbitalia in British Columbia samples. *American Journal of Physical Anthropology* 66:161 (abstr.).

Davidson, L., H.J.W. Fullerton, J. Howie, J. Croll, J.B. Orr, and W. Godden. 1933. Nutrition in relation to anaemia. The *British Medical Journal* 8:685–690.

Davidson, L., R. Passmore, J.F. Brock, and A. Truswell. 1975. *Human Nutrition and Dietetics*. Edinburgh: Churchill Livingstone.

El-Najjar, M.Y., B. Lozoff, and D.J. Ryan. 1975. The paleoepidemiology of porotic hyperostosis in the American Southwest: Radiological and ecological considerations. *American Journal of Roentgenology and Radium Therapy* 25:918–924.

El-Najjar, M., D.J. Ryan, C.G. Turner, and B. Lozoff. 1976. The etiology of porotic hyperostosis among the prehistoric and historic Anasazi Indians of the Southwestern U.S. *American Journal of Physical Anthropology* 44:477–488.

Hamperl, H., and P. Weis. 1955. Uber die spongose on schadeln aus Alt-Peru. *Virchows Archiv* 327:629–642.

Hengen, O.P. 1971. Cribra orbitalia: Pathogenesis and probable etiology. *Homo* 22:57–75.

Henschen, P. 1961. Cribra cranii—a skull condition said to be of racial or geographical nature. 7th Conf. Intern. Scot. Geograph. Pathol., London, 1960. *Pathology and Microbiology* 24:724–729.

Hershkovitz, I., B. Ring, M. Speirs, E. Galili, M., Kislev, G. Edelson, and A. Hershkovitz. 1991. Possible congenital hemolytic anemia in prehistoric coastal inhabitants of Israel. *American Journal of Physical Anthropology* 85(1):7–14.

Hoffbrand, A.V., and S.M. Lewis. 1981. *Postgraduate Haematology*. London: William Heinemann Medical Books.

Hooton, E.A. 1930. *Indians of Pecos Pueblo*. New Haven, CT: Yale University Press.

Hrdlička, A. 1914. Anthropological work in Peru in 1913, with notes on pathology of ancient Peruvians. *Smithsonian Miscellaneous Collection* 61:1–69.

Kennedy, K. 1984. Growth, nutrition, and pathology in changing paleodemographic settings in South Asia. In *Paleopathology at the Origins of Agriculture*. M.N. Cohen and G.J. Armelagos, eds., pp. 169–192. New York: Academic Press.

Kent, S. 1986. The influence of sedentism and aggregation of porotic hyperostosis and anaemia: A case study. *Man* 21:605–636.

Koganei, Y. 1912. Cribra cranii and cribra orbitalia. *Mitt. med. Fak. Tokyo* 10/2:113.

Lallo, J., G.J. Armelagos, and R.P. Mensforth. 1977. The role of diet, disease and physiology in the origin of porotic hyperostosis. *Human Biology* 49(3): 471–483.

Larsen, 1987. Bioarchaeological interpretations of subsistence economy and behavior. In *Advances in Archaeological Method and Theory*, Volume 10. Michael B. Schiffer, ed., pp. 339–445. New York: Academic Press.

Masawe, A.F., and H. Nsanzumhire. 1973. Growth of bacteria in vitro in blood from patients with severe iron deficiency anemia and from patients with sickle cell anemia. *American Journal of Clinical Pathology* 59:706–711.

Masawe,A.E., J.M. Miundi, and G.B. Swai. 1974. Infections in iron deficiency and other types of anaemia in the tropics. *Lancet* ii:314–317.

Mieklejohn, C., C. Schentag, A. Venema, and P. Key. 1984. Socioeconomic change and patterns of pathology in the Mesolithic and Neolithic of Western Europe: Some suggestions. In *Paleopathology at the Origins of Agriculture*. M.N. Cohen and G.J. Armelagos, eds., New York: Academic Press.

Mensforth, R., C. Lovejoy, J. Lallo, and G. Armelagos. 1978. The role of constitutional factors, diet, and infectious disease in the etiology of porotic hyperostosis and periosteal reactions in prehistoric infants and children. *Medical Anthropology* 2(1):1–59.

Møller-Christensen, V. 1953. *Ten Lepers from Naestved in Denmark*. Copenhagen: Danish Science Press.

Moore, S. 1929. Bone changes in sickle cell anemia with note on similar changes observed in skulls of ancient Mayan Indians. *Journal of Missouri State Medical Association* 26:561–564.

Moseley, J.E. 1961. Skull changes in chronic iron deficiency anemia. *American Journal of Roentgenology* 85(4):649–652.

Moseley, J.E. 1966. Radiographic studies in hematologic bone disease: implications for palaeopathology. In *Human Palaeopathology*. S. Jarcho, ed., pp. 121–130. New Haven, CT: Yale University Press.

Müller, H. 1935. Osteoporosis of the cranium in Javanese. *American Journal of Physical Anthropology* 20:493.

Nathan, H., and N. Haas. 1966. 'Cribra orbitalia' A bone condition of the orbit of unknown nature. *Israel Journal of Medical Sciences* 2:171–191.

Oetteking, P. 1909. Cited in Nathan and Haas (1966).

Owen, R. 1859. Report on a series of skulls of various tribes of mankind inhabiting Nepal, collected and presented to the museum by B.H. Hodgson. Report British Association, London.

Picciano, M.F., and Deering, R. 1980. The influence of feeding regimens on iron status during infancy. The *American Journal of Clinical Nutrition* 33:746–753.

Reinhard, K. 1987. Porotic hyperostosis and diet: The coprolite evidence. *American Journal of Physical Anthropology* 72(2):246 (abstr.).

Robinson, C.H. 1972. *Normal and Therapeutic Nutrition*. New York: Macmillan.

Rokitansky, C. 1848. Cited in Nathan and Haas (1966).

Stuart-Macadam, P. 1982. A correlative study of a palaeopathology of the skull. Ph.D. thesis, Department of Physical Anthropology, Cambridge University.

Stuart-Macadam, P. 1985. Porotic hyperostosis: Representative of a childhood condition. *American Journal of Physical Anthropology* 66:391–398.

Stuart-Macadam, P. 1987a. New evidence to support the anemia theory. *American Journal of Physical Anthropology* 74:521–526.

Stuart-Macadam, P. 1987b. A radiographic study of porotic hyperostosis. *American Journal of Physical Anthropology* 74:511–520.

Stuart-Macadam, P. 1988. Nutrition and anaemia in past human populations. Proceedings of the 19th Annual Chacmool Conference, 1986. Diet and Subsistence: Current Archaeological Perspectives. Calgary: University of Calgary.

Stuart-Macadam, P. 1989. Porotic hyperostosis: Relationship between vault and orbital lesions. *American Journal of Physical Anthropology* 74:511–520.

Toldt, C. 1886. Cited in Nathan and Haas (1966).

Ubelaker, D. 1984. Prehistoric human biology of Ecuador: Possible temporal trends and cultural correlations. In *Paleopathology at the Origins of Agriculture*. M.N. Cohen and G.J. Armelagos, eds., pp. 491–513. New York: Academic Press.

Virchow, R. 1848. Cited in Nathan and Haas (1966).

Wadsworth, G.R. 1975. Nutritional factors in anemia. *World Review of Nutrition and Dietetics* 21:75–150.

Walker, P.L. 1986. Porotic hyperostosis in a marine-dependent California Indian population. *American Journal of Physical Anthropology* 69(3):345–354.

Weinberg, E. 1974. Iron and susceptibility to infectious disease. *Science* 184: 952–956.

Weinberg, E. 1978. Iron and infection. *Microbiological Review* 42:45–66.

Weinberg, E. 1984. Iron withholding: A defense against infection and neoplasia. *Physiological Reviews* 64:65–102.

Welcker, H. 1885. Cited in Nathan and Haas (1966).

Welcker, H. 1888. Cribra orbitalia, ein ethologischdiagnostisches merkmal am schadel mehrerer menschrassen. *Archiv Anthropologie* 17.

Williams, H. 1929. Human paleopathology. *Archiv Pathologie* 17:839.

Wintrobe, M. 1974. *Clinical Hematology*. Philadelphia: Lea & Febiger.

Wood-Jones, F. 1910. The pathological report. *Bulletin of the Archaeological Survey Nubia* 2.

Woodruff, C. 1958. Multiple causes of iron deficiency in infants. *Journal of American Medical Association* 167(6):715–720.

Zaino, E. 1964. Paleontologic thalassemia. *Annals of the New York Academy of Science* 119:402–412.

Zaino, E. 1967. Symmetrical osteoporosis, a sign of severe anemia in the prehistoric Pueblo Indians of the S.W. In *Miscellaneous Papers in Paleopathology 1*,

Technical Series No. 7:40–47. W.D. Wade, ed., pp. 40–47. Flagstaff: Museum of Northern Arizona.

Zucker, S. 1980. Anemia of chronic disease. In *Hematology and Oncology.* M.A. Lichtman, ed., pp. 27–28. New York: Grune & Stratton.

Part II

CASE STUDIES

Chapter 6

A Hematological Study of !Kung Kalahari Foragers: An Eighteen-Year Comparison

Susan Kent and Richard Lee

A complex relationship exists between iron metabolism, anemia, diet, and social and economic conditions. It is no longer valid to accept a few indices, such as hematocrit and hemoglobin, as reliable markers for the health or nutritional status of a population. This chapter presents examples of how contradictory and even counterintuitive results might be found in populations. Dobe !Kung ("Bushmen," San, Basarwa) tested in 1987 exhibit superficially improved levels of hemoglobin over Dobe !Kung tested in 1969, while all ethnographic and clinical observations point in the opposite direction (i.e., meat intake was roughly equivalent but morbidity was higher). We analyzed this apparent contradiction by evaluating the iron levels of both Dobe !Kung populations. The first study was conducted in 1969 (Metz et al. 1971) and the second in 1987 (Hansen et al. 1992). Data collected in 1981 from a !Kung settlement at Chum!kwe, Namibia, provide a third study population for further comparison (Fernandes-Costa et al. 1984; see Figure 1).

Other studies indicate that sedentism and aggregation increase the pathogen load of a population (Kent 1992). We wanted to evaluate the hypothesis that the body reacts to increased pathogen loads with a hypoferremic defense, wherein circulating iron levels are reduced. To test this, we compared the hematology of sedentary (1981, 1987) and nomadic (1969) !Kung populations from the Kalahari Desert. If the hypothesis that chronic threats of microorganism invasion as found in sedentary contexts trigger chronic hypoferremia is valid (Chapters 1 and 4, this volume), the recently sedentary 1981 and 1987 !Kung should be more anemic than the more nomadic 1969 !Kung.

Nomadic foragers have been characterized as relatively healthy, in part because of their diet and in part because of their mobility (e.g., Truswell and Hansen 1976). To assess whether this health is the result of the diet of nomadic hunter–gatherers or of their mobility, we examine diet, nutrition, and hematology from the changing perspective of anemia discussed in the theoretical explorations section of this book. We interpret health status and hematological values by taking into account all aspects of the !Kung life-style. This is accomplished by incorporating diachronic ethnographic studies (Lee 1979 and elsewhere) with diachronic medical research of the !Kung (Fernandes-Costa et al. 1984; Nurse and Jenkins 1977; Metz et al. 1971; Truswell and Hansen 1976; Hansen et al. 1992).

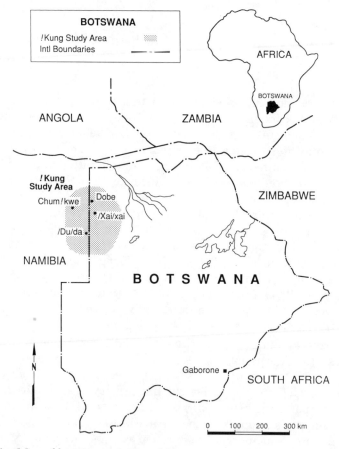

Figure 1. Map of locations mentioned in text.

The !Kung

Since the !Kung of the Dobe and Nyae Nyae areas (Figure 1) experienced rapid and dramatic changes between 1969 and 1987, a detailed description of the nature and magnitude of those changes is appropriate. The three study populations represented three very different circumstances. Although not exclusive or "pristine" hunter–gatherers, the earlier Dobe study group exhibited the least influence from contact with Bantu-speakers or Westerners. The 460 !Kung shared their waterholes with approximately 300 Herero pastoralists. In 1969 the !Kung community remained outside the cash economy (a few worked for wages but they did not fall into the study population). During this time, most pursued a subsistence based on seminomadic hunting and gathering combined with minor elements of pastoralism and horticulture.

By the time of the second Dobe study 18 years later, the situation had changed dramatically. By 1987 the !Kung had entered the cash economy through handicraft production. They received the bulk of their subsistence from mealie (maize) meal and soy milk that were either purchased at a store or distributed by the Botswana government as drought relief. However, meat was still acquired from hunting, although it was now sometimes done on horseback rather than by foot.

A more rapid change occurred among the Chum!kwe !Kung. In 1981 they had already adopted the social conditions of an African peasantry. They were the most aggregated and most sedentary. They also consumed the most commercial food and alcohol and the least meat. These factors separate the Chum!kwe !Kung from the earlier and later Dobe populations.

Changes in Diet

The Dobe area in 1969 supported a population of hunters and gatherers who relied primarily (though not exclusively) on wild plants and game for their subsistence. Food of domestic origins (crops, milk products, or meat from cows or goats) comprised a minor proportion of their diet, ranging by caloric content from less than 5% to not more than 30%, with an average of roughly 15%. Food obtained from stores or as government relief was of negligible significance (see Appendix).

Diet during the 1960s has been described in detail elsewhere (Lee 1979:159–249, 464–488). Though limited in calories, the composition of the diet was described as well-balanced in vitamins and minerals, high in proteins, and low in saturated fats (Truswell and Hansen 1976:180–194). Iron was available from both meat and wild plant sources (Wehmeyer et al. 1969). There was almost a complete absence of refined carbohydrates, alcohol, chemicals, or any kind of commercially processed foods. The broader implications of the traditional !Kung diet have been explored by Eaton et al. (1988).

By the 1987 restudy, this picture had undergone a fundamental shift. Wild plant foods had fallen to less than a third of the total, and government relief rations had become the primary vegetarian food source. Domesticated food, particularly cow's milk, was a prominent feature of most diets. However, store-bought foods still did not contribute substantially to the diet (see Appendix). Hunting continued to provide a generally adequate meat intake with a consumption rate of roughly twice a week.

Government relief foods began to supplement the diet in the early 1980s, with the onset of the latest in a series of long droughts occurring in Botswana in this century. Initially, the targeted population was families with young children and old people. By 1983, the distribution had expanded to include most of the Dobe peoples classified as remote area dwellers (RADs), i.e., people with few or no cattle and little or no cash income. The government distributed mealie meal (ground maize), cooking oil, and an American mixture of corn meal, soy flour, and powdered skim milk (CSM). Strong tea, heavily flavored with sugar and powdered milk, had become the major beverage, often substituting for a meal at midday. Alcohol consumption, in the form of home-brew beer, was of very minor importance in 1969, with less than 10% of the population consuming any alcohol at all. By 1987 the level of consumption had assumed greater significance. Most adults drank at least occasionally. Approximately 20% of all adults could be classified as moderate drinkers, and 10% as heavy drinkers. Thus, the most fundamental changes occurred in the vegetable part of the !Kung diet. Meat continued to be acquired through hunting, although the methods employed between 1969 and 1987 changed dramatically.

Chum!kwe in 1981 had experienced the most drastic changes in diet. Hunting and gathering had fallen to very low levels due to the high level of aggregation and reduced mobility of the population (see below). Commercial foods from a store and government rations, high in refined carbohydrates, formed the mainstay of the diet. They were supplemented with some milk and grain from home-grown sources. Meat was eaten less frequently than at Dobe in either 1969 or 1987. Canned soft drinks and heavily sugared tea were the main nonalcoholic beverages. Alcohol, in the form of home-brew and canned beer, as well as whiskey, brandy, rum, gin, and vodka, was widely consumed. Young children as well as adults drank beer (Marshall and Ritchie 1984:58). Mealie meal beer alone comprised approximately 21% of the diet. About 9% of the time no food was eaten for one or more meals, often for an entire day (Marshall and Ritchie 1984:60–61). In fact, by the 1980s, alcohol had become a major social problem, with Saturday night brawls often resulting in injury and death (Marshall and Ritchie 1984; Volkman 1982).

!Kung Settlement Patterns, Aggregation, and Mobility

The life-style of the Dobe population in 1969 can be described as tethered nomadism (cf. Binford 1983:341; Ingold 1987:184–185). Life revolved around the nine permanent waterholes in the !Kangwa and /Xai/xai valleys but all !Kung made summer forays to rainy season foraging areas in the hinterland. They built their characteristic beehive-shaped huts in circular camps during the summer and their ephemeral windbreaks during the winter. Camps were moved three to six times per year. Typically the !Kung would spend the winter months (May to September) at the pans or waterholes with permanent water, and the spring and summer months (October–April) moving around the hinterland. People spent up to 4 months a year at sites 10–30 km distant from the core areas. Since the 1950s some of these summer sites had become the locales of Herero cattle posts; thus many !Kung combined their summer foraging with work on the cattle posts. The 1960s was the last decade in which the Dobe !Kung retained this degree of mobility. After 1970, they settled increasingly into semipermanent villages, which were occupied for periods of 5 to 15 years. By 1987 the !Kung in the study group had experienced over a decade of semisedentary to sedentary living. At the Dobe waterhole the 1980s population had grown from 30 to 40 individuals during the 1960s to 165 residents, with over 400 head of cattle and small stock.

A typical village in the 1980s consisted of a fenced-in cluster of mud-walled huts facing the livestock kraal (Yellen 1985). A camp of 25 people, which in the 1960s might have occupied an area of 150–300 square meters, today spreads over an area of 1000–2000 square meters. Foraging trips for days or even weeks still occur, although some members of the village always remain behind to care for the animals. Thus all village sites are in continuous year-round occupation.

Sedentarization at Chum!kwe began in 1960 when the South African administration of the Namibia Territory decided to move all the !Kung of Nyae Nyae into a single settlement (presumably in order to watch them more closely). For the next 20 years the waterhole at Chum!kwe (augmented by boreholes), supported a standing population of 800–1000 people. These conditions of high aggregation, with its attendant social, nutritional, and alcohol-related stresses, were prevailing when the 1981 study was made (after 1981 some Chum!kwe !Kung began a "back to the land" movement and reoccupied their traditional hunting *n!ores* or territories).

Other Factors Affecting Health and Morbidity

In addition to sedentarization and nutritional changes, several other factors affected health. Tobacco use was common in all three study situations. In 1969 most of the tobacco was the strong leaf variety, smoked in pipes. In 1981 and 1987 commercial cigarettes accounted for between one-third and one-half of the tobacco consumed. It is difficult to discern whether levels of consumption varied significantly among the three studies. There are relatively few nonsmoking !Kung: probably over 90% of adults smoke, all who smoke inhale, and consumption per capita is in the range of 10–20 cigarette equivalents per day.

There was no bottle feeding in the Dobe area in 1969 or 1987, but there has been a decline in the length of breast feeding (Lee 1980, 1981). At Chum!kwe a few mothers bottle fed in 1981 (Fernandes-Costa et al. 1984). A marked decrease in birth intervals had been noted between 1963 and 1973 and this trend has continued into the 1980s. The mean birth interval of roughly 19–27 months in 1987 contrasts sharply with the mean birth interval of 44 months for nomadic women documented for the period 1968–1973 (Lee 1979:322).

Materials and Methods

The subjects of the 1969 study were populations inhabiting Mhopa, Goshi, Dobe, and /Xai/xai or Xoxgana (reported in Metz et al. 1971). The subjects of the 1987 study were comprised of persons residing in Dobe and Xangwa or /Xai/xai (Hansen et al. 1992). Each group is a subset of a homogeneous population and includes relatives living in Chum!kwe and /Du/da (Figure 1). A few Herero who are agropastoralists and are linguistically distinct from the !Kung were included in both studies. The Herero constitute a second population from which to compare results, although the small sample size precludes any definitive conclusions about their health status.

Blood samples were drawn at the end of the dry season in the latter part of September 1969. At that period, the nutritional status of the people would be expected to be at its poorest. The 1987 study occurred during the middle of the dry winter season in June, when nutritional status would be relatively similar. Mean age for male volunteers in 1969 was 39 (SD 13.7) and in 1987 was 48 (SD 15.9). The mean age for female volunteers in 1969 was 40 (SD 1.1) and in 1987 was 40 (SD 16.0).

Volunteers in both studies donated a blood sample collected from an antecubital vein by means of vacutainers. Samples for hemoglobin and red cell (erythrocyte) folate estimations were transferred into sequestrine (EDTA) tubes and stored at 4°C until tested. Hematocrit was measured in the field (with a generator-operated centrifuge), within 4–6 hours of collection. Clotted blood samples were centrifuged in the field; the serum was separated and stored at –170°C in liquid nitrogen until tested 3–7 days later in Johannesburg. Serum folate, serum vitamin B_{12} and B_{12} binders, together with serum iron and transferrin, were analyzed. Serum ferritin was measured only in the 1987 study.

Laboratory Methods

Hemoglobin concentration, red cell count, mean cell volume, and mean cell hemoglobin were measured in a Coulter Model S Senior using "4C" control in both studies. Hematocrit was measured by the microhematocrit method in the field in 1987 as it had been in the 1969 study. Blood smears were prepared at the time of blood collection. Thin films were fixed in the field but stained and examined in the laboratory for red cell morphology. Thick films were stained with Giemsa's stain and examined for malaria and other parasites. Serum ferritin was measured by radioimmunoassay (Amersham, U.K.), serum iron by a colorimetric method (Iron Test Roche) in a Microcentrifugal Analyzer III (Instrumentation Laboratories), and serum transferrin by an immunoturbidimetric method (Dako) using the Microcentrifugal Analzyer III.

During the 18-year interval between the two studies, some of the laboratory methods had changed. Serum iron was expressed in µg/100 ml in 1969 and normal limits were 70–150. In the 1987 study, serum iron was expressed in the System International as micromoles/liter. The current normal range is 12.5–26.9 µmol/liter. The 1969 values were converted to micromoles/liter for comparison. Red blood cell folate was measured in ng/ml in 1969. Today it is measured in micrograms/liter, but the values are numerically identical. Serum vitamin B_{12} was expressed as picograms/milliliter in 1969 and as nanograms/liter in 1987. Upper limits remained the same but lower normal limits changed from 250 pg/ml in 1969 to 200 ng/liter in 1987.

Test Results

Tables 1 and 2 illustrate the hematological findings of the two studies. Note that more individuals have elevated hemoglobin levels in 1987 than in 1969 (Figure 2). The difference between the two populations is statistically significant for females ($p = 0.047$) and for males ($p = 0.050$). At the same time there is a statistically significant decrease in the number of individuals with below normal hemoglobin values between 1969 and 1987 for males ($p = 0.030$) but not for females ($p = 0.152$). Another difference is the increase in individuals with subnormal serum iron and transferrin saturation levels in 1987 compared to 1969 (Figure 3). These differences are statistically significant for both males and females (serum iron males $p = 0.001$, females $p = 0.013$; transferrin saturation males $p = 0.004$, females $p = 0.000$). While hemoglobin means became significantly higher between 1969 and 1981 and 1987, with the exception of the Chum!kwe females, transferrin saturation means became significantly lower. Serum iron means are lower, but not at a statistically significant level (Table 3).

Subnormal serum iron levels are more common in 1987 than 1969. The percentage of !Kung and Herero with subnormal iron levels is similar. The number of subnormal and elevated occurrences of both red cell folate and serum folate is not statistically significant between the 1969 and 1987 studies. The folate values are also similar between ethnic groups and gender (Table 2). No children have any deficiencies or elevated values. A high number of elevated serum B_{12} levels were obtained. Some of these levels are quite impressive, including the highest, 3372 pg/ml, as well as some in the 2000 pg/ml level (upper normal limits are 1100 pg/ml). Very high B_{12} levels are found among both sexes and both ethnic groups in each study.

Discussion

Studies suggest that anemia, when not the result of diet or blood loss, is a physiological defense against disease rather than a pathological condition (see Kent, Chapter 1, and Weinberg, Chapter 4, this volume; Kent et al. 1990, 1992). The mechanism involved is the withholding of iron. Bacteria, fungi, and protozoa require iron for various metabolic functions but cannot store sufficient quantities of it in a nontoxic form (Weinberg 1984; also Chapter 4, this volume). As a consequence, they are forced to extract iron directly from their host. In defense, the body sequesters iron through a variety of mechanisms. For example, a malabsorption syndrome and fever that are associated with a number of disorders impair the ability of invading microorganisms to obtain iron (see Kent, Chapter 1, this volume).

It has been proposed that mild chronic hypoferremia, or low circulating iron levels, is an adaptation to cycles of continuous disease in areas of high pathogen loads (Kent and Weinberg 1989; Kent 1992; Stuart-Macadam 1988). In the face of cyclic infectious insults, the body maintains a lowered iron level to retard microbial proliferation. This is manifested in low serum iron and transferrin saturation values. The iron-withholding defense system is thwarted by iron overload; hyperferremic individuals tend to be more susceptible to disease (Weinberg, Chapter 4, this volume).

It is important to note that we are *not* referring to either blood loss as occurs from some parasitic infections such as hookworm or starvation diets where there are insufficient calories, vitamins, protein, and minerals, i.e., true iron deficiency. However, we, as other authors in this volume, suggest that anemia of chronic disease, wherein the body has adequate iron stores, is a nonspecific defense against pathogens. A comprehensive review of *in vivo* and *in vitro* research on animals and humans questions the traditional link between anemia and increased vulnerability to infection and finds serious faults with those studies claiming such a connection. The conclusion is that there "is, however, *no* evidence to suggest that individuals with iron deficiency suffer the devastating infective complications of the well-defined immunodeficiency syndromes either congenital or acquired. It seems likely therefore that despite the fun-

Table 1. Comparison of 1969 and 1987 Hematological Values

	Hemoglobin[a]		Hematocrit[b]		Serum Iron[c]		Serum Ferritin[d]		Transferrin[e]		Transferrin Saturation[f]	
	n	%	n	%	n	%	n	%	n	%	n	%
1969 !Kung												
Males												
Normal	30	(83.3)	33	(91.7)	28	(77.8)					31	(81.6)
Below	6	(16.7)	3	(8.3)	4	(11.1)					1	(2.8)
Above	—	—	—	—	4	(11.1)					4	(11.1)
Females												
Normal	107	(90.7)	109	(92.4)	77	(67.5)					101	(89.3)
Below	9	(7.6)	9	(7.6)	28	(24.6)					6	(5.3)
Above	2	(1.7)	—	—	9	(7.9)					6	(5.3)
1969 Herero												
Males												
Normal	1	(100.0)	1	(100.0)	—	—					—	—
Below	—	—	—	—	—	—					—	—
Above	—	—	—	—	1	(100.0)					1	(100.0)
1987 !Kung												
Males												
Normal	37	(90.2)	39	(95.1)	14	(36.8)	34	(81.0)	38	(97.4)	25	(65.8)
Below	1	(2.4)	—	—	17	(44.7)	—	—	—	—	10	(26.3)
Above	3	(7.3)	2	(4.9)	7	(18.4)	8	(19.0)	1	(2.6)	3	(7.9)

	Hemoglobin[a]		Hematocrit[b]		Serum iron[c]		Transferrin[d]		Serum ferritin[e]		Transferrin saturation[f]	
Females												
Normal	46	(90.2)	48	(94.1)	25	(50.0)	48	(96.0)	48	(96.0)	29	(58.0)
Below	1	(2.0)	1	(2.0)	22	(44.0)	—	—	1	(2.0)	21	(42.0)
Above	4	(7.8)	2	(3.9)	3	(6.0)	2	(4.0)	1	(2.0)	—	—
Children (under 15)												
Normal	13	(81.3)	13	(81.3)	11	(68.8)	16	(100.0)	14	(87.5)	10	(62.5)
Below	1	(6.3)	3	(18.8)	3	(18.8)	—	—	1	(6.3)	6	(37.5)
Above	2	(12.5)	—	—	2	(12.5)	—	—	1	(6.3)	—	—
1987 Herero												
Males												
Normal	4	(57.1)	7	(100.0)	7	(100.0)	6	(60.0)	9	(90.0)	7	(70.0)
Below	1	(14.3)	—	—	3	(30.0)	—	—	1	(10.0)	3	(30.0)
Above	2	(28.6)	—	—	—	—	4	(40.0)	—	—	—	—
Females												
Normal	4	(100.0)	4	(100.0)	3	(42.9)	7	(100.0)	7	(100.0)	1	(20.0)
Below	0	(0.0)	—	—	3	(42.9)	—	—	—	—	3	(60.0)
Above	0	(0.0)	—	—	1	(14.3)	—	—	—	—	1	(20.0)

Notes: Normal values used in this study:

[a] Hemoglobin: children, 11.0–15.5 g/dl; males, 13.5–18.0 g/dl; females, 12–16.0 g/dl.

[b] Hematocrit: males, 41–54%; females, 37–49%.

[c] Serum iron: 1969 values 70–150 μg/ml; 1987 values 12.6–27 μg/ml.

[d] Transferrin: 1.9–4.3 g/liter.

[e] Serum ferritin: 12–240 ng/gl.

[f] Transferrin saturation: 16–50%.

Table 2. Comparison of Folate and Vitamin B$_{12}$ Studies

	Red Cell Folate[a]		Serum Folate[b]		Serum B$_{12}$[c]	
	n	%	n	% of subgroup	n	%
1969 !Kung						
Males						
Normal			27	(79.4)	32	(97.1)
Below			4	(11.8)	—	—
Above			3	(8.8)	1	(2.9)
Females						
Normal			96	(84.2)	104	(90.4)
Below			7	(6.1)	—	—
Above			11	(9.7)	11	(9.6)
1969 Herero						
Males						
Normal						
Below						
Above						
1987 !Kung						
Males						
Normal	34	(82.9)	37	(90.2)	37	(86.0)
Below	3	(7.3)	2	(4.9)	—	—
Above	4	(9.8)	2	(4.9)	6	(14.0)
Females						
Normal	45	(88.2)	48	(94.1)	43	(84.3)
Below	2	(3.9)	1	(2.0)	—	—
Above	4	(7.8)	2	(3.9)	8	(15.7)
Children (under 15)						
Normal	14	(87.5)	16	(100.0)	12	(76.5)
Below	2	(12.5)	—	—	—	—
Above	—	—	—	—	4	(23.5)
1987 Herero						
Males						
Normal	6	(85.7)	6	(85.7)	6	(60.0)
Below	—	—	1	(14.3)	—	—
Above	1	(14.3)	—	—	4	(40.0)
Females						
Normal	2	(50.0)	5	(71.4)	7	(100.0)
Below	1	(25.0)	2	(28.6)	—	—
Above	1	(25.0)	—	—	—	—

Notes: Normal values used in this study:
[a] Red cell folate: 160–600 ng/ml.
[b] Serum folate: 3–14 ng/ml.
[c] Serum vitamin B$_{12}$: 250–1100 pg/ml.

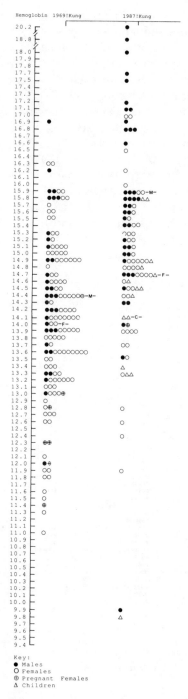

Figure 2. Comparison of 1969 and 1987 hemoglobin values.

damental importance of iron in maintaining the integrity of immune function, humans can tolerate the extremes of deficiency and excess and survive in a relatively healthy state" (Farthing 1989:44; emphasis added).

The hypoferremic response to disease seems to become chronic in environments of continual infection, such as sedentary settlements with poor sanitation (Kent and Weinberg 1989). It follows that anemia, specifically the anemia of chronic disease/inflammation, should be more prevalent among the 1987 sedentary study group. Serum iron and transferrin saturation values characteristically decrease in the anemia of chronic infection (e.g., Cook 1989; G. Lee 1983). "Serum iron concentration in the anemia of chronic disease is characteristically low despite adequate tissue stores of iron; and it appears as if infection, inflammation, or neoplastic disease impair the transfer of iron from cellular ferritin" (Reizenstein 1983:43). Low serum iron and transferrin saturation levels

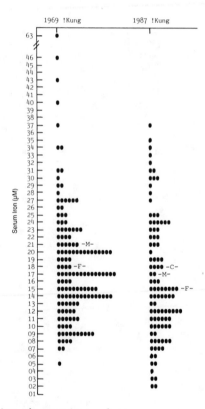

Figure 3. Distribution of serum iron values.

Table 3. Diachronic Comparison of !Kung Hematological Means (Excluding Pregnant Women)[a]

Year/Group	Hemoglobin (g/dl)		Serum Iron % (μM)		Saturation (%)		Transferrin (g/dl)		Serum Ferritin (ng/ml)	
1969 !Kung[b]										
Males[c]	14.4	(0.2)	20.9	(1.2)	36.8	(2.4)	—	—	—	—
Females[d]	14.0	(0.1)	17.5	(1.1)	29.5	(1.1)	—	—	—	—
1981 !Kung[e]										
Males	14.7	(0.2)	17.0	(1.6)	35.0	(1.2)	2.4	(0.1)	127	(9.0)
Females[f]	13.3	—	13.9	—	26.5	—	2.6	—	80	—
Children	12.9	(0.2)	13.2	(0.4)	26.0	(0.9)	2.5	(0.3)	53	(11.0)
1987 !Kung[g]										
Males	15.9	(0.3)	16.7	(1.4)	24.8	(2.4)	2.7	(0.1)	145	(13.7)
Females	14.7	(0.2)	15.3	(1.4)	19.7	(1.5)	3.0	(0.9)	89	(9.1)
Children	14.1	(0.3)	17.8	(2.6)	21.8	(2.6)	3.3	(0.2)	57	(6.4)

[a] All values are means with SD in parentheses.

[b] Data from Metz et al. (1971).

[c] Sample sizes (n): 1969 males = 37–38; 1969 females = 67–68; 1969 postmenopausal females = 45; 1981 males = 72; 1981 females = 82–90; 1981 postmenopausal females = 14; 1981 children = 30–32; 1987 males = 38–41; 1987 females = 31; 1987 postmenopausal females = 20; 1987 children = 16.

[d] Pregnant females' means for 1969 are Hb = 12.5 (0.3); iron = 17.6; % Sat = 27.4 (3.2).

[e] Data from Fernandes-Costa et al. (1984).

[f] Pregnant females' means for 1981 are Hb = 12.9 (0.2); iron = 16.3 (2.2); % Sat = 26 (4); transferrin = 3.2 (1.1); serum ferritin = 62 (12).

[g] Data from Hansen et al. (1992).

are the body's attempt to limit iron availability. We postulate that the high incidence of subnormal serum iron and transferrin saturation values in the 1987 population is a manifestation of the hypoferremic response wherein the body withholds iron during continual threats of microbial invasion.

The 1987 group had lower serum iron and transferrin saturation levels but higher hemoglobin levels, despite an increase in the mean age of males in 1987 compared to 1969 (hemoglobin levels tend to decrease with advancing age, Wadsworth 1989, personal communication). In the 1987 study, almost 45% of the males, 44% of the females, and nearly 19% of the children had below normal serum iron levels (Table 1). As noted above, this represents a significant increase of subnormal values in the same population tested 18 years before. Concomitant with the reduction of the serum iron levels is a substantial decrease in transferrin saturation levels (Figures 2 and 3).

Serum ferritin is normal (e.g., >50 ng/ml) or elevated in the anemia of chronic disease and depressed in iron deficiency anemia (Kent, Chapter 1, this volume). These values reflect the amount of storage iron in the body and indicate adequate stores in individuals with the anemia of chronic disease (Stein 1990; Worwood 1980). Serum ferritin values become elevated as the body attempts to reduce the availability of iron to microinvaders. Unfortunately serum ferritin was not measured in 1969. In 1987, no one had serum ferritin values below 12 ng/ml, the threshold value used to identify iron-deficiency anemia. However, between 4 and 19% of the adults had elevated serum ferritin levels above 240 ng/ml, the cutoff value used in Fernandes-Costa et al. (1984; no children in the 1987 study had elevated values; see Table 1). Even a larger number of individuals had serum ferritin values over 50 ng/ml, the threshold value used by most to infer the presence of the anemia of chronic disease/infection when in association with hypoferremia (e.g., Bothwell et al. 1979:53; Cash and Sears 1989; Cook and Skikne 1989; Stein 1990:1076). In 1987, 77% of hypoferremic adults and 43% of hypoferremic children had serum ferritin values above 50 ng/ml (34 individuals). Absolute eosinophil levels also were elevated in 1987, possibly due to parasites.

The hematological investigation of the Basarwa in 1969 revealed a very low incidence of anemia and iron deficiency. This finding is somewhat remarkable in that the subjects studied included numerous young females, many of whom were lactating, and others who were pregnant. Moreover, hookworm infection was present in 3 out of 18 fecal samples (Metz et al. 1971). It is unlikely that the iron in the food alone could maintain this level of iron nutrition, and it was suggested that the dietary iron intake was supplemented by iron derived from the cooking pots. Clinical and biochemical evidence of siderosis was not noted in the Basarwa and this is probably because, unlike Bantu-speakers, they do not brew beer in iron pots (Metz et al. 1971:240).

The reduction in the length of time children are breast-fed in 1987 compared to 1969 has made them more vulnerable to microorganisms. Breast milk is known to afford protection to young children, through the provision of lactoferrin, a powerful iron binder that makes iron less accessible to microinvaders (e.g., Clemens et al. 1986; Habicht et al. 1988; and others).

Analysis of subnormal values alone can be misleading. Equally illuminating as the below-normal values are the above-normal values. Notable increases in the above-normal hemoglobin and hematocrit values occur in the 1987 population compared to the 1969 group. These probably result from three different cultural practices—use of iron cooking pots, smoking, and alcohol consumption. All three practices are known to increase hemoglobin and hematocrit levels (Weinberg, Chapter 4, this volume).

Experiments have demonstrated that foods cooked in iron pots have a statistically significant higher level of iron than food cooked in noniron pots (Brittin and Nossaman 1986). Although it is widely acknowledged that iron is not as readily absorbed by individuals with chronic infections as by healthy individuals, oral iron is still absorbed by the former, though at a lower rate. In a classic study, the ingestion of 1 g of oral ferrous sulfate caused an increase in plasma iron in 14% of the subjects with chronic infection compared to 83% of normal subjects (Cartwright et al. 1946). The use of iron pots appears to mask what otherwise may have been lower hemoglobin/hematocrit levels, as well as lower serum iron and transferrin saturation levels. Alcohol has been shown to elevate hemoglobin levels (Rodriguez et al. 1986). Iron absorption is markedly enhanced in normal subjects (without liver damage) who drink alcohol because ethanol stimulates the secretion of hydrocholaric acid, which in turn increases iron absorption (Weinberg, Chapter 4, this volume; also see McLaren et al. 1983:225). Cigarette smoking has also been found to elevate hemoglobin levels, though not other iron indices (Forrest et al. 1987). According to the Centers for Disease Control (1989:402–403), "smoking increases Hb and Hct levels substantially. The higher Hb and Hct of smokers is a consequence of an increased carboxyhemoglobin from inhaling carbon monoxide during smoking. Because carboxyhemoglobin has no oxygen carrying capacity, its presence causes a generalized upward shift of the Hb and Hct distribution curves.... Therefore, a smoking-specific adjustment to the anemia cutoff is necessary for the proper diagnosis of anemia in smokers." We suggest that if it were not for these three cultural practices, hemoglobin values would have been much lower in 1987. In other words, the common association between anemia of chronic disease as evidenced by low serum iron and transferrin saturation values and slightly low hemoglobin levels is being masked by practices that inflate the latter, particularly smoking.

Above-normal vitamin B_{12} levels can be attributed to acute infectious diseases, among other conditions (e.g., Todd 1984:243). The increase in the occurrence of elevated vitamin B_{12} may be another measure of an increase in the morbidity of the 1987 !Kung, although it also could represent a genetic variation (Jenkins 1988, personal communication).

Chum!kwe: An Example of a Deficient Diet

If the proposition that iron withholding is a defense against chronic cycles of infections is valid, an increased incidence of hypoferremia ought to occur in sedentary aggregated communities. It should be possible to distinguish hypoferremia, a defense against disease, from iron-deficiency anemia, a pathological condition. Chum!kwe, Namibia, provides an interesting test. As discussed above, it is a sedentary !Kung and Herero community where, unlike the other groups investigated, the !Kung eat little meat.

The hematological difference between the 1969 !Kung data and the 1981 Chum!kwe data was attributed to the change in the Chum!kwe diet. Originally based primarily on wild plants and meat, the diet became one based primarily on agricultural produce and government distributed maize meal (Fernandes-Costa et al. 1984). However, these people not only had poor diets but were sedentary as well. The combination makes it difficult to distinguish anemia caused by diet from anemia caused by sedentism and the diseases associated with it.

Few males in 1981 had subnormal hemoglobin levels; children and women had the greatest percentage of subnormal values (Table 4). The health status of the Chum!kwe population was portrayed as poor. "The present study has shown that the change in lifestyle undergone by the San [!Kung] between 1969 and 1981 has been accompanied by a deterioration in their previously excellent iron and folate nutrition and in an increase in the incidence of anemia, most of which is almost certainly nutritional in origin" (Fernandes-Costa et al. 1984:1302–1303). The low

Table 4. Chum!kwe !Kung 1981 Hematology[a]

	Hemoglobin[b]		Serum Iron		Serum Ferritin		Transferrin		% Saturation		Serum Vitamin B_{12}		Serum Folate		Red Cell Folate	
	n	%	n	%	n	%	n	%	n	%	n	%	n	%	n	%
Males																
Normal	65?[c]	(90.0)	53	(73.6)	66	(91.7)	72	(100.0)	68	(94.4)	71?	(98.6)	38?	(52.8)	62	(86.1)
Subnormal	7	(9.7)	13	(18.1)	—	—	—	—	4	(5.6)	1	(1.4)	34	(47.2)	10	(13.9)
Above	?[d]	—	6	(8.3)	6	(8.3)	—	—	—	—	?	?	?	?	?	?
Females																
Normal	96?	(88.1)	70	(70.7)	97	(98.0)	99	(100.0)	85	(85.9)	103?	(94.5)	65?	(59.6)	99	(90.8)
Subnormal	13	(11.9)	28	(28.3)	2	(2.0)	—	—	14	(14.1)	6	(5.5)	44	(40.4)	10	(9.2)
Above	?	—	1	(1.0)	—	—	—	—	—	—	?	?	?	?	?	?
Children																
Normal	17?	(53.13)	18	(60.0)	20	(66.7)	30	(100.0)	20	(66.7)	27?	(100.0)	22?	(81.5)	21?	(77.8)
Subnormal	15	(46.9)	12	(40.0)	10	(33.3)	—	—	10	(33.3)	—	—	5	(18.5)	6	(22.2)
Above	?	—	—	—	—	—	—	—	—	—	?	?	?	?	?	?

[a] Data from Fernandes-Costa et al. (1984).

[b] Normal values used in this study. Hemoglobin: males: >13.5 g/dl; females: >12 g/dl (pregnant > 11 g/dl); children: >11 g/dl; serum iron: 12.6–27 μmol/liter; serum ferritin: 12–240 ng/ml; percent saturation: 16–50%; serum vitamin B_{12}: 400–1100 pg/ml; serum folate: 3–14 ng/ml; red cell folate: 160–600 ng/ml.

[c] Unknown number actually have normal values because of endnote 3.

[d] Above normal values either not encountered or not noted.

serum folate levels were probably the result of the heavy alcohol consumption at Chum!kwe (Fernandes-Costa et al. 1984:1302). This is substantiated by the presence of round, macrocytic red cells and target cells, indicating liver damage (Fernandes-Costa et al. 1984).

The results of the 1981 study are shown in Table 4 and can be contrasted with Tables 1 and 2. Approximately 47% of Chum!kwe !Kung children had subnormal hemoglobin levels, whereas only 10% of adult males and 12% of adult females had subnormal levels (Fernandes-Costa et al. 1984:1297). This differs significantly from the 6% of children, 2% of adult females, and 2% adult males with subnormal hemoglobin values in 1987 (unfortunately no children were tested in 1969). It is interesting to note that fewer adult males at Chum!kwe have subnormal hemoglobin levels than 1969 Dobe males, despite profound dietary differences that would suggest otherwise.

The Chum!kwe Basarwa suffered from extremely poor, at times starvation, diets. In addition, a large number of individuals were plagued by infectious diseases. Parasites were identified in 23% of the fecal samples. Some samples contained more than one species; most common were hookworm (*Necator americanus*) and *Giardia lamblia* (Fernandes-Costa et al. 1984:1302). Despite the documented extremely impoverished diet, only 6% of the adult women, no adult men, and 33% of the children had subnormal serum ferritin levels. Significantly, 20% of hypoferremic children, 65% of the hypoferremic adult females, and 70% of hypoferremic adult males have serum ferritin levels above 50 ng/ml, which is the threshold value to define the anemia of chronic disease. Unfortunately the ages of those afflicted with parasites were not published. However, many of the subnormal serum ferritin levels can be accounted for by the hookworm and other parasite infections that are known to cause gross gastrointestinal bleeding. This bleeding, along with the parasites' competition with the host for iron, produces low serum ferritin and hemoglobin levels regardless of diet. Chum!kwe children have subnormal serum ferritin values at a higher rate than adults. This distribution of subnormal values is consistent with the increased tendency of children to acquire parasites and to also have a heavier parasite load than adults in the same situation (Hern 1991).

In 1981, the Chum!kwe population was clearly not a healthy one and anemia was common. We believe the prevalence of anemia is a result of a generalized defense against a heavy pathogen load and in that respect Chum!kwe resembles the 1987 Dobe population more than it does the 1969 Dobe population. A poor diet and high levels of alcohol consumption at Chum!kwe have created other health problems, as reflected in low folate levels. Many of the subnormal serum ferritin levels seen in children are likely attributable to three factors: parasitic infections known to cause gross blood loss and competition with the host for nutrients, a truly deficient diet, and a shorter period of breast-feeding. It is significant that Chum!kwe adults were less anemic than children (only 10% men and 12% women, Fernandes-Costa et al. 1984). If diet were primarily responsible for the anemia in children, then it would have to be demonstrated that adults ate a significantly different and better diet than children. More likely causes for the difference are (1) the adults' use of alcohol and tobacco, both of which tend to raise iron absorption and hemoglobin levels, and (2) a possible difference in parasite load (iron cooking pots were not used at Chum!kwe).

Anemia and Morbidity among the !Kung

What appears to be occurring in 1987 at Dobe and in 1981 at Chum!kwe is the activation of the iron-withholding defense against chronic cycles of disease. However, in the 1987 Dobe population, the defense appears to be thwarted by cultural practices that elevate iron levels. Bantu siderosis caused by ingestion of exogenous iron from the use of metal pots for brewing beer is a common condition in southern Africa (Bothwell et al. 1964; McLaren et al. 1984). The absence of Bantu siderosis among the Dobe !Kung might be the result of the presence of hypoferremia that is being masked by the ingestion of iron from cast iron pots. Hemoglobin/hematocrit levels, then, may be potentially misleading, i.e., they make a relatively unhealthy population appear superficially healthier than it is. The researchers at Chum!kwe (Fernandes-Costa et al. 1984) acknowledged the high morbidity present partly because it was so pronounced in the most common blood indices used to determine general well-being (i.e., hemoglobin and hematocrit of children). The Chum!kwe !Kung diet was obviously poor and alcoholism was prevalent. Therefore the population was easily recognized as nonhealthy, despite the relatively low number of adults with subnormal hemoglobin or serum ferritin levels. Much more subtle are the 1987 Dobe !Kung population parameters. Their diet was at least minimally adequate and alcoholism was not as common as at Chum!kwe. Figures 3 and 4 show, however, a greater percentage of the 1987 population have subnormal serum iron and transferrin saturation levels than the more obviously unhealthy 1981 Chum!kwe population with a deficient diet. Both groups represent populations with high morbidity levels.

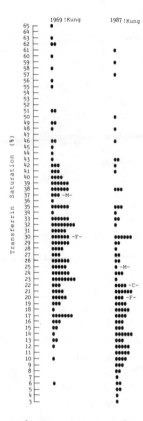

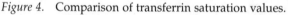

Figure 4. Comparison of transferrin saturation values.

If our hypothesis is valid, then how can we explain the fact that the Chum!kwe population had fewer subnormal serum iron and transferrin saturation levels than did the 1987 !Kung? Both groups drink homemade alcohol, and a large portion of the Chum!kwe population is and has been for some time alcoholic. Alcoholism at Chum!kwe can be inferred from "the large number of subjects having a high MCV or a raised serum μ-GT level, or both. Raised MCV and raised μ-GT levels are fairly sensitive indicators of alcoholism and the likelihood of alcoholism in an individual is increased if both indices are raised" (Fernandes-Costa et al. 1984:1302). Alcohol enhances the absorption of iron from food, resulting in abnormally high levels of iron and transferrin saturation, even in those without liver damage (Weinberg, Chapter 4, this volume). We suggest that high iron status often present in alcoholics is absent because of pathogen-induced hypoferremia. Hypoferremia results in low iron levels and alcoholism, and in the absence of gastrointestinal bleeding, results in high iron levels. In combination, the two can result in relatively normal levels. So few adults at Chum!kwe had subnormal serum ferritin values that they indicate that gastrointestinal bleeding, which can cause anemia in alcoholics, was not a factor.

Every population contains a certain proportion of ill individuals. A few, 14%, of the nomadic 1969 !Kung, for example, had parasites, including hookworm. Hookworm was present in 20% of the fecal samples examined from Chum!kwe (Fernandes-Costa et al. 1984). We do not have data on hookworm for the 1987 Dobe population. What few health problems did exist in 1969, such as hookworm, were masked by the ingestion of iron from the use of cast iron pots (Metz et al. 1971). Nevertheless, the 1969 group can be viewed as a generally healthy population, and used as a baseline for later studies.

Smoking, the consumption of alcohol, and the use of iron pots are all important practices among the 1987 !Kung that should be reflected in their iron levels. Although the diet has changed between 1969 and 1987, the later diet is not necessarily deficient in iron (Table 2 shows that only a few people had a folate deficiency). Considering the aforementioned practices that elevate iron levels and the fact that the 1987 population, depending on the subgroup, had the same or elevated hemoglobin levels as the 1969 population, it should follow that a higher percentage of the 1987 population would have similar serum iron and transferrin saturation levels. As they do not, something must be reducing these iron levels. We suggest that hypoferremia as a defense against disease is responsible for the lowered levels and for the absence of siderosis. The hypoferremic response is thwarted by the aforementioned cultural practices that would, in the absence of chronic infection, result in hyperferremia. We suggest that neither the 1987 Ngamiland !Kung nor the 1981 Chum!kwe !Kung represent healthy populations and that infectious diseases are serious problems in both groups. Chum!kwe !Kung morbidity is further complicated by alcoholism and a poor diet.

The high frequency of the anemia of chronic disease and absence of dietary iron-deficiency anemia is not restricted to the 1987 Dobe Basarwa. Similar studies among a different recently sedentary Basarwa group located outside the Khutse Game Reserve to the east and south of Dobe revealed the same pattern of morbidity and the anemia of chronic disease (Kent and Dunn 1992). This study shows that the Dobe !Kung are not an isolated or unusual case. The anemia of chronic disease appears to go along with sedentism and aggregation.

Conclusions

Superficially, the !Kung appear to be hematologically healthier in 1987 than in 1969 inasmuch as their hemoglobin/hematocrit and serum folate levels are higher. However, their hemoglobin levels may be elevated because of the combined effects of cooking in cast iron pots, smoking, and alcoholism. Other hematological indices suggest that the !Kung are in fact less healthy in 1987 than in 1969. Transferrin saturation, serum iron, and serum ferritin measurements indicate a hypoferremic response to microbial invasion. An indirect measure of hypoferremia in operation is the fact that the 1987 Dobe population had more individuals with subnormal serum iron and transferrin saturation values than did the Chum!kwe population with an acknowledged deficient diet. The incidence of iron-deficiency anemia appears to be very low in 1987 but the anemia of chronic disease is very high.

We have shown that it is not diet alone that keeps nomadic foragers healthy, as is sometimes inferred. Both the 1969 !Kung and the 1987 Dobe Basarwa have a diet sufficient in iron. However, a number of hematologic parameters suggest very different levels of morbidity between the two groups. The number of hypoferremic individuals with serum ferritin levels above 50 ng/ml in contrast to those with serum ferritin levels below 12 ng/ml attests to the prevalence of the anemia of chronic disease and the absence of dietary iron-deficiency anemia. Chum!kwe !Kung, who had a deficient diet, had a lower percentage of adults with subnormal serum iron and transferrin saturation values. The opposite should be the case if diet were responsible for the lowered iron levels. The deterioration of health at Dobe over the 18-year period seems to be directly attributable to increasing sedentism.

This study shows that it may be misleading to interpret medical data independent of anthropological data. It also indicates that percentages of normal, subnormal, and elevated iron values must be interpreted in context with the morbidity of a population. As pointed out by Garn in Chapter 2 (this volume), hemoglobin/hematocrit can be influenced by a number of spurious factors and are not, by themselves, reliable indicators of health or disease. Fewer than expected cases of hyperferremia were observed; some factor must therefore have been intervening. Because of the iron-withholding defense, hemoglobin values were normal in most adults, masking a higher level of morbidity than the figures alone suggest. The combination of serum iron and transferrin saturation and particularly serum ferritin levels provides a good indication of the level of morbidity in a population. The increase in aggregation and reduction of mobility resulted in a higher morbidity for both the 1981 Chum!kwe and the 1987 Dobe !Kung populations. Thus we conclude that in spite of a rise in hemoglobin values, a higher morbidity exists in the 1987 Dobe population than in the 1969 population.

Appendix

Estimated Percentage of Diet Provided by Different Food Sources for Subjects in Dobe Area Medical Surveys, 1969 and 1987

Year	Wild Food Plant/Animal		Domesticates Plant/Animal		Store-Bought Foods	Gov't	Total Sources
1969	58	27	5	5			
Total		85		10	*	*	100
1987	15	15	5	15			
Total		30		20	5	45	100

Acknowledgments

We are most grateful to Trefor Jenkins who participated in much of the data collection and initial analyses, and who also provided the published and unpublished raw data used in this paper. We appreciate the useful comments and suggestions made on various drafts by Drs. Gene Weinberg, Trefor Jenkins, Patty Stuart-Macadam, Steve Kent, Nancy Rikalo, R. Stuart, and George Wadsworth. Dr Henry Harpending kindly looked up 18-year-old field notes to give us information on the gender and age of individuals in the 1969 study. Finally we are indebted to the !Kung for volunteering to participate in these and other studies and to the government of Botswana for granting researchers permission to work in their country. An Old Dominion University College of Arts and Letters research grant paid for the entry of data on the mainframe computer and the ODU Graphics Department drafted the figures.

References

Binford, L. 1983. *Working at Archaeology*. New York: Academic Press.
Bothwell, T.H., H. Seftel, P. Jacobs, J. Torrance, and N. Baumslag. 1964. Iron overload in Bantu subjects. *The American Journal of Clinical Nutrition* 14:47–51.

Brothwell, T., R. Charlton, J. Cook, and C. Finch. 1979. *Iron Metabolism in Man.* Oxford: Blackwell Scientific Publications.

Brittin, H., and C. Nossaman. 1986. Iron content of food cooked in iron utensils. *Journal of the American Dietetic Association* 86(7):897–901.

Cartwright, G., G.A. Lauritsen, S. Humphries, P.J. Jones, I.M. Merrill, and M.M. Wintrobe. 1946. The anemia of infection. *Journal of Clinical Investigation* 25: 65–80.

Cash, J., and D. Sears. 1989. The anemia of chronic disease: Spectrum of associated diseases in a series of unselected hospitalized patients. *American Journal of Medicine* 87:683–644.

Center for Disease Control. 1989. CDC criteria for anemia in children and childbearing-aged women. *Morbidity and Mortality Weekly Report* 38(22):400–404.

Clemens, J., B. Stanton, B. Stoll, N. Shahid, H. Banu, and A.K. Chowdhury. 1986. Breast feeding as a determinant of severity in shigellosis. *American Journal of Epidemiology* 123:710–720.

Cook, James (ed.). 1980. *Iron.* New York: Churchill Livingston.

Cook, J.D. and B.S. Skikne. 1989. Iron deficiency: Definition and diagnosis. *Journal of Internal Medicine* 226:349–355.

Eaton, S.B., M. Konner, and M. Shostak. 1988. Stone agers in the fast lane: Chronic degenerative disease in evolutionary perspective. *American Journal of Medicine* 84(4):739–749.

Farthing, M.J. 1989. Iron and immunity. *Acta Paediatric Scandinavia Supplemental* 361:44–52.

Fernandes-Costa, F., J. Marshall, C. Ritchie, S. van Tonder, D. Dunn, T. Jenkins, and J. Metz. 1984. Transition from a hunter-gatherer to a settled lifestyle in the !Kung San: Effect on iron, folate, and vitamin B^{12} nutrition. *The American Journal of Clinical Nutrition* 40:1295–1303.

Forrest, R., C. Jackson, and J. Yudkin. 1987. The epidemiology of the haemoglobin level—A study of 1057 subjects in general practice. *Postgraduate Medical Journal* 63:625–628.

Habicht, J-P., J. DaVanzo, and W. Butz. 1988. Mother's milk and sewage: Their interactive effects on infant mortality. *Pediatrics* 18:456–461.

Hansen, J.D., R. Lee, J. van der Westerhuizen, T. Jenkins, and D. Dunn. 1992. The health of the hunter-gatherers: Twenty years on. Manuscript in preparation.

Harpending, H., and L. Wandsnider. 1982. Population structures of Ghanzi and Ngamiland !Kung. In *Current Developments in Anthropological Genetics*, Vol. 2. M. Crawford and J. Mielke, eds., pp. 29–50. New York: Plenum Press.

Hern, W. 1991. Epidemiologic issues in studying anemia. Paper presented at the Annual Meeting of the American Physical Anthropology Conference, Milwaukee, Wisconsin.

Ingold, T. 1987. *The Appropriation of Nature.* Iowa City: Iowa University Press.

Kent, S. 1986. The influence of sedentism and aggregation on porotic hyperostosis and anaemia: A case study. *Man* 21:605–636.

Kent, S. 1992. Iron deficiency and other acquired anemias. In *The Cambridge His-

torical, Geographical, and Cultural Encyclopedia of Human Nutrition. K. Kipple,
ed. Cambridge: Cambridge University Press.

Kent, S., and D. Dunn. 1991. A hematological study of a recently sedentary
Kalahari community. Manuscript submitted for publication.

Kent, S., and E. Weinberg. 1989. Hypoferremia: Adaptation to disease? *New
England Journal of Medicine* 672.

Kent, S., E. Weinberg, and P. Stuart-Macadam. 1990. Dietary and prophylactic
iron supplements: Helpful or harmful? *Human Nature* 1(1):55–81.

Kent, S., E. Weinberg, and P. Stuart-Macadam. 1992. The etiology of the anemia
of chronic disease. Manuscript submitted for publication.

Lal, H., K. Agarwal, M. Gupta, and D. Agarwal. 1973. Protein and iron sup-
plementations by altering cooking practices in community. *Indian Journal of
Medical Research* 61(6):918–925.

Lee, G.R. 1983. The anemia of chronic disease. *Seminar in Hematology* 20:61–80.

Lee, R. 1979. *The !Kung San: Men, Women, and Work in a Foraging Society*.
Cambridge: Cambridge University Press.

Lee, R. 1981. Politics, sexual and nonsexual, in an egalitarian society: The !Kung
San. *Social Inequality: Comparative and Developmental Approaches*. Gerald Ber-
reman, ed., pp. 83–102. New York: Academic Press.

Lee, R. 1980. Lactation, ovulation, infanticide, and women's work: A study of
hunter-gatherer population regulation. In *Biosocial Mechanisms of Population
Regulation*. M. Cohen, R. Malpass, and H. Klein, eds., pp. 321–348. New
Haven: Yale University Press.

Marshall, J., and C. Ritchie. 1984. Where are the Ju/wasi of Nyae Nyae? Changes
in a Bushman Society: 1958–1981. *University of Cape Town Center for African
Studies* 9:1–187.

McLaren, G., W.A. Muir, and R. Kellermeyer. 1983. Iron overload disorders:
Natural history, pathogenesis, diagnosis and therapy. *CRC Critical Reviews in
Clinical Laboratory Sciences* 19(3):205–266.

Metz, J., D. Hart, and H.C. Harpending. 1971. Iron, folate, and vitamin B^{12} nutrition in a hunter-gatherer people: A study of the !Kung Bushmen. *The
American Journal of Clinical Nutrition* 24:229–242.

Nurse, G.T., and T. Jenkins. 1977. *Health and the Hunter-Gatherer: Biomedical Studies
on the Hunting and Gathering Populations of Southern Africa*. London: S. Karger.

Reizenstein, P. 1983. *Hematologic Stress Syndrome: The Biological Response to Disease*.
New York: Praeger.

Rodriguez, M.C., M.S. Henriquez, A.F. Turon, F.J. Novoa, J.G. Diaz, and P.B.
Leon. 1986. Trace elements on chronic alcoholism. *Trace Elements in Medicine*,
3:164–167.

Stein, J. 1990. *Internal Medicine*. Boston: Little, Brown.

Stuart-Macadam, P. 1988. Nutrition and anaemia in past human populations. In
Diet and Subsistence: Current Archaeological Perspectives. B. Kennedy and G.
LeMoine, eds. The Archaeological Association of the University of Calgary.

Todd, J. 1984. *Clinical Diagnosis and Management by Laboratory Methods*, 17th ed.
Philadelphia: W.B. Saunders.

Truswell, A.S., and J. Hansen. 1976. Medical research among the !Kung. In *Kalahari Hunter-Gatherers*. R. Lee and I. DeVore, eds. Cambridge: Harvard University Press.

Wehmeyer, A.S., R. Lee, and M. Whiting. 1969. Nutrient composition and dietary importance of some vegetable foods eaten by the !Kung Bushmen. *South African Medical Journal* 43:1528–1540.

Wienberg, E. 1984. Iron withholding: A defense against infection and neoplasia. *Physiological Reviews* 64:65–102.

Worwood, M. 1980. Serum Ferritin. In *Iron*. J. Cook, ed., pp. 59–89. New York: Churchill Livingstone.

Volkman, T.A. 1982. The San in transition, Vol I. *Cultural Survival* 9:1–56.

Yellen, J. 1985. Bushmen. *Science 85* 41–48.

Chapter 7

Porotic Hyperostosis in Prehistoric Ecuador

Douglas H. Ubelaker

After decades of careful archaeological research, scholars of Ecuadorean prehistory have documented many aspects of the great geographic diversity and complex evolution of culture within Ecuador. Such complexity is manifest in the diverse ceramic and other artifact styles and methods of manufacture that characterize the late prehistoric periods, as well as in dynamic shifts of social systems, settlement patterns, and population demography evident throughout Ecuador for the last several thousand years. Generally, the story is one of growing regional variation, as well as increasing population growth, sedentism, and urbanism.

Since 1973, I have attempted to augment the cultural panorama described above with detailed information about the biology of the people themselves. Through study of carefully excavated and well-documented human remains from many sites within Ecuador, data on disease, demography, and physical characteristics are now available to be correlated with cultural information in an overall assessment of the dynamics of the interrelationship of biology and culture within several thousand years of Ecuador's past.

This essay focuses primarily on one aspect of the biological information gleaned from this study, porotic hyperostosis, and how it may relate to the emerging biocultural framework within Ecuador. Evidence presented in this essay suggests that, within Ecuador, porotic hyperostosis may be interpreted in a novel manner as a product of anemia brought on by the increased morbidity associated with growing population density and sedentism.

Evidence of Porotic Hyperostosis

In recent years, many skeletal biologists have gathered data on what Angel (1966) termed "porotic hyperostosis" as a measure of skeletal response to stress. As noted by Goodman et al. (1984) and Huss-Ashmore et al. (1982), porotic hyperostosis represents an expansion of the spongy diploë with associated thinning of the outer cortical bone and increased outer surface porosity. In the extreme, the outer surface is obliterated and covered with dense trabecular bone resembling "honeycomb." With time, these bony changes are remodeled and result in abnormally thick, but otherwise normally appearing exterior surfaces. The condition also has been described as porous periosteal bone deposition (Ortner and Putschar 1981) or "cribra orbitalia" when occurring in the orbital roof (Suzuki 1987).

Bony changes such as these have been attributed to a variety of conditions, including mumps, infection of the lacrimal gland (orbits only), rickets, chronic infection, scurvy, leprosy (or poor nutrition of individuals with leprosy), and anemia (Ortner and Putschar 1981). The anemia-related conditions include various forms of thalassemia, sickle-cell disease, and hereditary nonspherocytic hemolytic anemia as well as hereditary spherocytosis, hereditary elliptocytosis, cyanotic congenital heart disease, polycythemia, vera and iron-deficiency anemia (Huss-Ashmore et al. 1982; Ortner and Putschar 1981). In short, porotic hyperostosis results from pathological conditions that demand an increase in red blood cell production within the medullary cavities of long bones and diploë of the cranial bones.

Using radiographic comparisons, Stuart-Macadam (1987a,b) elucidated seven criteria that successfully correlated lesions in ancient remains with skeletal manifestations of anemia documented clinically. These criteria for the cranium include a "hair-on-end" pattern of trabeculation, thinning, or disappearance of the outer table, coarse, granular, stippled, and more radiolucent cranial vault trabeculae, diploic thickening, orbital roof thickening, thinning, flattening, and loss of definition of the orbital rim, and lack of frontal sinus development. Stuart-Macadam notes that "hair-on-end" pattern of trabeculation and orbital roof thickening greater than 3 mm (apparently indicative of cribra orbitalia) are absolutely diagnostic of anemia, whereas the other traits are less diagnostic. Elsewhere, Stuart Macadam (1985) has argued that porotic hyperostosis reflects childhood episodes of anemia.

Since there is no other evidence for the presence of the hereditary anemias in aboriginal New World populations, many scholars have concluded that porotic hyperostosis results from iron-deficiency anemia caused by inadequate nutrition. Such interpretation is strengthened in populations known to rely heavily on maize. Maize is a poor source of dietary iron and, furthermore, contains phytates that can inhibit the absorption of iron (El-Najjar et al. 1976; Lallo et al. 1977). However, most scholars note that the extent of iron-deficiency anemia may be augmented by parasitism, other diseases, and cultural factors such as methods of food preparation (Walker 1985, 1986).

Kent (1986) notes the nearly worldwide distribution of porotic hyperostosis and questions the popular tendency to attribute New World examples to dietary stress. Kent (1986) cites a wide literature arguing that diet even among the corn-eating Southwestern Indians was sufficiently varied to produce an adequate supply of iron. Although she does not exclude dietary factors altogether, Kent argues that disease, stimulated by increased sedentism and population density, is the primary factor. She suggests the problem is most likely brought on by poor sanitation associated with increased sedentism and population density. A variety of viral, bacterial, and parasitic infections are then easily spread, producing iron-deficiency anemia, especially in children, through blood loss and chronic diarrhea. Such a model would help explain the relatively high frequency of porotic hyperostosis among meat-eating Eskimo (Nathan 1966) or other groups with varied iron-rich diets (Cohen and Armelagos 1984).

Porotic Hyperostosis in Ecuador

My long-term study of prehistoric skeletal biology in Ecuador offers an opportunity to view the incidence and frequency of porotic hyperostosis within a broad, complex cultural–temporal framework (Ubelaker 1988a). Since 1973, I have collaborated with officials of the museum system of the Banco Central in Ecuador in a long-term study of biocultural variability and change in Ecuadorean prehistory (Ubelaker 1988a). This effort has resulted in the excavation and published analysis of skeletal samples from eight key sites (Ubelaker 1980a,b, 1981, 1983, 1987, 1988b,c,d) and ongoing study of material from three others. All but one (Cotocollao) of these sites are located on the Ecuadorean coast (Figure 1) and collectively span nearly 8000 years. The extended time dimension represented by these sites and the relatively large size of most of the individual samples

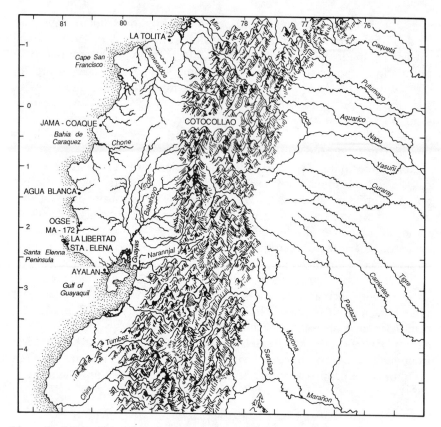

Figure 1.   Map of Ecuador showing location of sites discussed.

enable documentation of various biological variables within a chronological context.

The chronological range of this sample (Table 1) spans the shift from
hunting and gathering/horticultural subsistence at the Vegas Complex
site at Sta Elena (Ubelaker 1980a) to the relatively late agricultural based
cultures represented at Ayalán (Ubelaker 1981), and Agua Blanca
(Ubelaker 1988b). This over 7000 year time span witnessed not only extensive changes in subsistence, but also in settlement pattern, population
size and density, and cultural innovation. Undoubtedly, through time,
population size and density increased with increased sedentism man-
dated by growing reliance on agriculture. These temporal changes seem
correlated with changing patterns of skeletal manifestations of chronic

Table 1. Published Samples of Human Skeletal Remains from Ecuador

Sample	Date	Location (Province)	Culture	Number in Sample
Agua Blanca	800–1500 A.D.	Manabi	Manteno	7
Ayalán Urn	730–1730 A.D.	Guayas	Milagro	384
Ayalán Nonurn	500 B.C.–1155 A.D.	Guayas	Milagro	51
Jama-coaque	200 B.C.–800 A.D.	Manabi	Jama-coaque	1
La Tolita	90–190 A.D.	Emeraldas	Tolita Tardio	18
OGSE-MA-172	100 B.C.	Guayas	Guangala	30
La Libertad (OGSE-46)	900–200 B.C.	Guayas	Engory	24
Cotocollao	540 B.C.	Pichincha	Cotocollao	199
Sta. Elena	6000 B.C.	Guayas	Vegas Complex	192

anemia, as evidenced by the frequency of porotic hyperostosis. Such patterns can be detected because of the unusually large size and temporal depth of the sample. The frequency of porotic hyperostosis in ancient Ecuador appears to be associated with indirect indicators of disease such as life expectancy and dental hypoplasia, as well as such direct indicators as periosteal new bone formation. Significantly, increases in porotic hyperostosis are not entirely associated with dietary changes and reliance on corn agriculture.

The earliest site at Sta. Elena surely lacked agriculture, although there is some evidence for plant cultivation. Faunal analysis indicated reliance on local terrestrial animals, marine fish, and shellfish inhabiting mangrove swamps (Stothert 1985). Soil phytoliths indicated the possibility of primitive maize cultivation and Stothert (1985) speculated the diet may have been supplemented by squash, beans, and root crops.

Maize agriculture contributed to the diet of the populations represented by all other samples, however, the extent of reliance on other foods is not known. To at least some extent, diet included quinoa, white carrot, squash, beans, and potato in the highlands and marine and brackish-water fish and mollusks, manioc, sweet potato, achira, arrowroot, New World yam, and peanuts on the coast. Terrestrial mammals were, of course, available in both areas.

To date, 16 (2%) of 906 skeletons from 9 prehistoric archeological sites in Ecuador display porotic hyperostosis of the cranial vault and/or orbits (Table 2). These 16 individuals originate from the Guangala site of OGSE-MA-172 (Ubelaker 1983) (Figure 2) both components of the Ayalán

Table 2. Individuals in Ecuadorean Skeletal Samples with Porotic Hyperostosis

Site	Feature	Age (years)	Comments
OGSE-MA-172	47	1.0	Active deposits and porosity both temporals, occipital (Figure 2) and both orbits
OGSE-MA-172	77/166	1.5	Active porosity both parietals
OGSE-MA-172	122	3.0	Active fine perforations left orbit (right orbit absent)
Ayalán urn	2	Adult	Seven cranial vault fragments with extensive active and partially remodeled deposits (Figure 3) "Hair-on-end appearance
Ayalán urn	5	1.0	Active deposits and porosity both orbits and active porosity near the lambdoidal suture
Ayalán urn	5	10.5	Active deposits both parietals (Figure 4), active porosity near the lambdoidal suture
Ayalán urn	8	Adult	Three parietal fragments with well-remodeled deposits
Ayalán urn	10	4.5–5.0	Active porosity both orbits
Ayalán urn	21	1.0–3.0	Slight active porosity, right orbit and occipital
Ayalán urn	25	0.0–0.5	Active porosity, parietals
Ayalán urn	50	1.0–2.0	Active porosity both orbits, occipital and parietals
Ayalán urn	56	Adult	Active porosity and deposits on occipital and parietals
Ayalán urn	56	3.0	Active porosity near lambdoidal suture.
Ayalán nonurn	37A	20–25	Well-remodeled deposits, both parietals
Ayalán nonurn	37D-E	3–4	Active deposits, two parietal fragments
Jama-coaque		28–34	Active porosity and deposits, both orbits (Figure 5) of male cranium

sample (Ubelaker, 1981), (Figures 2, 3, 4), and the Jama-coaque cranium from Manabí (Ubelaker 1987) (Figure 5).

As Table 3 shows, in the overall sample, lesions on the vault are only slightly more common (13) than those on the orbits (7). Alterations on 13 of the individuals were active at the time of death. The well remodeled inactive alterations were all deposits on the cranial vaults of mature adults. Only five of the affected individuals were adults. All but one of the remaining 11 were under 5 years of age, the exception being under 10 years of age.

Study of the spatial–temporal patterning of the lesions reveals that the alterations are confined to relatively recent coastal sites. None of the 192 individuals examined from the earliest site of Sta. Elena showed evidence of porotic hyperostosis. Evidence was also lacking entirely among the 199

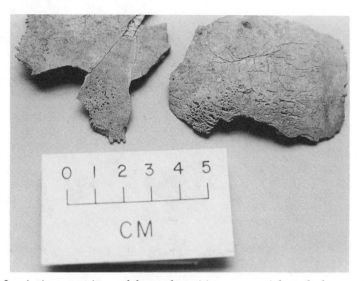

Figure 2. Active porosity and bone deposition on cranial vault fragments of infant from feature 47, OGSE-MA-172.

individuals of the Cotocollao sample, the only highland site in the series, as well as in the coastal La Libertad, La Tolita, and Agua Blanca samples (Figure 1). Recent unpublished research conducted by the author in 1988 detected at least one example of orbital porotic hyperostosis in a sample of newly excavated human remains from La Tolita, however, the overall frequency at that site remains very low. The earliest expression of porotic hyperostosis is found in the Guangala sample from OGSE-MA-172 (Figure 2), where 3 of the 30 individuals were affected.

Evidence for porotic hyperostosis in Ecuador loosely follows a temporal trend, but does not correlate as positively with increasing time or reliance on maize agriculture as suspected earlier (Ubelaker 1984). The data available continue to show absence in the preagricultural sample of Sta. Elena. However, absence at Cotocollao, La Libertad, and the small sample from Agua Blanca suggests that factors other than maize agriculture may be involved, since subsistence of the populations represented at these sites certainly included maize as a major component.

The relatively high frequency of porotic hyperostosis at OGSE-MA-172 also indicates that nondietary factors may be operating. Although maize as well as yucca, beans, and squash undoubtedly contributed to the diet of populations at that site, the proximity to the ocean and large amounts

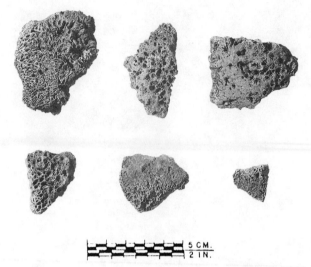

Figure 3. Remodeled deposition and porosity on cranial vault fragments of mature adult from feature 2, Ayalán urn component.

of fish bones recovered during excavation all suggest that diet included at least a substantial amount of iron-rich seafood (Karen Stothert 1988, personal communication).

Porotic hyperostosis was present in both Ayalán samples. At this last site, maize agriculture undoubtedly contributed to the diet, but faunal analysis suggests heavy reliance on brackish water oysters and clams as well as utilization of reptiles, birds, deer, and rodents (Ubelaker 1981). The relative proportions of various dietary elements are difficult to discern from the data available, although certainly midden shell frequencies indicate oysters and clams were a major component.

Skeletal evidence for infectious disease represents another relevant indicator of morbidity in these samples. In the Ecuadorean samples, evidence of infection usually consists of well-remodeled periosteal swellings on long bone shafts, usually from the tibia or fibula. The specific organism usually cannot be diagnosed, but the frequency of such lesions in the population offers a valuable indicator of morbidity. Previous studies have expressed this frequency as the ratio of the number of adult bones with periosteal lesions to the number of adults in the sample. This expression was chosen over the normally preferable percentage of affected

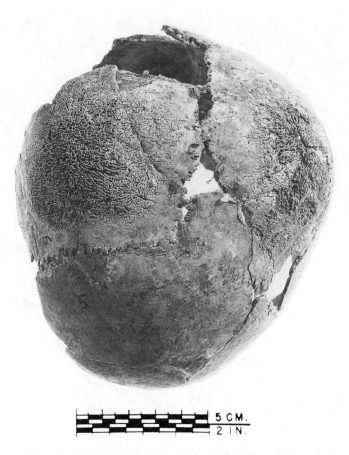

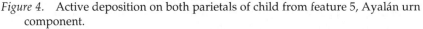

Figure 4. Active deposition on both parietals of child from feature 5, Ayalán urn component.

individuals, since many of the bones in these samples were from secondary deposits and could not be related to single individuals. The highest value for this ratio (0.47) comes from the La Tolita sample, followed closely by OGSE-MA-172 (0.44), La Libertad (0.29), Agua Blanca and Ayalán urns (0.14), Sta. Elena (0.07), and Cotocollao and Ayalán nonurns (0.04). Temporally, these data suggest early low levels of infectious disease, a rapid increase at the time of Engoroy and Guangala to La Tolita, followed by a rapid decline with the Ayalán nonurn sample and subsequent increase with Ayalán urn and Aqua Blanca.

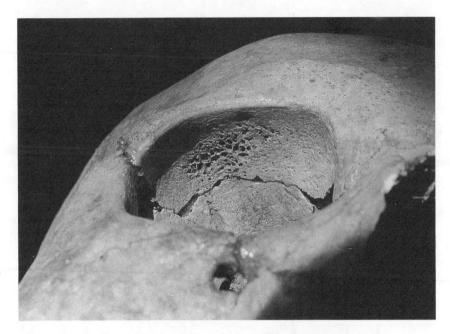

Figure 5. Active porosity in orbit of adult male Jama-coaque cranium.

Temporal trends of other data contribute to this interpretation. Estimates of living stature and frequencies of trauma show some regional
variation, but little temporal change.

Life expectancy at birth decreased with increasing time, apparently
reflecting an increase in infant and immature mortality. Life expectancy
at birth decreases in spite of the fact that adult maximum longevity and
adult life expectancy increase with time. Presumably, the increase in immature mortality results from increased frequency of infectious disease
brought on by increased sedentism and population density.

Dental hypoplasia occurs at low levels from 6000 B.C. to 500 B.C., increases rapidly to about 550 B.C., followed by a rapid decline and subsequent rapid increase. Similarly, dental alveolar abscesses and antemor-
tem loss of teeth show a gradual increase to about the time of Christ with
subsequent declines. Dental caries shows a general increase through time
with exceptions of low late frequencies from the small samples of Agua
Blanca and La Tolita.

Table 3. Summary Statistics on Porotic Hyperostosis in Ecuador

Sample	Number in Sample	With Lesions on Vault and/or Orbits		With Lesions on Vault		With Lesions in Orbits	
		No.	Percent	No.	Percent	No.	Percent
Agua Blanca	7	0	0	0	0	0	0
Ayalán Urn	384	10	3	9	2	4	1
Ayalán Nonurn	51	2	4	2	4	0	0
Jama-coaque	1	1	100	0	0	1	1
La Tolita	18	0	0	0	0	0	0
OGSE-MA-172	30	3	10	2	7	2	7
La Libertad	24	0	0	0	0	0	0
Cotocollao	199	0	0	0	0	0	0
Sta Elena	192	0	0	0	0	0	0
Total	906	16	2	13	1	7	1

Discussion

Temporal and spatial variation in the frequency of porotic hyperostosis in ancient Ecuador must be interpreted within the overall pattern of morbidity, subsistence, and settlement pattern. The data available now suggest that factors contributing to elevated levels of porotic hyperostosis in Ecuador are complex and perhaps variable. Increasing sedentism and population density with associated increases in infectious disease and parasitism probably are major contributing factors. The Ecuadorean data summarized above seem to suggest that elevated frequencies of porotic hyperostosis correlate with increased levels of periosteal lesions, dental hypoplasia, and subadult mortality. During the later time periods (excluding the early site of Sta. Elena) porotic hyperostosis shows an irregular correlation with heavy reliance on maize in subsistence, although, even at these later sites, the evidence suggests that maize was supplemented with a variety of iron-rich food sources.

Collectively, the above data suggest that porotic hyperostosis in Ecuador was largely confined to coastal sites beginning shortly before the time of Christ. The data closely fit the model proposed by Kent (1986) that the lesions reflect anemia, brought on by chronic levels of infectious disease resulting from the poor sanitation associated with increased sedentism and population density. The high frequency of porotic hyperostosis in infants and children as well as other evidence for high morbidity and mortality among this age group suggest that they were especially hard hit by pathogens. As Kent (1986) points out, the literature clearly demonstrates that diarrheal diseases are the major cause of childhood morbidity and mortality in third world countries today and chronic prolonged dysentery can result in significant blood loss and anemia. Many studies (Cartwright and Wintrobe 1952; May et al. 1952; de Gruchy 1978; Reizenstein 1983) demonstrate that extreme anemia also can result from severe, long-lasting nongastrointestinal infections, through decreased production of red blood cells, shorter red blood cell life survival, or any disturbance in hemoglobin synthesis. Such conditions can produce anemia in the absence of actual direct blood loss. Augmented anemia may result if coupled with blood loss.

Parasitism may be another important contributing factor in the manifestation of porotic hyperostosis/anemia since it can produce both severe diarrhea and direct blood loss. Hookworm, in particular, can produce a significant loss of blood resulting in anemia. In discussing anemia in the tropics, Woodruff (1982:141) mentions that the "most common conditioning factor is the effect of blood loss due to hookworm disease." Blood loss can be as much as 0.21 ml of blood per worm per day in infected individuals. Today in Ecuador, hookworms creating blood loss are limited to two species, *Necator americanus* (most common) and *Ancylostoma duodenale.* Both of these species require moisture and sustained high temperature to complete their life cycle and thus are confined to the coast. Contemporary clinicians report that hookworm infection is common and a major health problem on the Ecuadorean coast, but is nonexistent in the highlands (Frank Weilbauer, 1988, personal communication). In fact, those individuals in highland areas who are rarely found to be infected with hookworm inevitably represent recent migrants from coastal areas.

According to Gillman (1982) hookworms can reach a length of 1 cm. *Ancylostoma* produces about 25,000 eggs per day and *Necator* about 7000 per day. The eggs hatch in the soil within 48 hours. The larvae molt twice to become infective filariform larvae, which can survive as long as several months in the soil. The larvae climb grass and penetrate the feet of humans that come in contact with them. They then enter the venous circulation system and are carried to the lungs where they migrate across the alveolar capillary walls, and are eventually swallowed. Subsequently, they attach themselves to the wall of the intestine and can live in the intestines from 2 to 6 years. Both species are assumed to be historically imported from the Old World, *Necator* from sub-Saharan Africa and *Ancylostoma* from the Mediterranean basin and Asia (Blumenthal 1985). However, the Old World origin of the blood letting hookworms discussed above has been disputed by the archeological recovery of hookworms associated with precolumbian human remains from coastal South Carolina in the United States, possibly Brazil, (Araujo 1986) and from coastal Peru.

Rathbun et al. (1980) report cribra orbitalia in the orbits of two males and two females from a sample of eight individuals recovered from a shell midden on Daw's Island (38BU9) in Beaufort County, South Carolina. Radiocarbon dating and chronological comparison with material from other sites suggest a date between 3300 and 3700 years ago. Rathbun et al. (1980) rule out a dietary explanation of the cribra orbitalia since "varieties of oysters present are relatively high in iron, red meats were eaten, and hickory nuts contain as much iron as certain cuts of beef" (Rathbun et al. 1980:61). They suggest parasitism may have been a causal factor since the hard exoskeleton of an undetermined species of hookworm was microscopically identified from a partially mineralized coprolite recovered from the pelvic area of one of the skeletons.

The strongest evidence for Pre-Columbian New World hookworm infestation comes from the discovery by Allison et al. (1974) of *Ancylostoma duodenale* in the small intestine of a Peruvian mummy. Several worms were found attached to the intestinal lumen within a Tiahuanaco mummy from coastal southern Peru dating from about 890 to 950 A.D. Allison et al. (1974) used measurements of various anatomical parts of the worms to support an identification of *Ancylostoma duodenale*.

The above discussion is relevant to the interpretation of the Ecuadorean data, since all of the published examples of porotic hyperostosis originate from the coast. Also noteworthy is the absence of porotic hyperostosis from the large highland site of Cotocollao, even though the site represents a high density population with a subsistence including substantial maize consumption. These data suggest that parasitism, particularly the hookworm *Ancylostoma duodenale,* may have been an important causal factor.

Summary and Conclusions

Analysis of skeletal samples from different areas and time periods within Ecuador suggests that porotic hyperostosis appeared shortly before the time of Christ and was largely confined to the coast. A high frequency of porotic hyperostosis at the coastal site of OGSE-MA-172, where iron-rich seafood was consumed and the lack of porotic hyperostosis at the highland site of Cotocollao, where maize was a major dietary constituent argue against a dietary explanation. The cumulative evidence suggests that, although dietary factors may have been involved in some areas and time periods, porotic hyperostosis in Ecuador mostly results from chronic anemia produced by a temporal increase in viral, bacterial, and parasitic diseases. The increasing frequency of disease was stimulated by increasing sedentism, population density, and sanitation problems.

This interpretation contrasts with many studies from other areas suggesting a largely dietary cause of porotic hyperostosis (Cohen and Armelagos 1984). It also contributes to the growing evidence for a New World origin of blood-letting hookworms. Such interpretation echoes that offered by Trinkaus (1977) for porotic hyperostosis in the Alto Salaverry Child from coastal Peru, dating between 1700 and 2000 B.C. Trinkaus noted the child originated from a predominantly nonagriculturist population and thus suggested that the condition might have been produced by severe anemia caused by loss of blood from hookworm infestation, rather than dietary factors.

These interpretations also indicate that the dynamics of Ecuadorean biocultural prehistory may have been more complex than previously believed. The data suggest a close and perhaps fragile relationship among such factors as population density, mortality, diet, disease, and sedentism. Additional research on well-documented human skeletal remains should further elucidate the temporal and geographic variation in this relationship.

References

Allison, M.J., A. Pezzia, I. Hasegawa, and E. Gerszten. 1974. A case of hookworm infestation in a precolumbian American. *American Journal of Physical Anthropology* 41(1):103–106.

Angel, J.L. 1966. Porotic hyperostosis, anemias, malarias, and marshes in the prehistoric Eastern Mediterranean. *Science* 153:760–763.

Araujo, A. 1986. Microscopia de varredura de larvas de Ancilostomideos encontradas em coprolitos humanos datados de 3490 ± 120 A 430 ± 70 anos. Apresentado ao *Simp. Tec. Esp. Microscopia Eletronica aplicadas as Ciencias Biomedicas*, Caxambu, 10-11-1986.

Blumenthal, D.S. 1985. Hookworm Disease. No. 352 in *Cecil Textbook of Medicine.* J.B. Wyngaarden and L.H. Smith, Jr., eds., pp. 1766–1767. Philadelphia: W.B. Saunders.

Cartwright, G.E., and M.M. Wintrobe. 1952. The anemia of infection—a review. In *Advances in Internal Medicine,* Vol. 5. W. Dock and I. Snapper, eds., pp. 165–226. New York: The Year Book Publishers.

Cohen, M., and G. Armelagos (eds.). 1984. *Paleopathology at the Origins of Agriculture.* New York: Academic Press.

de Gruchy, G.C. 1978. *Clinical Haematology in Medical Practice,* 4th ed. D. Penington, B. Rush, and P. Castaldi, eds., Oxford: Blackwell Scientific Publications.

El-Najjar, M.Y., D.J. Ryan, C.G. Turner II, and B. Lozoff. 1976. The etiology of porotic hyperostosis among the prehistoric and historic Anasazi indians of southwestern United States. *American Journal of Physical Anthropology* 44: 477–487.

Gillman, R.H. 1982. Hookworm Disease: Host-pathogen biology. *Review of Infectious Disease* 4:824.

Goodman, A.H., D.L. Martin, G.J. Armelagos, and G. Clark. 1984. Indications of stress from bone and teeth. In *Paleopathology at the Origins of Agriculture.* M.N. Cohen and G.J. Armelagos, eds., Chapter 2, pp. 13–49, New York: Academic Press.

Huss-Ashmore, R., A.H. Goodman, and G.J. Armelagos. 1982. Nutritional inference from paleopathology. *Advances in Archaeological Method and Theory* 5:395–474.

Kent, S. 1986. The influence of sedentism and aggregation on porotic hyperostosis and anaemia: A case study. *Man* 21(4):605–636.

Lallo, J.W., G.J. Armelagos, and R.P. Mensforth. 1977. The role of diet, disease, and physiology in the origin of porotic hyperostosis. *Human Biology* 49: 471–483.

May, C., C.T. Stewart, A. Hamilton, and R.J. Salmon. 1952. Infection as cause of folic acid deficiency and megaloblastic anemia. *American Journal of Diseases of Children* 84:718–728.

Mensforth, R.P., C.O. Lovejoy, J.W. Lallo, and G.J. Armelagos. 1978. The role of constitutional factors, diet, and infectious disease in the etiology of porotic hyperostosis and periosteal reactions in prehistoric infants and children. *Medical Anthropology* 2:1–59.

Nathan, H., and N. Haas. 1966. "Cribra orbitalia." A bone condition of the orbit of unknown nature: Anatomical study with etiological considerations. *Israel Journal of Medical Science* 2:171–191.

Ortner, D.J., and W.G.J. Putschar. 1981. Identification of pathological conditions in human skeletal remains. *Smithsonian Contributions to Anthropology,* 28. Washington, D.C.: Smithsonian Institution Press.

Rathbun, T.A., J. Sexton, and J. Michie. 1980. Disease Patterns in a Formative Period South Carolina Coastal Population. *Tennessee Anthropological Association. Miscellaneous Paper* No. 5:52–74.

Reizenstein, P. 1983. *Hematologic Stress Syndrome: The Biological Response to Disease.* New York: Praeger.

Stothert, K.E. 1985. The preceramic Las Vegas culture of coastal Ecuador. *American Antiquity* 50:613–637.

Stuart-Macadam, P. 1985. Porotic hyperostosis: Representative of a childhood condition. *American Journal of Physical Anthropology* 66(4):391–398.

Stuart-Macadam, P. 1987a. A radiographic study of porotic hyperostosis. *American Journal of Physical Anthropology* 74:511–520.

Stuart-Macadam, P. 1987b. Porotic hyperostosis: New evidence to support the anemia theory. *American Journal of Physical Anthropology* 74:521–526.

Suzuki, T. 1987. Cribra orbitalia in the early Hawaiians and Mariana Islanders. *Man and Culture in Oceania* 3:95–104.

Trinkaus, E. 1977. The Alto Salaverry child: A case of anemia from the Peruvian Pre-ceramic. *American Journal of Physical Anthropology* 46:25–28.

Ubelaker, D.H. 1980a. Human skeletal remains from site OGSE-80, a preceramic site on the Sta. Elena Peninsula, coastal Ecuador. *Journal of the Washington Academy of Sciences* 70(1):3–24.

Ubelaker, D.H. 1980b. Prehistoric human remains from the Cotocollao site, Pichincha Province, Ecuador. *Journal of the Washington Academy of Science* 70(2):59–74.

Ubelaker, D.H. 1981. The Ayalán cemetery: A late integration period burial site on the south coast of Ecuador. *Smithsonian Contributions to Anthropology* 29. Washington, D.C.: Smithsonian Press.

Ubelaker, D.H. 1983. Human skeletal remains from OGSE-MA-172 an early Guangala cemetery site on the coast of Ecuador. *Journal of the Washington Academy of Sciences* 73(1):16–27.

Ubelaker, D.H. 1984. Prehistoric human biology of Ecuador: Possible temporal trends and cultural correlations. In *Paleopathology at the Origins of Agriculture.* M.N. Cohen and G.J. Armelagos, eds., Chapter 19, pp. 491–513. New York: Academic Press.

Ubelaker, D.H. 1987. Dental alteration in prehistoric Ecuador a new example from Jama-coaque. *Journal of the Washington Academy of Sciences* 77(2):76–80.

Ubelaker, D.H. 1988a. Skeletal biology of prehistoric Ecuador: An ongoing research program. *Journal of the Washington Academy of Sciences* 78(1)1–2.

Ubelaker, D.H. 1988b. Human remains from OGSE-46 La Libertad, Guayas Province, Ecuador. *Journal of the Washington Academy of Sciences* 78(1):3–16.

Ubelaker, D.H. 1988c. A preliminary report of analysis of human remains from Agua Blanca, a prehistoric Late Integration site from coastal Ecuador. *Journal of the Washington Academy of Sciences* 78(1):17–22.

Ubelaker, D.H. 1988d. Prehistoric human biology at La Tolita, Ecuador, a preliminary report. *Journal of the Washington Academy of Sciences* 78(1):23–37.

Walker, P.L. 1985. Anemia among prehistoric indians of the American Southwest. In *Health and Disease in the Prehistoric Southwest.* C.F. Merbs and R.J. Miller, eds., Chapter 13, pp. 139–164. *Arizona State University, Anthropological Research Papers* No. 34.

Walker, P.L. 1986. Porotic hyperostosis in a marine-dependent California Indian population. *American Journal of Physical Anthropology* 69:345–354.

Woodruff, A.W. 1982. Recent work concerning anemia in the tropics. *Seminars in Hematology* 19(2):141–147.

Chapter 8

Patterns of Diet, Parasitism, and Anemia in Prehistoric West North America

Karl J. Reinhard

Introduction

Anemia in the prehistoric desert west in North America has been associated with dietary and disease changes linked to the developments of horticulture, sedentism, and population aggregation. Nutrition and parasitism may be two key etiological factors of prehistoric anemia. Using the theoretical perspective established by El-Najjar et al. (1976), the role of dietary specialization and infectious disease among horticultural peoples is explored. Coprolite data are used to evaluate the impact of diet and disease on the development of anemia.

The Data Base

The analysis of coprolites provides detailed information regarding macroparasitism (helminth and arthropod infection) and diet (Bryant 1974a,b; Faulkner 1991; Fry 1985; Reinhard 1988a; Reinhard and Bryant 1992; Reinhard et al. 1987). The helminth data can also be used to indirectly estimate the general level of microparasitism (protozoal, bacterial, and viral infection) among archaeological peoples. Microparasitism can have a pronounced health impact, but evidence of microparasites is rarely directly preserved in archaeological remains. When incorporated with other archaeological data, coprolites can be used to help reconstruct details of ancient parasite ecology (Reinhard 1988a).

Coprolite analysis is a time-intensive process. It is a procedure that at very least requires identification of plant and animal residues, as well as the recovery of helminth remains. Until very recently, too few coprolites from the Southwest had been examined to allow comparative analysis of diet and parasitism between sites and subsistence strategies. Although the actual number of coprolites analyzed are still small, the growing body of coprolite data in the western United States is sufficient to begin comparative analysis of diet and parasitism (Minnis 1989; Reinhard 1988a).

The history and theory of coprolite analysis have recently been summarized (Reinhard and Bryant 1992). Typically, macroscopic analysis (both floral and faunal) and pollen analysis are applied in coprolite study (Bryant 1974a,b, 1986; Bryant and Williams-Dean 1975; Fry 1985; Reinhard 1985a, 1988a). Helminth analysis has relatively recently become consistently applied in coprolite analysis, although helminth analysis has a long history with certain researchers (Dunn and Watkins 1970; Fry 1977; Fry and Hall 1969, 1975; Moore et al. 1969, 1974). The fact that so many coprolites from the western United States have been analyzed for helminth remains ($n = 1,018$) is largely due to the efforts of a small number of parasitologists in the 1980s (Gardner and Clary n.d.; Hevly et al. 1979; Reinhard 1988b, 1992; Reinhard and Clary 1986; Reinhard et al. 1987, 1988) building on previous work of anthropologists and parasitologists in the 1960s and 1970s (Dunn and Watkins 1970; Fry 1977, 1980; Fry and Hall 1969, 1975; Fry and Moore 1969; Hall 1972; Moore et al. 1969, 1974).

Hunter–gatherer coprolites have been recovered from the Great Basin (Lovelock Cave, Danger Cave, Hogup Cave), the Colorado Plateau (Dust Devil Cave), the western portion of the Mojave Desert (Bighorn Cave), and the lower Pecos of western Texas (Hinds Cave and Baker Cave) (Figure 1). Macroscopic component analysis has been completed for 433 coprolites (Table 1), pollen analysis for 339 coprolites (Table 2), and helminthological analysis for 401 coprolites (Table 3). All of these sites are dry caves and most are in desert environments with the exception of Lovelock Cave, which is in a lakeside environment. The preservation of pollen and macroscopic components is excellent for all sites. The hunter–gatherer coprolites are ideal for the preservation of helminth remains because all sites are located in dry caves. Quantification of macroscopic remains is available in terms of presence/absence per coprolite for all sites. Weight quantification is available for Bighorn Cave, Danger Cave, and Hogup Cave. Pollen data are based on 200 grain minimum counts for all sites. Parasitological data are presented in terms of the number of coprolites containing helminth eggs of given species.

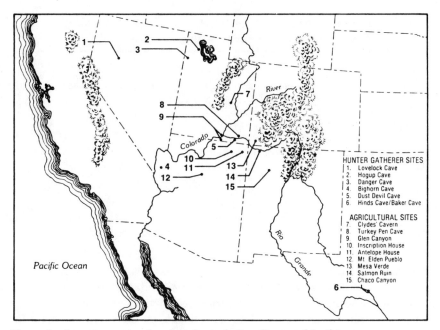

Figure 1. Location map of archaeological sites discussed in this paper.

Coprolites from horticultural sites on the Colorado Plateau have been studied (Figure 1). Two main cultural groups are represented, the Anasazi and the San Rafael Fremont. For the Anasazi, both Basketmaker and Pueblo Periods are represented in the coprolite series. To date, 538 coprolites from horticultural sites have been examined for macroscopic remains (Table 4), 319 for pollen (Table 5), and 617 for helminths (Table 6). Both cave sites and open sites are represented in the horticultural coprolite collection. Coprolites from the cave sites are ideal for the preservation of all types of data. The open sites in Chaco Canyon and at Salmon Ruin show poor preservation of macroscopic floral components, and for that reason macroscopic floral data from these sites are not used in the following analyses. Pollen is well preserved from the open sites, and parasite eggs are well preserved at Salmon Ruin. Macroscopic faunal remains were well preserved in coprolites from all sites. Macroscopic presence/absence data are available for all coprolites from all horticultural sites. Weight quantification is available from Glen Canyon Fremont sites, Glen Canyon Anasazi sites, Antelope House, and Turkey Pen Cave, but the poor preservation of Salmon Ruin and Chaco Canyon coprolites

Table 1. Sites Used in This Study for Which Macroscopic Analyses
Have Been Completed from Hunter–Gatherer Contexts

Sites	Reference	Number of Coprolites Studied
Lovelock Cave	Heizer and Napton (1969)	50
Danger Cave	Fry (1977)	46
Hogup Cave, Archaic	Fry (1977)	51
Hogup Cave, Shoshoni		3
Dust Devil Cave	Reinhard (1985a)	50
Bighorn Cave	Reinhard (1988a)	20
Hinds Cave	Reinhard (1988a);	25
	Williams-Dean (1978);	100
	Stock (1983)	50
Baker Cave	Sobolik (1988)	38

renders meaningful weight quantification impossible. Pollen and parasite
data are quantified in the same manner as for hunter–gatherer coprolites.

As can be seen in Tables 1–6, sample size varies from site to site. One
must determine what is a suitable sample size for comparative analysis.
In the determination of suitable sample sizes, the author records the
number of components that accumulate with each coprolite during the
course of analysis. Eight components might be found in the first coprolite
from a hypothetical site, five different components in the second, three
different components in the third, etc. At some point the number of accumulating components becomes negligible. It is at that point that the
sample size is considered sufficient to characterize a prehistoric diet.

Usually, 80–90% of identifiable plant components are found after 15–20

Table 2. Sites Used in This Study for Which Pollen Analyses Have Been
Completed from Hunter–Gatherer Contexts

Site	Reference	Number of Coprolites Studied
Lovelock Cave	Napton and Kelso (1969)	50
Danger Cave	Kelso (1970)	8
Hogup Cave, Archaic	Kelso (1970)	33
Dust Devil Cave	Reinhard (1988a)	20
Bighorn Cave	Reinhard (1988a)	20
Hinds Cave	Reinhard (1988a)	20
	Williams-Dean (1978);	100
	Stock (1983)	50
Baker Cave	Sobolik (1988)	38

Table 3. Sites Used in This Study for Which Helminthological Analyses Have Been Completed from Hunter-Gatherer Contexts

Site	References	Number of Coprolites Studied
Lovelock Cave	Dunn and Watkins (1970)	50
Danger Cave	Fry (1977)	46
Hogup Cave, Archaic	Fry (1977)	51
Hogup Cave, Shoshoni	Fry (1977)	3
Dust Devil Cave	Reinhard et al. (1985)	100
Bighorn Cave	Reinhard (1988a)	35
Hinds Cave	Reinhard (1988a);	39
	Reinhard (current research);	40
	Williams-Dean (1978);	13
	(Stock)	7
Baker Cave	Reinhard (1988a)	17

coprolites have been examined. For example, in the analysis of Bighorn Cave, 20 coprolites were quantified by weight and an additional 15 coprolites were surveyed for components not found in the first 20. Eleven different identifiable plant components were found. After 15 coprolites were studied, 10 of these components had been found and after the study

Table 4. Sites for Which Macroscopic Analyses Are Available from Horticultural Contexts[a]

Site	Reference	Number of Coprolites Studied
Hogup Cave[a]	Fry (1977)	6
Clyde's Cavern[a]	Hall, (1972)	16
Glen Canyon[a]	Fry (1977)	10
Glen Canyon	Fry (1977)	30
Antelope House	Fry and Hall (1986)	90
Antelope House	Reinhard (1985a)	62
Inscription House	Fry and Hall (1986)	16
Turkey Pen Cave	Reinhard (1988a)	24
Turkey Pen Cave	Aasen (1984)	28
Step House BM III	Stiger (1977)	20
Step House Pueblo	Stiger (1977)	17
Hoy House	Stiger (1977)	56
Lion House	Stiger (1977)	4
Salmon Ruin	Reinhard (1985a)	112
Chaco Canyon	Clary (1984)	47

[a] *Fremont culture sites; all others Anasazi sites.*

Table 5. Sites for Which Pollen Analyses Are Available from Anasazi
Horticultural Contexts

Site	Reference	Number of Coprolites Studied
Glen Canyon	Martin and Sharrock (1964)	31
Antelope House	Williams-Dean (1986)	92
Antelope House	Reinhard (1988a)	27
Turkey Pen Cave	Reinhard (1988a)	24
Turkey Pen Cave	Aasen (1984)	28
Hoy House	Scott (1981)	59
Salmon Ruin	Reinhard (1988a)	30
Chaco Canyon	Clary (1984)	28

of 17 coprolites, all 11 components had been found. Continued analysis of the remaining 18 coprolites revealed no additional dietary components. Therefore 91% of the components were found by the study of only 15 coprolites and all components were found in the analysis of 17.

In the case of the 30 Glen Canyon Anasazi coprolites (Fry 1977), 90%

Table 6. Sites for Which Helminthological Analyses Are Available from Horticultural Contexts[a]

Site	Reference	Number of Coprolites Studied
Hogup Cave[a]	Fry (1977)	6
Clyde's Cavern[a]	Hall (1972)	16
Glen Canyon[a]	Fry (1977)	10
Glen Canyon	Fry (1977)	30
Antelope House	Fry and Hall (1986)	90
Antelope House	Reinhard et al. (1987)	49 human 13 dog
Antelope House	Reinhard (1988a)	180
Inscription House	Fry and Hall (n.d.)	16
Turkey Pen Cave	Reinhard (1988a)	24
Step House	Samuels (1965)	20
Hoy House	Stiger (1977)	56
Lion House	Stiger (1977)	4
Salmon Ruin	Reinhard (1985a)	112
Chaco Canyon	Reinhard and Clary (1984)	20
Bighorn Sheep Ruin	Gardner and Clary (n.d.)	20
Elden Pueblo	Hevly et al. (1979)	b

[a] Fremont culture sites; all others Anasazi sites.
[b] Soil samples, not coprolites, were studied from Elden Pueblo.

of the components (19 of 21) were found in the study of 20 coprolites. In the case of 56 coprolites from Hoy House (Stiger 1977) and 50 coprolites from Dust Devil Cave (Reinhard 1988a), all components had been found by the time the twentieth coprolite was analyzed. Twenty of 25 components (80%) were found in the study of 20 of 92 coprolites from Antelope House (Fry and Hall 1986). In general, most components were found after the study of 20 coprolites. This trend is even more obvious when components that occur in only one coprolite are excluded. Component increment curves are depicted in Figure 2 for sites for which 40 or more coprolites were studied. Only in the case of Hinds Cave (Figure 3) did the curve not reach plateau in the analysis of 20 coprolites or less.

Based on these cases and others, it is probable that analysis of 20 coprolites from a site is sufficient for the recovery of most identifiable plant components and tracing trends in dietary specialization, providing that the coprolites do not all come from the same locus in a site. Certainly no less than 15 coprolites should be studied to characterize a diet. A sample size of 15 to 20 coprolites is marginal and should be interpreted with caution.

Various sample sizes are represented in Southwest coprolite studies. Some are too small for consideration, such as from Lion House (four coprolites), Hogup Cave Fremont (six coprolites), Hogup Cave Shoshoni

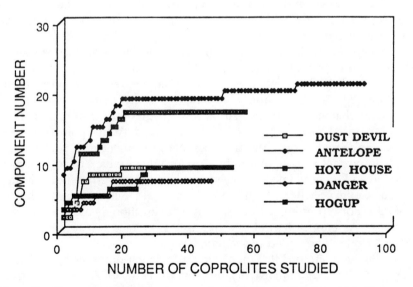

Figure 2. Component increment curves for prehistoric sites for which 40 or more coprolites have been analyzed.

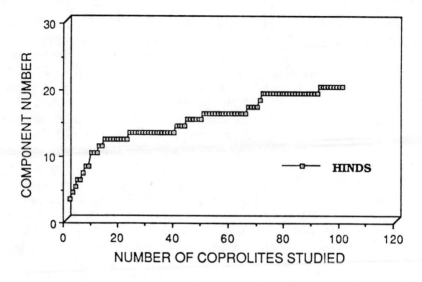

Figure 3. Component increment curve for Williams-Dean's (1978) study of Hinds Cave coprolites.

(three coprolites), and Glen Canyon Fremont (10 coprolites). Three analyses are marginal with respect to sample size: Inscription House (16 coprolites), Clyde's Cavern (16 coprolites), and the Pueblo Period occupation of Step House (17 coprolites). The remainder of the studies are based on 20 or more coprolites and are suitable for comparative analysis.

The preceding comments regarding sample size refer to dietary reconstruction only. In the author's experience, many more coprolites are needed to characterize parasitism at any given site. A minimal sample size for parasite analysis has not been determined. At this point, it is wise to analyze as many coprolites from distinct proveniences as possible.

It is important to note that only sites for which there are both parasitological and dietary data are considered here. Thus, certain notable sites such as Conejo Shelter (Bryant 1974a) and Caldwell Shelter (Holloway 1985) are not represented in this analysis even though dietary data are available. As parasitological analyses are completed on these sites and others, they will be added to the data base.

The Sinagua site of Mt. Elden Pueblo, Arizona deserves special note (Hevly et al. 1979; Reinhard 1988b; Reinhard et al. 1987). Privy deposits were found in this open site, but no distinct coprolites were found. The fecal deposits were represented by dark, organic-rich strata in several

Table 7. Incidence of Porotic Hyperostosis among Subadult Skeletons from Sites for Which Corprolite Data Are Available

Site	Reference	Porotic Hyperostosis/ Total Subadults
Chaco Canyon	El-Najjar et al. (1976)	10/12
Chaco Canyon	Akins (1986)	22/36
Inscription House	El-Najjar et al. (1976)	7/11
Canyon de Chelly, Pueblo Period	El-Najjar et al. (1976)	15/17
Canyon de Chelly, Basketmaker Period	El-Najjar et al. (1976)	36/50
Salmon Ruin	Berry (1983)	14/33

rooms. Helminth remains were well preserved in the deposits and are presented in Table 6. Because helminth prevalence could not be quantified for this site in the same way as for sites from which coprolites were excavated, helminthological data from Elden Pueblo are not conducive for most statistical evaluations.

Skeletal pathology studies are available for five horticultural areas for which coprolite data are available (Table 7). Four of these are presented by El-Najjar et al. (1976), although Antelope House is incorporated in the skeletal pathology for the general region of Canyon de Chelly. Two analyses are available for Chaco Canyon: El-Najjar et al. (1976) and Akins (1986). Although Akins' study is more desirable than El-Najjar's with respect to sample size, her criteria for diagnosing porotic hyperostosis were more conservative than those used by El-Najjar et al. (1976). In the interest of maintaining consistency for statistical evaluation, I chose to use El-Najjar's data in this study. Finally, Berry (1983) presents a study of pathology at Salmon Ruin including a treatment of porotic hyperostosis.

Skeletal pathology data for Mesa Verde are presented by Miles (1975). He differs from most paleopathologists by classifying the lesions of porotic hyperostosis as erythroblastosis fetalis. Unfortunately, his report does not indicate the number of crania studied and for that reason his analysis could not be included for study.

The Nature of Hunter–Gatherer Diet

As reviewed by Walker (1985) and others (Cohen and Armelagos, 1984), anemia was more common among horticultural peoples than hunter–gatherers. The skeletons of Southwestern horticultural people exhibit a higher prevalence of porotic hyperostosis (Walker 1985) than those of hunter–gatherer populations in the Great Basin of Nevada (Stark and Brooks, 1985) and lower Pecos of Texas (Marks et al. 1985).

It is instructive to compare the coprolite data for the two groups to evaluate the possibility of a dietary explanation. In general, the utilization of maize as a Southwestern horticultural dietary staple is thought to replace a diverse Archaic hunter–gatherer diet (El-Najjar et al. 1976). The coprolite evidence indicates that Archaic dietary diversity was not pronounced and was specialized around a small group of dietary staples. For this chapter, dietary staples are defined as plant genera that are available for harvest throughout the year or genera that predictably produce an abundance of fruit that can be parched and stored for the later months.

Macroscopic floral data for hunter–gatherer sites are presented in Tables 8 and 9 and Figure 4. The tables present the direct counts of identifiable components in coprolites from each site. The figures are based on percentage expressions of the data presented in the tables. As can be seen, most diets include a large variety of components, but relatively few components were eaten with great frequency. Thus, most diets were specialized around a core of frequently consumed plant foods with additional plants that were occasionally eaten.

Archaic hunter–gatherer sites reflect different types of occupation. Danger and Hogup Caves represent seasonal and temporary occupations. Both Danger and Hogup caves probably represent the fall seasonal round when people came to harvest the chenopod *Allenrolfea* (pickleweed). *Opuntia* was also harvested at Hogup Cave (Fry 1977). Fry (1980) suggests that during other parts of the year, peoples from the caves exploited plant remains in mountain and bog habitats. In contrast, a sedentary hunter–gatherer population is represented at Lovelock Cave (Fry 1980), which subsisted largely on wetland species of plants and animals with specialization on *Scirpus* and *Typha*.

Coprolites from Archaic sites in the lower Pecos of Texas indicate a late spring through fall occupation (Reinhard 1988a). Shafer (1986) suggests that the three staples in the area that were harvested year-round were *Agave*, *Opuntia*, and *Dasylirion*, but at the onset of spring and into the summer and fall, other foods were harvested such as *Yucca* flowers, *Allium*, cactus flowers, cactus fruits, and *Diospyros* fruit. This is certainly true of coprolites from the early Archaic studied by Williams-Dean (1978) (Table 9). Coprolites from the late Archaic studied by Reinhard (1988a) show a decrease in consumption of *Allium*, *Juglans*, and *Sporobolis*. Whether this is due to climate change or difference in dietary preference

Table 8. Direct Counts of Identifiable Plant Components Recovered from Hunter–Gatherer Coprolites Used in This Study[a]

Taxon	LC	DC	HC	DDC	BC
Allenrolfea		44	50		
Allium				1	
Amaranthus	2				
Asteraceae		2			
Atriplex	13	8	3	1	
Artemisia			3		
Celtis			3		
Chaenactus	1				
Chenopodium				17	1
Chrysothamnus		1			
Cornus		1			
Cucurbitaceae					1
Cycloloma				2	
Descurania (?)				1	3
Distichlis	11				
Eleocharis	2				
Elymus	15				
Equisetum	1				
Juglans				1	
Juncus	1				
Juniperus				1	1
Mentzelia	1			2	
Lepidium			1		
Opuntia		7	30	22	13
Panicum	1				
Phlox		1			
Phragmites	1				
Pinus	4	2			
Poaceae			2	6	2
Prosopis					13
Rumex	2				
Salsola	1				
Scirpus	50	3	1		
Sporobolus	1			30	
Stellaria	3				
Suaeda	8				
Typha	35				
Yucca				20	
Diversity[b]	0.71	0.58	0.58	0.74	0.73

[a] LC, Lovelock Cave ($n = 50$); DC, Danger Cave ($n = 46$); HC, Hogup Cave ($n = 51$); DDC, Dust Devil Cave ($n = 50$); BC, Bighorn Cave ($n = 20$).
[b] Shannon's diversity index, *J* values presented.

Table 9. Direct Counts of Identifiable Plant Components Recovered
from Hunter–Gatherer Coprolites from the Lower Pecos Area[a]

Taxon	GW	KJR	KDS
Acacia		1	
Agave	51	15	5
Allium	40	2	11
Amaranthus	1		
Brassicaceae			3
Carex	8	1	
Celtis	4	2	1
Cenchrus	2		
Chenopodium	3	2	1
Dasylirion	7		9
Descurania		5	
Diospyros	14	2	
Echinocereus		2	
Helianthus		3	
Juglans	23	1	2
Juniperus			2
Mammillaria		1	3
Opuntia	88	20	19
Panicum	7		
Poaceae	2	6	
Prosopis	13	1	1
Quercus			1
Sporobolus	42		
Vitus	3		
Yucca	1	3	4
Diversity[b]	0.76	0.80	0.82

[a] GW, Hinds Cave, Williams-Dean (1978) ($n = 100$); KJR, Hinds Cave, Reinhard
(1988a) ($n = 25$); KDS, Baker Cave, Sobolik (1988) ($n = 38$).
[b] Shannon's diversity index, J values presented.

is unknown. Winter would have been a time of limited resources when
people moved away from the site to concentrate on hunting with consumption of the staples noted above (Shafer 1986).

The coprolites from Dust Devil Cave on the Colorado Plateau represent
a cold season diet. *Opuntia, Chenopodium, Sporobolus,* and probably *Yucca*
were the year-round staples. *Yucca* is identified on the basis of phytoliths
in the coprolites (Reinhard 1985a). Apparently the cave was also used in
the warm season as indicated by fruits, seeds, and vegetative portions of
plants typically associated with the warm seasons found in the cave midden. At Dust Devil Cave, Archaic peoples probably augmented year-

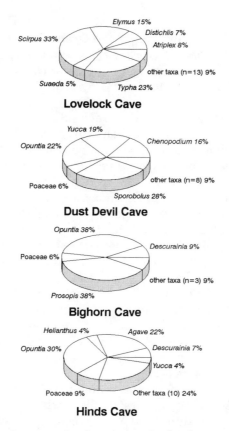

Figure 4. Relative importance of macroscopic floral components in hunter–gatherer diets. Values are percentage expressions of data presented in Tables 8 and 9.

round staples in the warm season with plants such as *Pinus edulis, Amelanchier, Celtis,* and *Allium* (Reinhard 1988a). These plants could be gathered at several localities within walking distance of the cave.

The coprolites from Bighorn Cave suggest a warm season diet during which *Opuntia* and *Prosopis* fruits were eaten (Table 9). Pollen analysis of Bighorn Cave coprolites, not included in Table 9, indicates that *Yucca* flowers were also eaten. It is very likely that these three genera were dietary staples.

One can characterize these diets by the dietary staples exhibited in the coprolite series. For example, the diet of Lovelock Cave is based on *Scirpus* and *Typha,* that of Danger Cave is based on *Allenrolfea* in the Chenopodiaceae, that of Hogup Cave is based on *Allenrolfea* and *Opuntia*, that of Bighorn Cave is based on *Prosopis* and *Opuntia*, and that of Dust Devil Cave is based on *Opuntia*, *Sporobolus*, *Yucca*, and *Chenopodium*. For Hinds Cave, the diet favored *Opuntia*, *Agave*, and *Sporobolus* in the Early Archaic (Williams-Dean 1978) and *Opuntia* and *Agave* in the Late Archaic (Reinhard 1988a).

The diversity indices presented in Tables 8 and 9 provide an idea of relative specialization at the sites. The diversity indices (*J*) reflect the evenness of distribution of observations per category. In a situation in which every category contains the same number of observations (diversification), the index is 1.0. When observations are concentrated in only a few categories (specialization), the index approaches 0.0. Thus, higher dietary diversity result in *J* values closer to 1.0 while less diverse samples produce lower *J* values. Statistical significance in diversity cannot be determined by the diversity index. The index simply shows comparative variation in relative specialization between samples. Maximum specialization is seen in the values for Hogup and Danger Caves but reduced specialization is evident in the warm season diets of Hinds Cave, Lovelock Cave, and Bighorn Cave and the winter diet of Dust Devil Cave. This is not surprising since the coprolites from Hogup and Danger Caves probably represent seasonal occupations of very short duration. However, in examining the direct count data (Tables 8 and 9), it is apparent that even warm season diets are specialized.

Specialization on dietary staples is more pronounced among short-term occupations. Dietary staples of the Archaic diet were *Opuntia*, chenopods, *Sporobolus*, *Agave*, and *Yucca* where *Agave* was not available. The species of *Agave* most commonly used by Archaic peoples are not indigenous to the Colorado Plateau and, consequently, *Yucca* replaces *Agave* as a dietary staple on the Plateau. Chenopods and grasses such as *Sporobolus* became available in fall for harvesting, parching, and storage. Vegetative portions of *Agave*, *Yucca*, and *Opuntia* are available year-round, although evidence of consumption of fruits and flowers of these plants appears only in warm season diets. In the author's opinion, based on the analysis of many coprolites, it is highly probable that these plant genera formed a nucleus for the Archaic diet.

It is noteworthy that many of the plants that formed the nucleus of Archaic diet (*Agave*, *Yucca*, *Opuntia*, *Chenopodium*) are C-4 or CAM plants that are high carbohydrate producers. Some of the other plants, although not necessarily C-4 or CAM plants, are also high carbohydrate producers (*Sporobolus*, *Allenrolfea*). This suggests that desert Archaic hunter–gatherers selected high carbohydrate-producing plants as dietary staples.

The Nature of Horticultural Diet

Macroscopic floral data for horticultural sites are presented in Table 10 and Figure 5. The horticultural sites probably represent sedentary occupations, and therefore the coprolites probably reflect the sorts of food eaten throughout the year. For example, Williams-Dean (1986) was able to distinguish warm season dietary components among the coprolites from Antelope House. Other coprolites from that site represent what she identifies as "year-round" dietary components that could be stored and consumed in winter. Similarly, Reinhard (1988a) argues that Salmon Ruin was occupied year-round.

Maize horticulture appeared relatively rapidly on the Colorado Plateau. Previous researchers had suggested that there was a gradual increase in maize consumption from early Basketmaker peoples to Puebloans, a notion that can be tested with the coprolite data. From Pueblo occupations, 209 coprolites from five sites have been examined of which 181 (88%) contain maize. From Basketmaker occupations, 72 coprolites from 2 sites have been examined of which 63 (88%) contain maize. An insignificant chi square value of 0.000 was obtained (χ^2 $_{0.5,1}$ = 3.841). The coprolite data do not reflect any significant difference in maize consumption between Basketmaker and Pueblo times, but rather demonstrate that maize horticulture was well established by Basketmaker times. Minnis (1989) in an independent analysis of Anasazi coprolites came to the same conclusion.

This point deserves some emphasis. It is generally thought that horticultural practices had a gradual growth among the earlier phases of Anasazi culture, the Basketmaker II and Basketmaker III phases. Analysis of Basketmaker III coprolites (Stiger 1977; Minnis 1989) shows that during that phase, maize horticulture was firmly established. Analysis of coprolites from the earliest Anasazi phase, Basketmaker II, also shows heavy reliance on maize (Aasen 1984; Reinhard 1988a). This indicates that the adoption of maize horticulture on the Colorado Plateau did not represent a smooth transition from hunting–gathering to horticulture. Instead, it appears that maize horticulture may have been an abrupt dietary change for Anasazi peoples.

Although maize horticulture was widely practiced in the Southwest, maize consumption was less important in some Southwestern horticulturalist diets. This is especially true of the Fremont culture. Fremont coprolites from Clyde's Cavern, Utah show evidence of reduced consumption of maize in comparison to Anasazi sites. Fremont coprolites from Glen Canyon show that squash was commonly consumed, but

Table 10. Direct Counts of Identifiable Plant Components from Horticultural Sites[a]

Taxa	CCF	GCF	GCA	TPC	AH
Allium					2
Amaranthus		6	10	2	9
Amelanchier		2			
Artemisia		1			
Asteraceae	6	3	8		
Atriplex				1	1
Cactaceae					38
Celtis			5		
Chenopodium		5	16	10	4
Cheno Am	7			4	
Cleome			5	4	14
Cryptantha			1		
Cucurbita		9	20	6	26
Descuranea				3	
Elymus	2				1
Ephedra			1		
Equisetum		1			6
Franseria				3	
Gossypium			9		16
Helianthus				5	4
Juniperus		1		5	
Lepidium	1	1	5	2	1
Opuntia		6	16	7	11
Oryzopsis			5	9	2
Panicum					1
Phaseolus		1		1	1
Physalis				1	14
Pinus	1		1	19	26
Poaceae		4	14	3	1
Polygonum			1		
Portulaca			2	6	19
Rhus					6
Scirpus	1	1	1		
Solanum				1	
Sporobolus	12				1
Vitus					2
Yucca		2		1	1
Zea	7	3	18	50	82
Diversity[b]	0.83	0.890	0.87	0.77	0.69

Table 10. (Contd.)

Taxa	IH	HH	SH	CC[c]	SR[c]
Amaranthus		5	3	1	6
Artemisia		1	1		
Atriplex		10			
Cactaceae	8				
Celtis	3				
Chenopodium		6	11		14
Cleome		3	3		2
Corispermum			2		
Cucurbita		11	13	2	
Cycloloma					1
Descurainea					4
Echinocereus					1
Erigonum		1			
Gossypium	4				
Helianthus	3	1	1	2	
Juniperus			1		
Lepidium	9				
Opuntia		14	19		1
Oryzopsis	5	2	2	1	
Panicum	1				
Phaseolus	4	10	3		11
Physalis	2	15	8		1
Pinus		7	10	11	6
Poaceae	1	1	2		
Portulaca	1	10	9	7	6
Prunus		2	2		
Rhus	1		3		23
Shepherdia		3			
Solanum				1	
Sporobolus	3			2	
Zea	10	56	28		43
Diversity[b]	0.89	0.78	0.86	—	—

[a] CCF, Clyde's Cavern Fremont (*n* = 16); GCF, Glen Canyon Fremont (*n* = 10); GCA, Glen Canyon Anasazi (*n* = 30); TPC, Turkey Pen Cave (*n* = 25); AH, Antelope House (*n* = 90); IH, Inscription House (*n* = 16); HH, Hoy House (*n* = 56); SH, Step House (*n* = 37); CC, Chaco Canyon (*n* = 47); SR, Salmon Ruin (*n* = 112).
[b] Shannon's diversity index, *J* values.
[c] Results effected by poor preservation.

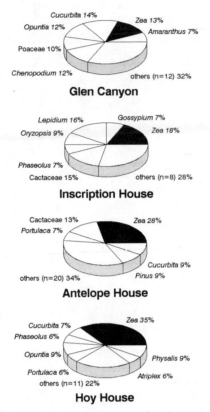

Glen Canyon

Cucurbita 14%
Opuntia 12%
Poaceae 10%
Chenopodium 12%
Zea 13%
Amaranthus 7%
others (n=12) 32%

Inscription House

Lepidium 16%
Oryzopsis 9%
Phaseolus 7%
Cactaceae 15%
Gossypium 7%
Zea 18%
others (n=8) 28%

Antelope House

Cactaceae 13%
Portulaca 7%
others (n=20) 34%
Zea 28%
Cucurbita 9%
Pinus 9%

Hoy House

Cucurbita 7%
Phaseolus 6%
Opuntia 9%
Portulaca 6%
others (n=11) 22%
Zea 35%
Physalis 9%
Atriplex 6%

Figure 5. Relative importance of macroscopic floral components in horticultural diets. Values are percentage expressions of data presented in Table 10.

maize was a minor dietary component. *Opuntia* pads, seeds of *Amaranthus* and *Chenopodium*, and wild grass seed were also commonly consumed. It is probable that in this region maize cultivation was tenuous and Fremont peoples relied on alternate dietary staples, including those used by previous Archaic peoples.

Maize clearly plays an important role in most Anasazi diets. At all Anasazi sites except for Glen Canyon, maize occurs in more coprolites than any other plant taxon. Squash, *Chenopodium*, and *Opuntia* were major dietary components along with maize at Glen Canyon.

Maize consumption at Anasazi sites is universal but variable. Of Glen

Canyon Anasazi corpolites, 60% contain maize remains and of Inscription House coprolites, 63% contain maize remains. This is in contrast to 91% for Antelope House, 96% for Turkey Pen Cave, 100% for Hoy House, and 88% for the Pueblo occupation of Step House (Table 10). The small sample of 16 coprolites from Inscription House reflects a more diverse diet with representation of many wild plant foods (Table 10). The variability of maize consumption is evident when all plant foods are considered. Of all components found in coprolite series, maize composes only 13% of Glen Canyon coprolite components, 18% of Inscription House components, 28% of Antelope House components, and 35% of Hoy House components.

Weight quantification provides a better base for evaluating the importance of maize in diet in relation to other plants. Of identifiable plant components, on the average 61% by weight of coprolites from Antelope House and 65% from Turkey Pen Cave consist of maize. In contrast, only 25% by weight of Glen Canyon Anasazi coprolites and a scant 12% of Glen Canyon Fremont coprolites consist of maize (Reinhard 1988a). The weights bear strong testimony to the variability of maize consumption at horticultural sites. The weight and frequency data cast doubt on the speculation of El-Najjar and Robertson (1976:143) that in Canyon de Chelly, Chaco Canyon, and Inscription House "maize constituted over 75% of the diet."

Although many gathered plant species were consumed at these sites, certain species stand out as being more dominant. *Opuntia* and *Pinus edulis* were important at Antelope House, *Chenopodium* and *Pinus edulis* were important at Turkey Pen Cave, *Chenopodium*, *Physalis*, and *Opuntia* were commonly consumed at Step House, *Physalis*, *Chenopodium*, and *Pinus edulis* were important foods at Hoy House, and *Rhus* was important at Salmon Ruin.

For some wild plant species, frequency data may provide an inaccurate idea of their relative importance. Often wild plant foods occur in many coprolites, but only in trace amounts that probably represent spices and condiments. For example, *Cleome*, and *Portulaca* were consumed in historic times as spices (Whiting 1939) and the small amounts of these plants in coprolites represent a similar use in prehistory. The nutritional value of these plants when used in small amounts as spices is probably minimal.

The diversity indices for horticultural sites (Table 10) are more consistent than those for hunter–gatherer sites. This may be due to season-specific diets reflected in the hunter–gatherer coprolites, which would result in more variable values. Alternatively, the more consistent values among horticulturalists may reflect the fact that all sites are located on the Colorado Plateau and there is consequently little difference in plant species availability due to ecological differences. The value for Antelope House is lower than the majority of horticultural sites and reflects a stronger trend in dietary specialization. This is based, however, on macroscopic remains only. At Antelope House, the pollen evidence indicates that *Typha* and *Equisetum* were very important dietary components (Reinhard, 1988a). Among Anasazi sites, the consumption of these plants is unique to Antelope House.

One of the most surprising dietary observations is that horticultural peoples consumed a greater variety of plants than did hunter–gatherers. On the average, 12 genera are present in the hunter–gatherer sites and 17 in horticultural sites. There are several explanations for the increased diversity of plants consumed in horticultural times. First, horticultural peoples may have supplemented a diet of horticultural foods with a diversity of collected plants to augment the nutritional value of their diets. Second, as horticultural sites are probably more sedentary, the diets may reflect year-round use of plants, which results in more genera being recovered from the coprolites. Third, horticulture may broaden the range of available food plants by encouraging the growth of weedy genera such as *Cleome, Portulaca, Amaranthus,* and *Chenopodium.* Fourth, horticultural peoples may have exploited more species to spice a relatively bland maize-dependent diet. Finally, population growth associated with horticulture may stress the subsistence base with resultant utilization of a broad range of gathered plants. Continued research will hopefully indicate which combination of these explanations, and possible others, is correct.

There is a substantial amount of component variation among Anasazi diets, represented in both wild and cultivated foods. This contradicts previous research in which Anasazi diet has been characterized as relatively uniform (Clary 1984). Comparison of Anasazi dietary components in Table 10 clearly demonstrates that utilization of wild plant foods varied both in kind and amount from site to site.

Fry (1980:332) characterized the Anasazi as "foraging specialists who practiced horticulture of maize, beans, and squash but did not depend exclusively on these cultivars." It is now clear that maize had a consistent and important role in most Anasazi diets. I would therefore modify Fry's characterization slightly and say that the Anasazi were maize horticulturalists who practiced both broad spectrum foraging and horticulture of other cultivars such as beans, cotton, and squash.

Comparison of Archaic and Horticultural Plant Use

With respect to change in plant consumption from Archaic to horticultural times, maize specialization largely replaced specialization on carbohydrate-rich collected plants. The change was simply a substitution of a carbohydrate-rich cultivar in the place of carbohydrate-rich wild plants. The impact of this change with respect to anemia may have been significant. As described by El-Najjar et al. (1976), maize is high in phytic acid, which binds with iron, making iron unavailable for intestinal absorption. Thus, the switch to maize may have been a factor in the increase of anemia. It is of interest to note that some of the Archaic dietary staples persisted among horticultural peoples. *Opuntia* is still eaten as is *Chenopodium,* although they occur with much less frequency than maize.

The iron availability in desert food plants must be considered as this directly affects dietary iron availability for prehistoric peoples. Nutritional values have been determined for some Southwestern food plants (Winkler 1982), allowing qualitative inferences about iron availability in prehistoric diets. Iron levels vary between the food plants. Sunflower seeds (*Helianthus*) and cactus flowers contain high levels of iron. Prickly pear pads contain moderate amounts of iron but *Agave* flowers and prickly pear fruit contain less iron than the other plants for which there are nutritional values.

Cactus fruit, as evidenced by seeds in coprolites, was eaten by hunter–gatherers, especially at Hogup Cave, Bighorn Cave, and Hinds Cave. Although *Opuntia* is abundant in Dust Devil Cave coprolites, the remains are of prickly pear pads, not fruit. However, this is a winter diet and it is likely that the fruits were eaten when in season. *Opuntia* continued to be consumed in horticultural times by the Anasazi and Fremont peoples. However, prickly pear remains are not as abundant in Anasazi and Fremont coprolites as they are in Archaic coprolites. Thus, there appears to have been a decline in the consumption of *Opuntia* fruit after the introduction of horticulture. Considering that resources of uncultivated flowers and fruit remained constant through the prehistory of the Southwest but that human populations increased in size and density with horticulture, it is likely that flower and fruit availability decrease on a per capita basis among horticulturalists.

It is important to note that iron in desert plants occurs in bound form that is liberated for intestinal absorption in the presence of ascorbic acid (Winkler 1982). Ascorbic acid is present in various desert flowers and in *Opuntia* fruit. Pollen analysis documents the consumption of cactus flowers (*Opuntia* and *Mammillaria*), *Agave* flowers, *Yucca* flowers, and *Dasylirion* flowers among hunter–gatherers (Bryant 1974a,b, 1986; Bryant and Williams-Dean 1975; Reinhard 1988a,b; Williams-Dean 1978). Although Anasazi peoples continued to eat cactus flowers, there is an overall decline in flower consumption once horticulture is introduced into the Southwest.

Flowers would have been available only during the spring and early summer months. *Opuntia* fruit would have been most abundant in late summer and fall, although some cactus fruit can be harvested earlier. Because such plant foods high in ascorbic acid are available only seasonally, the dietary availability of bound iron may have reduced during the late fall, winter, and early spring.

Nutritional data are gradually becoming available for many more aboriginal plant foods. The nutritional value of diets represented in coprolites will be an important facet of future research into dietary involvement in anemia. At this point, however, one can only suggest that a decrease in ascorbic acid in combination with an increased reliance on maize among horticulturalists contributed to anemia at some prehistoric villages. However, there is variation in the level of maize dependence exhibited at horticultural sites. This suggests that maize dependence is an inadequate explanation for iron-deficiency anemia as proposed by El-Najjar et al. (1982). However, on a site-specific basis, when many aspects of local ecology are considered, maize dependency may have contributed to anemia as discussed by El-Najjar et al. (1976).

Role of Meat Prehistoric Diets

The importance of small animal consumption has been largely ignored in the zooarchaeological literature, yet it is obvious from the coprolite data that small animals (from mouse size to racoon size) were an important source of protein for both horticultural and hunter–gatherer peoples (Reinhard et al., 1993). Indeed, the importance of small animals may have outweighed that of large animals in the diet. Unfortunately, the comparative importance of the two classes of animal cannot be assessed by the coprolite data. Large animal bones (deer size) are only occasionally found in coprolites (Williams-Dean 1978; Reinhard 1985a). Undoubtedly, because of the difficulty of ingesting large animal skeletal elements, large animals are underrepresented in the coprolite data.

Small animal consumption, as indicated by animal remains in coprolites, differs between horticulturalists and hunter–gatherers (Tables 11
and 12). The main difference between these subsistence types is the
greater consumption of small animals at hunter–gatherer sites. From
hunter–gatherer sites, 50–100% of the coprolites contain small animal
remains and from horticultural sites 14–50% of the coprolites contain
animal remains. Overall, of 357 hunter–gatherer coprolites, 73% contain
bone in comparison to 29% of 425 horticultural coprolites. A chi-square
value of 13.0 was derived and is highly significant ($\chi^2_{1,0.0005} = 10.6$). This
indicates that fewer meals among horticultural peoples included small
animals in comparison to hunter–gatherers.

As pointed out previously, iron is in bound form in desert plants. It is
likely, then, that animal consumption served as the major source of iron
for prehistoric peoples. It is clear that Archaic peoples with a pronounced
dietary component from small animals were obtaining large amounts of
iron. However, animal consumption among horticulturalists is variable,
and inadequate meat consumption at some villages may have contributed to anemia.

The coprolite data can adequately address the consumption of only
small animals. Whether this reflects the general level of prehistoric meat
consumption is debatable. It is possible that the hunting of large animals
by horticulturalists may have made up the deficit in meat consumption
that resulted from decreased small animal consumption. However, this

Table 11. Frequency of Bone Remains from Horticultural Sites
Expressed as Percentages

Site	Coprolites w/bone (%)	n
Clyde's Cavern	19	3/16
Glen Canyon Fremont	50	5/10
Glen Canyon Anasazi	50	15/30
Antelope House	34	33/96
Inscription House	19	3/16
Salmon Ruin	24	27/112
Hoy House	14	8/56
Step House BM II	35	7/20
Step House P III	35	6/17
Turkey Pen Cave	31	16/52
Total	29	123/425

Table 12. Frequencies of Bone Recovered from Hunter–Gatherer Sites Expressed as Percentages

Site	w/bone (%)	n
Lovelock Cave	61	31/51
Hogup Cave	70	36/51
Danger Cave	67	31/49
Great Basin Fremont	50	3/6
Great Basin Shoshoni	100	3/3
Dust Devil Cave	58	58/100
Hinds Cave	97	97/100
Total	73	259/357

is, in the author's opinion, an unlikely possibility. In all likelihood, the practice of horticulture increased the availability of small animals (Reinhard et al. 1993). Support for this notion is found in Emslie's (1981) study of bird bones from Puebloan sites. Some species of bird were apparently attracted by an increased rodent population on which they preyed. The rodents in turn were attracted by maize fields. In the author's opinion, it is likely that the consumption of small animals reflects the general level of meat consumption of both hunter–gatherers and horticulturalists.

Comparative Analysis of Helminth Parasites among Desert Hunter–Gatherers and Horticulturalists

The notion that parasite infection was less common among hunter–gatherers than horticulturalists is discussed by several authors (Reinhard 1988b). Parasitism is limited by hunter–gatherer behavior and is promoted by poor sanitation and larger populations of horticultural peoples. It can be hypothesized that horticulture should lead to increased prevalence of parasitic infection among horticulturalists and to increased diversity and richness of parasite fauna. The coprolite data can be used to assess these factors.

Virtually all of the coprolite data derived from analyses of hunter–gatherer and horticultural sites discussed in this research (Tables 13 and 14) are used in statistical analysis with some exceptions. Because taeniid eggs are dubious evidence of true human parasitism (Reinhard 1990), taeniid remains are not included in the evaluations. Also excluded are the acanthocephalan eggs from Clyde's Cavern since it is unclear that these

Table 13. Parasite Finds from Hunter-Gatherer Sites

Site Name with Number of Coprolites Studied	Number of Coprolites Positive for Specified Taxa
Lovelock Cave (*n* = 50)	1 Fascioloid trematode
(Dunn and Watkins 1970)	1 Charco-Leyden crystals
Hogup cave (*n* = 51)	
(Fry 1977)	4 *Enterobius vermicularis*
	2 *Moniliformis clarki*
	5 taeniid cestode
Danger Cave (*n* = 46)	1 *E. vermicularis*
(Fry 1977)	6 *M. clarki*
	1 taeniid cestode
Hinds Cave early Archaic (*n* = 13)	Negative
(Williams-Dean 1978)	
Hinds Cave early Archaic (*n* = 7)	Negative
(Stock 1984)	
Hinds Cave middle Archaic (*n* = 39)	Negative
(Reinhard 1988a)	
Dust Devil Cave (*n* = 100)	Negative
(Reinhard et al. 1985)	
Baker Cave (*n* = 17)	Negative
(Reinhard 1988a)	
Bighorn Cave (*n* = 35)	Negative
(Reinhard 1988a)	

are human parasites, remains of an adult nematode from Clyde's Cavern since its taxonomic place is obscure, and rhabditid larvae from Inscription House. These larvae are not described in sufficient detail to indicate whether they are actually parasites rather than free living nematodes. Several studies are now available from Antelope House (Fry and Hall 1986; Reinhard 1985a,b,c; Reinhard et al. 1987). Because the analysis of 180 coprolites by Reinhard (1988a) is most exhaustive, it is included in the evaluation presented below.

Species Richness

Species richness refers to the number of species present in the samples. In the hunter–gatherer sample, three species are represented, *Moniliformis clarki, Enterobius vermicularis,* and a fascioloid trematode. In horticultural coprolites six species are present: *E. vermicularis, M. clarki, Strongyloides* spp., hymenolepidid cestodes, strongylate nematodes, and an unknown trematode. When the soil samples from Elden Pueblo are considered, two

Table 14. Parasite Finds from Horticultural Sites[a]

Site Name with Number of Coprolites Studied	Number of Coprolites Positive for Specified Taxa
Human Coprolites	
Antelope House (*n* = 1980)	45 *Enterobius vermicularis*
(Reinhard 1988a)	2 *Strongyloides* sp.
	4 strongylate eggs
	1 hymenolepidid cestode
Antelope House (*n* = 49)	9 *E. vermicularis*
(Reinhard et al. 1987)	1 *Strongyloides* sp.
	1 strongylate eggs
	1 hymenolepidid cestode
Antelope House (*n* = 90)	14 *E. vermicularis*
(Fry and Hall 1986)	8 rhabditid (?) larvae
Bighorn Sheep Ruin (*n* = 20)	
(Gardner and Clary n.d.)	2 *E. vermicularis*
Chaco Canyon (*n* = 19)	
(Reinhard and Clary 1986)	4 *E. vermicularis*
Glen Canyon (*n* = 30)	1 *Moniliformis clarki*
(Fry 1977)	3 taeniid cestode
(Moore et al. 1974)	1 unidentified trematode
Hoy House, Mesa Verde (*n* = 56)	
(Stiger 1977)	4 *E. vermicularis*
Inscription House (*n* = 16)	3 *E. vermicularis*
(Fry unpublished data)	1 unidentified nematode egg
	1 rhabditid (?) larvae
Salmon Ruin (*n* = 112)	
(Reinhard 1985a)	9 *E. vermicularis*
Step House, Mesa Verde (*n* = 20)	
(Samuels 1965)	1 *E. vermicularis*
Turkey Pen Cave (*n* = 24)	
(Reinhard 1988a)	7 *E. vermicularis*
Elden Pueblo (*)	*Trichuris trichiura* present
(Hevly et al. 1979)	*Ascaris lumbricoides* present
	E. vermicularis present
	taeniid cestodes present
	hymenolepidid cestodes

[a] The three notations for Antelope House represent three separate coprolite samples.
* Asterisk indicates latrine soils without distinct coprolites.

additional species, *Trichuris trichiura* and *Ascaris lumbricoides,* can be added to the list of prehistoric helminths of Southwestern horticultural peoples. Clearly a greater species richness is exhibited by the sample of coprolites from horticultural sites.

Prevalence

Three of six hunter–gatherer site coprolite collections contained helminth remains, whereas 10 of 11 horticultural sites provided evidence of helminth parasitism. A chi-square value of 6.24 indicates significance beyond the 95% confidence limit ($\chi^2_{0.025,1} = 3.841$).

The prevalence of helminth remains in the total samples also differs between the hunter–gatherer and the horticultural samples. Of 357 coprolites in the hunter–gatherer sample, 14 (4%) contain helminth remains. Of 513 coprolites from horticultural sites, 89 (17%) contain helminth remains. Again the difference between prevalence between the subsistence types is significant beyond the 95% confidence interval. A chi-square value of 35.09 is obtained ($\chi^2_{0.001,1} = 10.83$).

Because the Antelope House collection is so large (180 coprolites) and has one of the largest prevalence values of any site (29%), there was concern this site would skew the overall prevalence of horticultural coprolites upward. However, calculation excluding the Antelope House data also showed a statistically significant increase in prevalence among coprolites from horticultural sites. The value obtained was 11.98, still significant beyond the 95% confidence interval ($\chi^2_{0.001,1} = 10.83$).

It is noteworthy, however, that prevalence data from both subsistence types is highly variable and that there is a degree of overlap in prevalence between the two subsistence groups. Hunter–gatherer sites at Danger Cave and Hogup Cave exhibit high prevalence. The helminth prevalence at these sites (15% for Danger Cave and 12% for Hogup Cave) approaches the overall prevalence for the horticultural sample (17% with the inclusion of Antelope House and 11% with the exclusion of Antelope House). However, the nature of parasitism at these sites is different than that of horticultural sites in that most of the Hogup and Danger Cave infections were zoonotic, the infective organism being *Moniliformis clarki*. Some of the horticultural sites exhibit very low prevalence as evidenced by helminth remains in coprolites. For example, none of the 10 coprolites from Glen Canyon that are attributed to the Fremont culture contained helminth remains. In this case, the lack of helminths may be attributed to a small sample size. However, some sites with larger samples exhibit relatively low prevalence. For example, Step House exhibits a 5% prevalence, Hoy House and the Glen Canyon Anasazi exhibit a 7% prevalence, and Salmon Ruin exhibits a 8% prevalence.

Because there is overlap in prevalence between hunter–gatherer and agricultural sites, it would be inappropriate to state that coprolites from any horticultural site will exhibit a higher prevalence than coprolites excavated from any hunter–gatherer site. However, given the data at hand, there is a probability that a sample of horticultural coprolites will exhibit a higher prevalence of helminth parasitism than a sample of hunter–gatherer coprolites.

Diversity

The diversity of parasite fauna was evaluated using Shannon's index, which is adapted to nominal data (Zar 1981). Parasite taxa were used as categories in the analysis. The evaluation was based on the number of sites exhibiting evidence of each category. Thus, for the horticultural sample, two sites each exhibited evidence of parasitism with hymeno-lepidids, *Strongyloides*, and strongylate worms. One site each exhibited evidence of *M. clarki*, trematode, *A. lumbricoides*, and *T. trichiura*. Nine horticultural sites provided evidence of *E. vermicularis* parasitism. For the hunter–gatherer sites, two exhibited parasitism with *M. clarki* and *E. vermicularis*. One exhibited evidence of trematode infection.

The *J* values calculated for the hunter–gatherer and horticultural samples were 0.9602 and 0.8102, respectively. This is contrary to the prediction that the horticultural sample would be more diverse than the hunter–gatherer sample. In reviewing the data it was observed that while many parasite taxa appeared in the horticultural sample, the number of observations of *E. vermicularis* was very high and was perhaps lowering the diversity index. To test this, diversity indices were calculated excluding the *E. vermicularis* data. The resulting *J* values were 0.9183 for hunter–gatherers and 0.9696 for horticulturalists. The similarity of these values leads to the conclusion that helminth diversity did not change very much with the advent of horticulture in spite of the increase in richness.

Parasitological Inferences

It is probable that horticultural life-style allowed more species to be established in human populations (Reinhard 1988a). However, most species established themselves at low prevalence levels. The greatest change in prevalence occurred with *E. vermicularis*, which was present in some Archaic hunter–gatherer populations at low levels. Horticultural life apparently allowed this species to proliferate. In the hunter–gatherer sample, *E. vermicularis* was present in 1.4% of the coprolites. Among horticultural coprolites, *E. vermicularis* is present in 15.0% of the coprolites. Thus, it appears that pinworm infection underwent an explosive proliferation in the sedentary, crowded, and unhygienic conditions of Southwest horticultural pueblos.

Causal Factors of Anemia: The Role of Diet and Parasitism

The survey of dietary data and parasite data presented above suggests that among horticulturalists, limited meat consumption, reliance on maize as a dietary staple, and increased parasitism could all have had an effect on the increase in anemia at some horticultural villages. Now we explore whether these factors individually had causal relationships with anemia among horticulturalists. To evaluate possible causal relations, skeletal data of porotic hyperostosis are correlated with coprolite evidence of maize consumption, small animal consumption, and parasite prevalence. The analysis is limited to Canyon de Chelly (Antelope House), Chaco Canyon, Salmon Ruin, and Inscription House. These Anasazi sites are the only ones for which coprolite and skeletal data are available.

Diet as a Cause of Anemia

If maize consumption is a cause of prehistoric anemia, one would predict that for those sites for which both coprolite data and skeletal data are available (Salmon Ruin, Antelope House, Inscription House), the prevalence of porotic hyperostosis in the skeletal series will covary with the prevalence of maize in the coprolites. This will be evaluated by testing the null hypothesis that no significant covariance will be present. Maize pollen frequency data will be used in the analysis.

The null hypothesis is not refuted statistically. The percentage of coprolites containing maize pollen and the percentage of skeletons exhibiting porotic hyperostosis from Salmon Ruin, Antelope House, and Chaco Canyon were used in the calculation of the correlation coefficient. The calculated r value of 0.6363 and r^2 value are insignificant ($r^2_{0.05(2),1} = 0.997$: $t=1.0692$, $t_{0.05(2),1}=12.706$) and suggest that maize frequency in coprolites varies independently of porotic hyperostosis frequency in skeletons.

If meat consumption is a cause of prehistoric anemia, one would predict that for those sites for which both coprolite data and skeletal data are available, the prevalence of porotic hyperostosis in the skeletal series will covary with the prevalence of bone in the coprolites. This will be evaluated by testing the null hypothesis that no significant covariance will be present.

The percentage of coprolites containing animal residue and the percentage of skeletons exhibiting porotic hyperostosis from Salmon Ruin, Antelope House, Inscription House, and Chaco Canyon are used in the calculations. When all data for all sites are used in the calculations, the r value is 0.7114 and the r^2 value is 0.5062. This value is insignificant at the 95% confidence interval (t=2.8825, $t_{0.05(2),2}$=4.303). Therefore, it appears that meat consumption varies independently of porotic hyperostosis frequency.

There is no significant covariance of dietary data, either maize or animal residue, with skeletal evidence of anemia. This suggests that individual aspects of diet such as maize consumption and meat consumption have no causal relationship with anemia.

Parasitism as a Cause of Anemia

In general, parasitism among southwestern horticulturalists increased in comparison to that of hunter–gatherers (Tables 13 and 14). This increase especially affected the prevalence of pinworm (*Enterobius vermicularis*), a species transmitted in conditions of poor hygiene and crowding.

At Anasazi sites, pinworm is often the only helminth parasite found and its prevalence in coprolites is variable, ranging from 29% at Turkey Pen Cave to 5% at Step House. Occasionally, other helminth taxa have been found (Table 14), but their numbers are small relative to *E. vermicularis* (Reinhard 1988b; Reinhard et al. 1987).

An important question is whether parasitism had an impact on prehistoric anemia. This question can be addressed statistically by comparison of sites for which parasite data from coprolites and porotic hyperostosis data from skeletal series are available. These sites include Chaco Canyon, Antelope House, Inscription House, and Salmon Ruin.

Correlation coefficients (r) and correlation indices (r^2) were calculated on the basis of the percentage prevalence of coprolites containing parasite remains and the percentage incidence of porotic hyperostosis in skeletons of subadults. The r^2 values indicate how much of the variability in one data set can be accounted for by correlation with the second data set. The calculations were made in two ways. The first pair of calculations include all helminth data for Salmon Ruin, Chaco Canyon, Antelope House, and Inscription House correlated with incidences of porotic hyperostosis. The r value obtained was 0.9545, and r^2 was 0.9111. The r values are significant at the 95% confidence limit ($r_{0.05(2)}$=0.95). The second pair of calculations included pinworm prevalence from all four sites and resulted in an *r* value of 0.9640 and an r^2 of 0.9293. The *r* value is also significant at the 95% confidence interval ($r_{0.05(2)}=0.95$)

The correlation indices are strikingly high. Based on the data at hand, 93% of the variation in porotic hyperostosis for all four sites is correlated with pinworm prevalence variation in coprolites (Figure 6). In the same way, 91% of the variability of porotic hyperostosis for all four sites correlates with prevalence of all helminth species in coprolites.

These data do not necessarily reflect a causal relationship between helminth parasitism and anemia. Pinworm accounts for the vast majority of observations and is the only organism found with consistency at Anasazi sites. Since pinworm is largely nonpathogenic and is not implicated as a cause of anemia by modern studies, there is no reason to believe that this species caused anemia in the Anasazi sites discussed here. Indeed, as discussed by Reinhard (1988b), outside the tropical and subtropical ranges of Ancylostomidae (hookworm) and *Strongyloides* (threadworm), and outside of the range of *Diphyllobothrium* (fish tapeworm), it is unwise to implicate helminth parasitism as a cause of prehistoric New World anemia. However, the strong correlations suggest that the factors that affect pinworm parasitism are linked with the factors that caused prehistoric anemia.

The correlation of pinworm prevalence in coprolites and porotic hyperostosis prevalence in skeletal series can be explained as a relationship

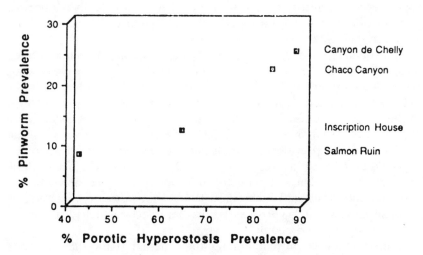

Figure 6. Prevalence of pinworm remains in coprolites vs. porotic hyperostosis frequency in skeletons for Anasazi sites.

with microparasitism (protozoal, bacterial, and viral infection). The conditions conducive to microparasitism were also conducive to high pinworm transmission, and therefore pinworm prevalence can be viewed as a general indicator of microparasitism resulting from poor sanitation. Microparasitism may have had a causal effect with respect to porotic hyperostosis by producing elevated levels of anemia. This is due either to direct damage done to the host's hematopoietic tissue or by host response to infection (Kent 1989). Microparasitic organisms associated with poor hygiene and crowding include several protozoa and bacteria.

Diarrhea is a likely pathogenic cause of prehistoric anemia. Diarrheal organisms that are likely to have been endemic among the Anasazi include *Entamoeba hystolitica*, *Salmonella*, *Escherichia coli*, and *Shigella*. With all of these organisms, poor sanitation and hygiene combined with concentrated populations would increase infection levels.

Fink (1985) notes that the dark, cramped quarters of Anasazi villages would also increase the chance of infection since bacteria could survive in these areas for prolonged periods of time without the killing and desiccating effects of sunlight. Protozoan cysts would also survive for prolonged periods in such conditions.

Other conditions that would promote infection by a variety of microparasites cited by Fink are the use of communal eating utensils, nonsegregation of sick individuals, and close association with domesticated turkeys and dogs. In such conditions, contamination of foodstuffs probably occurred in the fouled environment of prehistoric habitations. Fly pupae cases and puparia have been noted in coprolites indicating the presence of flies in feces and suggesting that fly-borne disease may have existed in these sites.

Unfortunately, evidence of microparasites has not yet been identified in coprolites from the Southwest and only a few organisms leave osseous traces. Therefore, the nature of Anasazi microparasitism is largely in the realm of speculation. However, osseous evidence of microparasitism is present in some Anasazi skeletons. Preliminary data from Black Mesa (Martin et al. 1985) show that periosteal infection was endemic in that Anasazi area. The prevalence of periosteal lesions increases from a low of 15% at A.D. 850–975 to over 45% by A.D. 1100–1150. On Black Mesa, however, the prevalence of periosteal infection does not covary with that of porotic hyperostosis. With respect to infectious disease, Martin et al. (1985) support Kunitz's (1970) assertion that infectious diarrhea was endemic among Anasazi peoples.

Tuberculosis was present among the Anasazi (Fink 1985; Sumner 1985). Fink presents an especially graphic description of the probable living conditions at Anasazi villages that might promote microparasitism. Fink points out that the main factor that predisposed Anasazi peoples to tuberculosis was a lack of understanding of contagions and their transmission. This would apply to water and fly-borne diseases as well.

Conclusions

In summary, it appears that the role of maize dependency as an etiologic factor has been overstated (El-Najjar 1976; El-Najjar et al. 1982). In contrast, the role of infectious disease has been understated. In both cases, the impact of diet and parasitism on anemia must be evaluated on a site by site basis (El-Najjar et al. 1976). Both the level of maize dependency and parasitism vary between sites.

The coprolite data indicate that the transition from hunting and gathering was probably abrupt for peoples on the Colorado Plateau. The adoption of maize horticulture was accompanied by an increase of phytic acid and possible decrease in ascorbic acid in the diet. Meat consumption also decreased. These changes potentially had negative impacts on both iron availability in the diet and physiological availability of iron to prehistoric horticulturalists. However, a causal relationship between maize consumption alone or meat consumption alone with anemia cannot be demonstrated. Thus, the coprolite data show that maize dependency and low meat consumption were aspects of Anasazi horticultural life. However, the role of these dietary factors in causing porotic hyperostosis has been exaggerated (El-Najjar 1976; El-Najjar and Robertson 1976; El-Najjar et al. 1982). In essence, single dietary factors cannot be demonstrated as having a causal relationship with anemia.

The coprolite data also show that helminth parasitism increased among horticultural peoples over hunter–gatherers. The most dramatic increase occurred with the essentially nonpathogenic species *Enterobius vermicularis* (pinworm). There is a statistically significant covariance of pinworm parasitism and porotic hyperostosis. Because pinworm is relatively nonpathogenic, a causal relationship between helminth parasitism and anemia cannot be inferred. However, it is proposed that the increase in pinworm and general helminth parasitism is a proxy indicator of increase in microparasitism. It is then proposed that microparasitic protozoal, bacterial, and viral disease directly caused anemia. It is important to emphasize that these conclusions and inferences apply only to the area under study, which is the arid west of North America. In the tropics, subtropics, and coastal regions parasite ecology is much different. In these areas, helminth infection could have a causal relationship with anemia (Allison 1974; Araujo et al. 1981, 1983; Callen and Cameron 1960; Ferreira et al. 1980, 1983, 1984; Horne 1985; Patrucco et al. 1983).

If pinworm parasitism is viewed as a gauge of microparasitic infectious disease, then the high correlation of pinworm prevalence in coprolites and porotic hyperostosis prevalence in crania could implicate microparasitic infections as a causal factor. This indicates that protozoal and bacterial infection by species transmitted in conditions of poor hygiene, poor sanitation, and crowding had a causal relationship with anemia. The organisms most likely involved are those that cause diarrhea (Kent 1986).

The application of dietary and parasitological data from coprolites to paleopathology is just beginning. With respect to porotic hyperostosis, continued study of coprolites must include thorough nutritional reconstruction. This aspect of coprolite analysis is still in its infancy. As this facet of coprolite study matures, the question of ascorbic acid consumption raised in this paper will be addressed more fully. New coprolite studies have revealed evidence of microparasitism (Faulkner 1991). The analysis of coprolites for bacterial, protozoal, and perhaps viral diarrhea-causing organisms must be developed. Once techniques are developed for the identification of microparasites in coprolites, then direct correlation of intestinal microparasitic disease with anemia can be done. A third emphasis in future coprolite studies must be the integration of skeletal and coprolite data on a large scale, a goal that has been attempted for the first time in this chapter. Future work must include the collection of dietary, parasitological, and porotic hyperostosis data for those areas for which both coprolites and skeletons are available. Mesa Verde and Glen Canyon are two specific areas that have the immediate potential of providing such data. At this point it is clear that coprolite data, both dietary and parasitological, have direct relevance to skeletal paleopathological problems such as the etiology of porotic hyperostosis. It is also clear that the integration of skeletal and coprolite data will bring fruitful results in the future.

The most important lesson to be learned from coprolite analysis is that diet and parasitism is highly variable on a site by site basis for both hunter–gatherers and horticulturalists. Thus, the evaluation of these variables as causal factors for anemia must be done on a site by site basis. Modern archaeological investigations are detailed enough to allow for the reconstruction of economy and parasite ecology (Reinhard 1988a). Further investigations of the relation of parasitism and diet to anemia in prehistory would be better focused on site-specific data rather than on broad stroke generalization to regional causes of anemia as presented others (El-Najjar 1976; El-Najjar and Robertson 1976). In essence, general environmental conditions of a large geographic area have little impact on parasitism and diet in comparison to local ecologies and economies of villages within the region. Thus, village level analyses will be more insightful in defining patterns of diet and disease for prehistoric peoples than examination of regional data.

References

Aasen, D.K. 1984. Pollen, macrofossil, and charcoal analyses of Basketmaker coprolites from Turkey Pen Ruin, Cedar Mesa, Utah. M.A. Thesis, Department of Anthropology, Washington State University, Pullman.

Akins, N.J. 1986. *A biocultural approach to human burials from Chaco Canyon, New Mexico.* Reports of the Chaco Center number 9. Sante Fe: National Park Service.

Allision, M.J., A. Pezzia, I. Hasigawa, and E. Gerszten. 1974. A case of hookworm infection in a pre-Columbian American. *American Journal of Physical Anthropology* 41:103–106.

Araújo, A.J.G., L.F. Ferreira, and U.E.C. Confalonieri. 1981. A contribution to the study of helminth findings in archaeological material in Brazil. *Revista Brasileira de Biologia* 41:873–881.

Araújo, A.J.G., L.F. Ferreira, U.E.C. Confalonieri, and L. Nuñez. 1983. Eggs of *Diphyllobothrium pacificum* in pre-Columbian human coprolites. *Paleopathology Newsletter* 41:11–13.

Berry, D. 1983. Disease and climactical relationship among P III–P IV Anasazi of the Colorado Plateau, Ph. D. Dissertation, Department of Anthropology, University of California–Los Angeles.

Bryant, V.M., Jr. 1974a. Prehistoric diet in southwest Texas: the coprolite evidence. *American Antiquity* 39:407–420.

Bryant, V.M., Jr. 1974b. The role of coprolite analysis in archaeology. *Bulletin of the Texas Archaeological Society* 45:1–48.

Bryant, V.M., Jr. 1986. Prehistoric diet: A case for coprolite analysis. In *Ancient Texans: Rock Art and Lifeways along the Lower Pecos.* H.J. Shafer, ed., pp. 132–139. Austin: Texas Monthly Press.

Bryant, V.M., and G. Williams-Dean. 1975. The coprolites of man. *Scientific American* 232:100–109.

Callen, E.O., and T.W.M. Cameron. 1960. A prehistoric diet revealed in coprolites. *New Scientist* 8:35–40.

Clary, K.H. 1984. Prehistoric coprolite remains from Chaco Canyon, New Mexico:

Inferences for Anasazi diet and subsistence. M.S. Thesis, Department of Biology, University of New Mexico, Albuquerque.

Cohen, M.T., and G.J. Armelagos. 1984. *Paleopathology at the Origins of Agriculture.* New York: Academic Press.

Dunn, F.L., and R. Watkins. 1970. Parasitological examination of prehistoric human coprolites from Lovelock Cave, Nevada. *Contributions of the University of California Archaeological Research Facility* 10:176–185.

El-Najjar, M.Y., 1976. Maize, malaria and the anemias in the Pre-Colombian New World. *Yearbook of Physical Anthropology* 20:329–337.

El-Najjar, M.Y., and A.L. Robertson, Jr. 1976. Spongy bones in prehistoric America. *Science* 193:141–143.

El-Najjar, M.Y., D.J. Ryan, C.G. Turner II, and B. Lozoff. 1976. The etiology of porotic hyperostosis among the prehistoric and historic Anasazi Indians of the southwestern United States. *American Journal of Physical Anthropology* 44:447–448.

El-Najjar, M.Y., J. Andrews, J. G. Moore, and D.G. Bragg. 1982. Iron deficiency anemia in two prehistoric American Indian skeletons: A Dietary hypothesis. *Plains Anthropologist* 44:447–448.

Emslie, S.D. 1981. Birds and prehistoric agriculture: the New Mexican Pueblos. *Human Ecology* 9:305–329.

Faulkner, C.T., 1991. Prehistoric diet and parasitic infection in Tennessee: Evidence from the analysis of desiccated human paleofeces. *American Antiquity* 56:687–700.

Ferreira, L.F., A.J.G. Araújo, and U.E.C. Confalonieri. 1980. The finding of eggs and larvae of parasitic helminths in archaeological material from Unai, Minas Gerais, Brazil. *Transactions of the Royal Society of Tropical Medicine and Hygiene* 74:798–800.

Ferreira, L.F., A.J.G. Araújo, and U.E.C. Confalonieri. 1983. The finding of helminth eggs in a Brazilian mummy. *Transactions of the Royal Society of Tropical Medicine and Hygiene* 77:65–67.

Ferreira, L.F., A.J.G. Araújo, U.E.C. Confalonieri, and L. Nuñez. 1984. The finding of *Diphyllobothrium* in human coprolites (4,000–1,950 B.C.) from northern Chile. *Memorias do Instituto Oswaldo Cruz* 79:175–180.

Fink, T.M. 1985. Tuberculosis and anemia in a Pueblo II–III (ca. AD 900–1300) Anasazi child from New Mexico. In *Health and Disease in the Prehistoric Southwest.* C.F. Merbs and R.J. Miller, eds., pp. 359–379. Tempe: Arizona State University Anthropological Research Papers 34.

Fry, G.F., 1977. *Analysis of Prehistoric Coprolites from Utah.* University of Utah Anthropological Papers 97. Salt Lake City: University of Utah Press.

Fry, G.F. 1980. Prehistoric diet and parasites in the desert west of North America. In *Early Native Americans.* D.L. Browman, ed., pp. 325–339. The Hague: Mouton Press.

Fry, G.F. 1985. Analysis of fecal material. In *The Analysis of Prehistoric Diets.* R.I. Gilbert and J.H. Mielke, eds., pp. 127–154. New York: Academic Press.

Fry, G.F., and H.J. Hall. 1969. Parasitological examination of human coprolites from Utah. *Proceedings of the Utah Academy of Science, Arts and Letters* 36: 102–105.

Fry, G.F., and H.J. Hall. 1975. Human coprolites from Antelope House: Preliminary analysis. *The Kiva* 47:87–96.

Fry, G.F., and H.J. Hall. 1986. Human coprolites. In *Archaeological Investigations at Antelope House*. D.P. Morris, ed., pp. 165–188. Washington, D.C.: National Park Service.

Fry, G.F., and H.J. Hall. n.d. The analysis of human coprolites from Inscription House. Unpublished m.s. on file with the Western Archaeological Center, National Park Service, Tucson.

Fry, G.F., and J.G. Moore. 1969. *Enterobius vermicularis:* 10,000 year old human infection. *Science* 166:1620.

Gardner, S.L., and K.H. Clary. n.d. Helminth remains of Anasazi period coprolites from Bighorn Sheep Ruin [42SA1563], Canyonlands National Park, Utah. Unpublished report prepared for Nickens and Associates, P.O. Box 727, Montrose, Colorado.

Hall, H.J. 1972. Diet and disease at Clyde's Cavern, Utah. M.A. Thesis, University of Utah, Salt Lake City.

Heizer, R.F., and L.K. Napton. 1969. Biological and cultural evidence from prehistoric human coprolites. *Science* 165:563–568.

Hevly, R.H., R.E. Kelly, G.A. Anderson, and, S.J. Olsen. 1979. Comparative effects of climate change, cultural impact, and volcanism in the paleoecology of Flagstaff, Arizona, A.D. 900–1300. In *Volcanic Activity and Human History*. P. Sheets and D. Grayson, eds., pp. 487–523. New York: Academic Press.

Holloway, Richard G. 1985. Diet and medicinal plant usage of a late Archaic population from Culberson County, Texas. *Bulletin of the Texas Archaeological Society* 54:319–329.

Horne, P.D. 1985. A review of the evidence of human endoparasitism in the pre-Columbian New World through the study of coprolites. *Journal of Archaeological Science* 12:299–310.

Kelso, G.K. 1970. Hogup Cave, Utah: Comparative pollen analysis of human coprolites and cave fill. In *Hogup Cave*. C.M. Aikens, ed., pp. 251–262. University of Utah Anthropological Papers 93.

Kent, S. 1989. Hypoferremia: Adaption to disease?. *The New England Journal of Medicine* 320: 672.

Kent, S. 1986. The influence of sedentism and aggregation on porotic hyperostosis and anemia: A case study. *Man* 21:605–636.

Kunitz, S.J. 1970. Disease and death among the Anasazi. *El Palacio* 76:1722.

Marks, M.K., J.C. Rose, and E.L. Buie. 1985. Bioarchaeology of Seminole Sink. In *Seminole Sink: Excavation of a Vertical Shaft Tomb*. S.A. Turpin, ed., Research Report 93, Texas Archaeological Survey, University of Texas, Austin.

Martin, D.L., C. Piacentini, and G.J. Armelagos. 1985. Paleopathology of the Black Mesa Anasazi: A biocultural approach. In *Health and Disease in the Prehistoric Southwest*. C.F. Merbs and R.J. Miller, eds., pp. 104–114. Tempe: Arizona State University Anthropological Research Papers 34.

Martin, P.S., and F.W. Sharrock. 1964. Pollen analysis of prehistoric human feces; new approach to ethnobotany. *American Antiquity* 30:168–180.

Miles, J.S. 1975. *Orthopedic Problems of the Wetherill Mesa Populations, Mesa Verde National Park, Colorado*. Washington, D.C.: U.S. Government Printing Office.

Minnis, P.E. 1989. Prehistoric diet in the northern Southwest: macroplant remains from Four Corners feces. *American Antiquity* 54:543–563.

Moore, J.G., G.F. Fry, and E. Englert. 1969. Thorny-headed worm infection in North American prehistoric man. *Science* 163:1324–1325.

Moore, J.G., A.W. Grundman, H.J. Hall, and G.F. Fry. 1974. Human fluke infection in Glen Canyon at AD 1250. *American Journal of Physical Anthropology* 41:115–118.

Napton, L.K., and G. Kelso. 1969. Preliminary palynological analysis of Lovelock Cave coprolites. *Kroeber Anthropological Society Special Publications*. 2:19–27.

Patrucco, R., R. Tello, and D. Bonavia. 1983. Parasitological finds of coprolites of pre-hispanic Peruvian populations. *Current Anthropology* 24:393–394.

Reinhard, K.J. 1985a. Recovery of helminths from prehistoric feces: the Cultural ecology of ancient parasitism. M.S. Thesis, Department of Biological Sciences, Northern Arizona University, Flagstaff.

Reinhard, K.J. 1985b. Parasitism at Antelope House, a Puebloan village in Canyon de Chelly, Arizona. In *Health and Disease in the Prehistoric Southwest*. C.F. Merbs and R.J. Miller, eds., pp. 220–223. Tempe: Arizona State University Anthropological Research Papers 34.

Reinhard, K.J. 1985c. *Strongyloides stercoralis* in the prehistoric Southwest. In *Health and Disease in the Prehistoric Southwest*. C.F. Merbs and R.J. Miller, eds., pp. 234–242. Tempe: Arizona State University Anthropological Research Papers 34.

Reinhard, K.J. 1988a. Diet, parasitism and anemia in the prehistoric southwest. Ph. D. Dissertation, Department of Anthropology, Texas A&M University, College Station.

Reinhard, K.J. 1988b. Cultural ecology of prehistoric parasitism on the Colorado Plateau as evidenced by coprology. *American Journal of Physical Anthropology* 77:355–366.

Reinhard, K.J. 1990. Archaeoparasitology in North America. *American Journal of Physical Anthropology* 82:145–163.

Reinhard, K.J., and V.M. Bryant, Jr. 1992. Coprolite analysis: A biological perspective on archaeology. In *Advances in Archaeological Method and Theory*, Vol. 4. M.B. Schiffer, ed., New York: Academic Press.

Reinhard, K.J., and K.H. Clary. 1986. Parasite analysis of prehistoric coprolites from Chaco Canyon, New Mexico. In *A Biocultural Approach to Human Burials from Chaco Canyon, New Mexico*. N.J. Akins, ed., pp. 214–222. Sante Fe: National Park Service.

Reinhard, K.J., J.R. Ambler, and M. McGuffie. 1985. Diet and parasitism at Dust Devil Cave. *American Antiquity* 50:819–824.

Reinhard, K.J., R.H. Hevly, and G.A. Anderson. 1987. Helminth remains from prehistoric Indian coprolites on the Colorado Plateau. *Journal of Parasitology* 73:630–639.

Reinhard, K.J., U.E. Confalonieri, B. Herrmann, L.F. Ferreira, and A.J.G. Araújo. 1988. Recovery of parasite eggs from coprolites and latrines: Aspects of paleoparasitological technique. *Homo* 37:217–239.

Reinhard, K.J., C. Szuter, and J.R. Ambler. 1993. Small animal exploitation as evidenced by coprolite analysis. *International Journal of Osteoarchaeology* (in press).

Samuels, R. 1965. Parasitological study of long dried fecal samples. *American Antiquity* 31:175–179.

Scott, L. 1979. Dietary inferences from Hoy House coprolites: A palynological interpretation. *The Kiva* 44:257–281.

Shafer, H.J. 1986. *Ancient Texans: Rock Art and Lifeways along the Lower Pecos.* Austin: Texas Monthly Press.

Sobolik, R.D. 1988. The prehistoric diet and subsistence of the Lower Pecos Region, as reflected in coprolites from Baker Cave, Val Verde County, Texas. M.A. Thesis, Department of Anthropology, Texas A&M University, College Station.

Stark, C., and S.T. Brooks. 1985. A survey of paleopathology in the Nevada Great Basin. In *Health and Disease in the Prehistoric Southwest.* C.F. Merbs and R.J. Miller, eds., pp. 65–78. Tempe: Arizona State University Anthropological Research Papers 34.

Steinbock, R.T. 1976. *Paleopathological Diagnosis and Interpretation.* Springfield: Charles C Thomas.

Stiger, M.A. 1977. Anasazi diet: The coprolite evidence. M.A. Thesis, Department of Anthropology, University of Colorado, Boulder.

Stock, J.A. 1983. The prehistoric diet of Hinds Cave: Val Verde County, Texas. M.A. Thesis, Department of Anthropology, Texas A&M University, College Station.

Sumner, D.R. 1985. a probable case of prehistoric tuberculosis from northeastern Arizona. In *Health and Disease in the Prehistoric Southwest.* C.F. Merbs and R.J. Miller, eds., pp. 340–346. Arizona State University Anthropological Research Papers 34.

Walker, P. 1985. Anemia among prehistoric Indians of the American Southwest. In *Health and Disease in the Prehistoric Southwest.* C.F. Merbs and R.J. Miller, eds., pp. 139–164. Tempe: Arizona State University Anthropological Research Papers 34.

Whiting, A.E., 1939. *Ethnobotany of the Hopi.* Museum of Northern Arizona, Bulletin 15. Flagstaff: Museum of Northern Arizona.

Williams-Dean, G. 1978. Ethnobotany and cultural ecology of prehistoric man in Southwest Texas. Ph.D. Dissertation, Department of Biology, Texas A&M University, College Station.

Williams-Dean, G. 1986. Pollen analysis of human coprolites. In *Archaeological In-*

vestigations at Antelope House. D.P. Morris, ed., pp. 189–205. Washington, D.C.: National Park Service.

Winkler, B.A. 1982. Wild plant foods of the desert gatherers of West Texas, New Mexico, and Northern Mexico: Some nutritional values. M.A. Thesis, Department of Anthropology, University of Texas at Austin.

Zar, J.H. 1974. *Biostatistical Analysis*. Englewood Cliffs, NJ: Prentice-Hall.

Part III

COMMENTARY

Chapter 9

Anemia Reevaluated: A Look to the Future

Patricia Stuart-Macadam

The importance of iron-deficiency anemia as a factor in human health is undeniable; it has done and does affect populations in every country around the globe from prehistoric times to the present. Its occurrence has been inextricably linked to health and disease of the human species throughout our evolutionary history. However, it is an issue that means different things to different people. For example, nutritionists, hematologists, microbiologists, and anthropologists view iron-deficiency anemia from their own perspective and source of data. A lack of interdisciplinary communication means that what may be common knowledge in one field is little known or understood in another. Here lies the strength of *Diet, Demography, and Disease: Changing Perspectives of Anemia*. For the first time perspectives, ideas, and data on iron-deficiency anemia from a number of fields are synthesized and presented in one volume. This provides a more comprehensive and holistic view of iron-deficiency anemia.

Three major issues are emphasized in this volume; one, the complexity of the role of iron in health and disease; two, the relative unimportance of diet compared with other factors in the etiology of iron-deficiency anemia; and three, the role of iron withholding as a defense against pathogens. Iron is an essential body mineral; both too much and too little can have detrimental effects. This, and the fact that iron is involved in maintaining body defenses as well as a number of metabolic processes, means that it plays a complex role in health and disease. The literature suggests that the fact that iron-deficiency anemia rarely occurs from dietary deficiency alone has been known by nutritionists for about 20 years. Nevertheless, researchers in a number of other fields are still under the impression that insufficient dietary iron is the most important contributing factor in the development of iron-deficiency anemia. Certainly many anthropologists, as well as the general public, would consider the amount of iron in the diet to be of paramount importance in the etiology of iron-deficiency anemia. The role of iron withholding as a defense against infection is an issue that has been explored by microbiologists for the past 25 years, but is only now becoming widely accepted by researchers in other fields. Anthropologists have been largely unaware of the implications and certainly the general public has been completely unaware of this aspect of iron physiology. Anthropologists have known of patterns in the occurrence of iron-deficiency anemia in the past that provide clues about its etiology in the present, but nutritionists, hematologists, and microbiologists have been unaware of this information. These differing perspectives and understanding will provoke different reactions to this book. To some it will represent a challenging, controversial volume, to others the concepts and ideas will be more readily accepted. However, all should benefit from the broadened outlook on iron-deficiency anemia achieved by the multidisciplinary approach.

The book is divided into two main sections, theoretical explorations and case studies, as well as a commentary section. The contributors to the section on theoretical explorations introduce the three major issues of the volume. The data that have been presented in the case study section explore these issues in more detail and illustrate the complexities involved in any discussion of iron-deficiency anemia.

In his chapter Garn presents a more traditional view, but emphasizes the problems associated with applying hematological standards that do not consider the considerable variability in "normal" values that occur. He states that fully 50% of boys, girls, and younger men and women and an even larger proportion of older adults evaluated in large nutritional surveys would be considered to be low in hemoglobin and hematocrit values if the commonly used textbook standards were adhered to. Garn emphasizes the importance of individual variability on hematological indices; he notes the myriad factors that can affect hemoglobin levels in normal individuals, including sex, age, maturation level, pregnancy, altitude, obesity, smoking, and fitness level, and cautions that textbook norms for hemoglobin and hematocrit must be used with extreme caution. Although he emphasizes the dietary factors involved in the development of iron-deficiency anemia, he also recognizes, along with others in his field, the importance of disease and parasitic infestation in contributing to anemia and presents a section on this topic.

Wadsworth sets the tone for viewing iron deficiency in a new light by emphasizing the lexibility and adaptability of iron metabolism.

He stresses the problems involved in interpreting hemoglobin and hematocrit values, and emphasizes the variability of "normality." He presents three "laws of erythrokinetics":

1. The body tends to conserve iron, so once iron enters the system very little is lost.
2. The amount of iron that enters from the intestine is directly related to the amount of iron in the tissues; as iron stores decrease the amount absorbed by the intestine increases.
3. The amount of iron entering from the intestine is directly related to the rate of erythropoeisis; the higher the rate the more iron is absorbed.

These "laws" and the fact that as the amount of iron in the diet decreases, the proportion absorbed increases, illustrate the plasticity and flexibility of iron metabolism and show how difficult it is to become anemic simply through a diet low in iron. This challenges the prevailing view that diet plays a major role in the development of iron-deficiency anemia. Wadsworth states that not even a broad association between the intake of iron and the prevalence of anemia has been established. He suggests that there is something inherent in the individual, not in the diet, that results in any one individual developing iron-deficiency anemia. He feels that iron-deficiency anemia is much more likely to result from a disruption in the internal transfer of iron, such as that which occurs with infections and parasitic diseases. These can be important causes of anemia due to interference with the normal turnover of iron within the body. He concludes by saying that iron is ubiquitous in our environment and it seems unlikely that humans have evolved without adapting to a wide range in availability of iron.

Weinberg's chapter highlights the adaptive nature of iron metabolism in the face of disease. He focuses on the ability of humans to withhold iron from microbial pathogens and neoplastic cells while allowing normal tissues access to physiological levels of iron. This iron-withholding capability is an important aspect of the body's immune response to disease. It is achieved by several mechanisms, including the stationing of iron-binding proteins around the areas of invasion, the reduction of dietary intake of iron, and the lowering of the amount of iron normally contained in the iron-binding protein, transferrin. Weinberg explains that evidence that humans develop a hypoferremic response to infection and chronic disorders began to accumulate six decades ago when Locke et al. (1932) observed that tubercular and cancerous patients lower their level of plasma iron. Apparently plasma iron levels begin to decline early in the incubation phase of disease, sometimes reducing to 70% of normal. With recovery, the level of plasma iron returns to normal.

Weinberg points out that this iron-withholding system can be compromised by excess iron, resulting either from interference with the synthesis of various iron-binding proteins, or the acquisition of exogenous or endogenous iron. The use of iron cookware to brew alcoholic beverages consumed by adult males in parts of Africa and high alcohol consumption are two examples of cultural practices that can compromise the iron-withholding system. Certain diseases such as thalassemia or hereditary spherocytosis, which are associated with an increase in bone marrow (erythroid hyperplasia), also lead to increased iron accumulation and a compromised immune response.

My own chapter challenges the traditional view that diet is an important factor in the development of iron-deficiency anemia in prehistoric populations. Signs of anemia in bone (known as porotic hyperostosis) occur in populations from almost every geographic area and time period. By examining the patterns of occurrence of porotic hyperostosis through time and space I have shown that certain factors are associated with higher levels of porotic hyperostosis, hence anemia. These factors can be generalized into three broad categories: temporal, geographic, and ecological, that cut across dietary differences. I also illustrate that in some cases where diet was considered to be a major factor in the development of anemia in prehistoric groups, new analyses or new data showed that this was not actually the case. When carefully examined, the pattern of porotic hyperostosis shows that the pathogen load of the immediate environment was probably a much more critical factor than diet in the development of anemia in prehistoric populations. A heavy pathogen load is associated with the anemia of chronic disease and with the iron-withholding accompanying episodes of acute infection, a situation that can compromise iron metabolism and, in some cases, produce the characteristic bone changes associated with anemia.

The case study section presents new data from diverse fields including archaeology, social, and physical anthropology. However, in each case the data support the concept of iron metabolism being actively involved in the body's defense system. Data from all three cases studies (Kent and Lee on the !Kung, Ubelaker on Ecuadorian skeletal populations, and Reinhard on Western U.S. skeletal populations based on coprolite data) support the hypothesis that diet, per se, plays a minor role in the development of iron deficiency. The authors show that other factors, particularly the occurrence and chronicity of pathogens, have a much greater effect on the occurrence of iron-deficiency anemia.

Kent and Lee's chapter tests the proposition that the hypoferremic defense is triggered by a heavy pathogen/and or disease load and that sedentism contributes to the heavy pathogen/disease load. They examine data collected over an 18-year-period from !Kung populations of the Kalahari desert. During that time the life-style of the !Kung changed from mainly seminomadic hunting and gathering to a fairly settled existence with the bulk of their subsistence coming from store-bought or relief supplies. This meant quite a radical change in diet from reliance primarily on wild plants and game to an increasing reliance on refined carbohydrates from government relief rations.

Analysis of hematologic values reveals an interesting story. The recent data show decreases in serum iron and percent saturation of transferrin, which are indicative of anemia of chronic infection, but increases in hemoglobin level, which was contradictory. However, by considering changes in cultural practices, such as increases in tobacco use, alcohol consumption, and the use of iron pots, all of which increase hemoglobin and hematocrit levels, the contradictions can be explained.

When interpreting signs of anemia in past human populations (porotic hyperostosis) the emphasis has frequently been on a dietary causation. Ubelaker's data on a range of sites in Ecuador within a broad, complex cultural-temporal framework indicate that diet was probably not a major factor in the development of anemia in those populations. His data come from coastal and highland sites that represent a span of nearly 8000 years and include a shift from hunting and gathering/horticulture to agriculture. Ubelaker found no evidence for anemia in earlier sites (i.e., hunting and gathering/horticulture) or highland areas, but found that porotic hyperostosis was confined to skeletal material from relatively recent coastal sites. He found that evidence for porotic hyperostosis in Ecuador loosely follows a temporal trend, but does not correlate as closely with time or reliance on maize agriculture as he had originally thought. There was a relatively high frequency of porotic hyperostosis at site OGSE-MA-172 where the large quantities of fish bones recovered indicated that the diet included a substantial amount of iron-rich seafood. Porotic hyperostosis also occurred at two later coastal sites, where faunal analysis indicates a heavy reliance on oysters and clams, as well as utilization of reptiles, birds, deer, and rodents.

When Ubelaker examined the frequency of porotic hyperostosis within the overall patterns of morbidity, subsistence, and settlement in prehistoric Ecuador he found an interesting picture. Elevated frequencies of porotic hyperostosis correlate with increased frequency of periosteal lesions (indicating infection of some type), dental hypoplasia (indicating stress that results in arrested growth of tooth enamel), and subadult mortality. He attributes this mainly to temporal increases in viral, bacterial, and parasitic diseases brought about by increasing sedentism, population density, and sanitation problems.

Reinhard's chapter is important because it illustrates how new data can provide a different perspective and alter interpretation of existing data. Previously, signs of anemia (porotic hyperostosis) seen in prehistoric Southwest Anasazi populations have been largely attributed to a dietary causation. It has been suggested that maize, since it contains phytates that inhibit absorption of iron, is a major factor in the development of anemia in some Southwest Anasazi groups (El-Najjar 1976; El-Najjar and Robertson 1976; El-Najjar et al. 1976, 1982). Reinhard, on the basis of coprolite data, shows that there was no relationship between maize consumption and the occurrence of anemia. He did find a very high correlation between pinworm prevalence in coprolites and porotic hyperostosis, which he felt provided evidence for a relationship between porotic hyperostosis and microparasitism (protozoal, bacterial, and viral infection). In conclusion, Reinhard noted that the role of dietary factors such as maize dependency and low meat consumption in contributing to anemia in the Anasazi has been exaggerated.

The present volume reveals the complexities involved in the story of iron-deficiency anemia. It demonstrates how different disciplines can contribute different perspectives and knowledge and thereby enhance the overall picture of an issue. In the past there has been a lack of appreciation for the flexibility and adaptability of iron metabolism, an overemphasis on the role of dietary iron in the etiology of iron-deficiency anemia, and a lack of awareness of the importance of iron withholding as a defense mechanism. A synthesis of data from nutrition, hematology, microbiology, and anthropology now offers a changing perspective, one that emphasizes the plasticity of iron metabolism and its role in the body's defense against microorganisms and deemphasizes the role of dietary iron in the development of iron-deficiency anemia. Iron withholding as a defense against microorganisms is a relatively new concept, and one that has not yet permeated scientific or popular literature. The idea of a relationship between iron withholding and infection originates with the work of Schade and Caroline in 1944. However, their observations were largely ignored for 20 years; it has only been in the past 25 years that the significance of iron in host defense has begun to be appreciated.

It is true that microorganism pathogenicity and host resistance involve a large number of interacting factors. The role of iron in the host–parasite relationship is only one of several mechanisms involved in this complex relationship. However, a large body of research indicates that the influence of iron metabolism is widespread and often crucial in deciding the outcome of an infection (Bullen and Griffiths 1987). It is important to emphasize that the human body must continually strive to maintain a balance between too much iron and too little. Too much iron results in fibrotic scarring and eventual failure of the liver, pancreas, heart, and endocrine system, whereas too little iron can result in severe anemia, which can affect the quality of life in a number of ways and lead to a failure of the cardiac and respiratory systems (Cook 1990). In both cases the immune system is compromised. The situation is complicated by the fact that a reduction of serum iron is one of the defense strategies of the body's immune system.

Throughout our evolutionary history we have been susceptible to developing iron-deficiency anemia; this could be related to the body's dilemma of maintaining a fine balance between too much and too little iron. As previously mentioned there are a number of problems associated with both excessive and insufficient iron, but perhaps from a long-term evolutionary perspective erring on the side of too little is less deleterious. In the past those individuals who were adequately nourished but had a lower iron status may have fared better in environments where there were high levels of disease organisms.

For some, this will be a controversial book; it compels the reader to reevaluate traditional views of health and disease. It illustrates the complexity of the body's response to physiological and environmental factors and shows that our interpretation of physiological status based on laboratory tests may be hindered by our lack of appreciation of this complexity. The fact that iron appears to be involved in the defense of the body against microorganisms as well as playing a vital role in physiological processes is a good example of this. The evaluation of an individual as "anemic" and in need of iron supplementation based on low hemoglobin/hematocrit values may be an oversimplification of a complex situation. One of the main goals of the book is to bring an awareness of the multiplicity of issues surrounding iron deficiency, regardless of whether there is acceptance of all of the ideas presented.

It is our hope that the book will provide the impetus for further discussion, and that it will stimulate the development of new ideas, research, and insights into the fascinating story of iron-deficiency anemia.

References

Bullen, J.J., and E. Griffiths. 1987. *Iron and Infection*. London: John and Wiley.
Cook, J. 1990. Adaptation in iron metabolism. *American Journal of Clinical Nutrition* 51:301–308.

El-Najjar, M.Y. 1976. Maize, malaria and the anemias in the Pre-Colombian New World. *Yearbook of Physical Anthropology*. 20:329–337.

El-Najjar, M.Y., and A.L. Robertson. 1976. Spongy bones in prehistoric America. *Science* 193:141–143.

El-Najjar, M.Y., D.J. Ryan, C.G. Turner II, and B. Lozoff. 1976. The etiology of porotic hyperostosis among the prehistoric and historic Anasazi Indians of the southwestern United States. *American Journal of Physical Anthropology* 44:447–448.

El-Najjar, M.Y., J. Andrews, J.G. Moore, and D.G. Bragg. 1982. Iron deficiency anemia in two prehistoric American Indian skeletons: A dietary hypothesis. *Plains Anthropologist* 44:447–448.

Locke, A., E.R. Main, and D.O. Rosbach. 1932. The copper and non-hemoglobinous iron content of the blood serum in disease. Journal of Clinical Investigation 11: 527–542.

Schade, A.L., and L. Caroline. 1944. Raw hen egg white and the role of iron in growth inhibition of *Shigella dysenteriae, Staphylococcus aureus, Escherichia coli* and *Saccharomyces cerevisiae*. Science, 100:14–15.

Biographical Sketches of the Contributors

Stanley M. Garn, A.B., A.M., Ph.D. 1922- Fellow of the Center for Human Growth and Development, University of Michigan Professor of Nutrition and Professor of Anthropology. Primary Interest; the interaction of nutrition and genetics on reproduction, growth and development and aging including body composition, mortality and morbidity.

Susan Kent received her Ph.D. in anthropology from Washington State University in 1980 and has taught in one year positions at University of New Mexico, Iowa State University, and University of Kentucky. She has been at Old Dominion University since 1986 where she is currently an associate professor. Her research interests are diverse and include past and present distributions of anemia, health, and morbidity, implications of the shift from nomadism to sedentism, hunter-gatherers, architecture and the use of space, and ethnoarchaeology. Her field research has been equally diverse and includes excavations of a paleo-Indian site from eastern Washington State, Ozette a proto-historic Northwest Coast village site on the Olympic Peninsula, Sinagua sites in Arizona, and archaic and Anasazi sites in New Mexico and Colorado. Her ethnographic research includes fieldwork among Tulalip Indians (Coastal Salish-speakers located on the coast of Washington State), Navajo Indians living in the northern part of the Navajo Reservation, Spanish-speaking Americans and Euroamericans from Oklahoma and Colorado, and, most recently, Basarwa ("Bushmen," San) and Bakgalagadi (Bantu-speakers) who live in the Kalahari Desert of Botswana.

Richard B. Lee is a professor of anthropology at the University of Toronto with long-term interests in ecology, nutrition, and social change. Since the early 1960s he has been conducting research on hunting and gathering societies, particularly the !Kung San or Ju/'hoansi of Botswana. His books include *Man the Hunter*, *Kalahari Hunter-Gatherers*, and *The !Kung San: Men Women and Work in Foraging Society*.

Karl Reinhard is Assistant Professor of Anthropology at the University of Nebraska, Lincoln. His major areas of research have been in the origins and evolution of human parasitism and variation in prehistoric human diet. Currently he is involved in studying historic and modern health patterns of the Omaha Indians. His recent publications are "Parasitology as an Interpretive Tool in Archaeology," *American Antiquity*, 1992 and "Coprolite Analysis: A Biological Perspective on Prehistory" in M. B. Schiffler (Ed.) *Advances in Archaeological Method and Theory* (1992).

Patricia Stuart-Macadam received her Ph.D. in physical anthropology from the University of Cambridge in 1983. Between 1983 and 1987 she was involved in part-time teaching at Cambridge and contract work at the British Museum (Natural History) and the Passmore Edwards Museum in London. She has been in the Department of Anthropology at the University of Toronto since 1987. Her research interests focus generally on an evolutionary perspective of health and disease in human populations, and more specifically on palaeopathology, palaeonutrition, and complementary medicine. She has participated in archaeological excavations in Canada, England, Ghana, Sudan, and Egypt and has a long-standing commitment to field research in Macedonia.

Douglas H. Ubelaker, received his Ph.D. degree from the University of Kansas in 1973. Since then as a Curator of Physical Anthropology at the National Museum of Natural History of the Smithsonian Institution in Washington, D.C., he has conducted research throughout the Americas, concentrating especially on archaeologically recovered human remains from Ecuador. Since 1977, he has also served as the exclusive consultant in forensic anthropology for the F.B.I. laboratories in Washington and has reported on nearly 400 cases. Dr. Ubelaker has authored over 100 scientific articles, books and monographs.

George R. Wadsworth is a medical graduate of the University of Liverpool, England and was a medical officer in West Africa and, in the British Army, in India and Malaya. He has held successive appointments in physiology or nutrition in the universities of Malaya, Liverpool, London and Singapore. He has undertaken assignments as an international consultant in Kenya, Turkey, Iran, Morocco, Philippines, Sarawak, Malaya, Sudan, India, Singapore, Zaire and Hong Kong.

E.D. Weinberg received his Ph.D. degree in Microbiology at the University of Chicago in 1950 and, since then, has been a faculty member at Indiana University in Bloomington. He has published over 140 full-length papers that mainly are concerned with interactions of microbial and host cell physiology in determining the outcome of infectious and neoplastic diseases. Two of these papers have been officially designated as Benchmark Papers in Microbiology. Dr. Weinberg is retired from the USPHS Commissioned Corps Reserve where he held the rank of Scientist Director.

Index